Radiation Oncology

Radiation Oncology
Difficult Cases and Practical Management

Editors

William Small, Jr., MD, FACRO, FACR, FASTRO
Professor and Vice Chairman
Department of Radiation Oncology
Associate Medical Director
Robert H. Lurie Comprehensive Cancer Center
Northwestern University Feinberg School of Medicine
Chicago, Illinois

Tim R. Williams, MD, FACR, FASTRO
Medical Director
Department of Radiation Oncology
Lynn Cancer Institute
Boca Raton Regional Hospital
Boca Raton, Florida

Eric D. Donnelly, MD
Assistant Professor
Department of Radiation Oncology
Robert H. Lurie Comprehensive Cancer Center
Northwestern University Feinberg School of Medicine
Chicago, Illinois

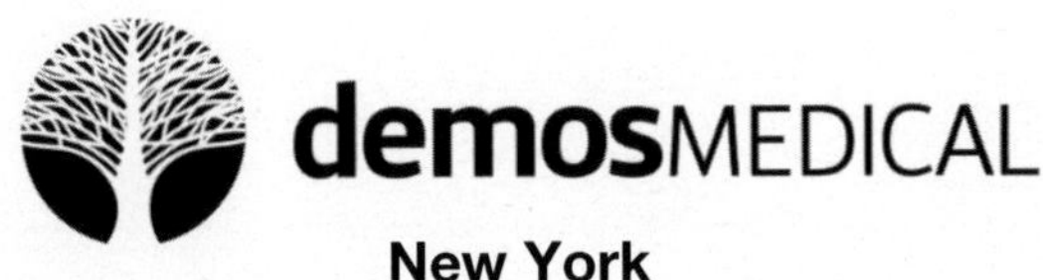

New York

Visit our website at www.demosmedpub.com

ISBN: 9781936287376
e-book ISBN: 9781617050725

Acquisitions Editor: Rich Winters
Compositor: Exeter Premedia Services Private Ltd.

Medicine is an ever-changing science. Research and clinical experience are continually expanding our knowledge, in particular our understanding of proper treatment and drug therapy. The authors, editors, and publisher have made every effort to ensure that all information in this book is in accordance with the state of knowledge at the time of production of the book. Nevertheless, the authors, editors, and publisher are not responsible for errors or omissions or for any consequences from application of the information in this book and make no warranty, express or implied, with respect to the contents of the publication. Every reader should examine carefully the package inserts accompanying each drug and should carefully check whether the dosage schedules mentioned therein or the contraindications stated by the manufacturer differ from the statements made in this book. Such examination is particularly important with drugs that are either rarely used or have been newly released on the market.

Library of Congress Cataloging-in-Publication Data
Radiation oncology : difficult cases and practical management / [edited by] William Small Jr., Tim R. Williams, Eric D. Donnelly.
    p. ; cm.
  Includes bibliographical references.
  ISBN 978-1-936287-37-6—ISBN 978-1-61705-072-5 (e-book)
 I. Small, William.   II. Williams, Tim R.   III. Donnelly, Eric D.
  [DNLM: 1. Neoplasms—radiotherapy—Case Reports. QZ 269]
  RC271.R3
  616.99′40642—dc23

                                                                    2013002905

Printed in the United States of America by Bradford and Bigelow.
13 14 15 / 5 4 3 2

*To our patients, who inspire and teach us to remain humble in our
pursuit of knowledge.*

*To our professional colleagues, who have been our sounding boards and continuously
challenge us with difficult cases.*

*To our families and friends for the continued love and support they have selflessly
given us through the years.*

Contents

SECTION 7: THORAX
Section Editor: Gregory Videtic

SECTION 8: CENTRAL NERVOUS SYSTEM
Section Editor: Minesh P. Mehta

Contributors

Matthew C. Abramowitz, MD
Assistant Professor of Radiation Oncology
Sylvester Comprehensive Cancer Center
University of Miami
Miami, FL

Paul D. Aridgides, MD
Department of Radiation Oncology
State University of New York
Syracuse, NY

Igor J. Barani, MD
Assistant Professor in Residence
Department of Radiation Oncology
University of California San Francisco
San Francisco, CA

William Blackstock, MD
Chair and Professor
Department of Radiation Oncology
Comprehensive Cancer Center
Wake Forest Baptist Medical Center
Winston-Salem, NC

Jeffrey A. Bogart, MD
Professor and Chair
Department of Radiation Oncology
State University of New York
Syracuse, NY

Kristin A. Bradley, MD
Associate Professor
Department of Human Oncology
University of Wisconsin School of Medicine and
    Public Health
Madison, WI

Thomas Carlson, MD
Wenatchee Valley Medical Center
Wenatchee, WA

Kimberly Creach, MD
Mercy Clinic
Springfield, MO

Laura A. Dawson, MD, FRCPC
Professor
Department of Radiation Oncology
Princess Margaret Hospital
University of Toronto
Toronto, Ontario
Canada

Jennifer F. De Los Santos, MD
Associate Professor
Department of Radiation Oncology
University of Alabama at Birmingham
Birmingham, AL

Thomas J. Dilling, MD
Moffitt Cancer Center
Tampa, FL

Jacob Estes, MD
Assistant Professor
Department of Obstetrics and Gynecology
Division of Gynecologic Oncology
University of Alabama at Birmingham
Birmingham, AL

Elizabeth Falkenberg, MD
Center for Cancer Care
Huntsville, AL

Steven J. Frank, MD
Associate Professor
Department of Radiation Oncology
The University of Texas MD Anderson
    Cancer Center
Houston, TX

David K. Gaffney, MD, PhD
Vice-Chair and Professor of Radiation Oncology
University of Utah School of Medicine
Huntsman Cancer Hospital
Salt Lake City, UT

Yolanda I. Garces, MD
Assistant Professor of Radiation Oncology
Mayo Clinic
Rochester, MN

Adam S. Garden, MD
Professor
Department of Radiation Oncology
The University of Texas MD Anderson
 Cancer Center
Houston, TX

Karyn A. Goodman, MD
Department of Radiation Oncology
Memorial Sloan-Kettering
 Cancer Center
New York, NY

Christopher L. Hallemeier, MD
Department of Radiation Oncology
Mayo Clinic
Rochester, MN

Eleanor E. R. Harris, MD
Professor and Chair
Department of Radiation Oncology
Leo Jenkins Cancer Center
Brody School of Medicine
East Carolina University
Greenville, NC

Joseph M. Herman, MD
Associate Professor
Department of Radiation Oncology
Johns Hopkins Hospital
Baltimore, MD

Andrew J. Hope, MD, FRCPC
Assistant Professor
Department of Radiation Oncology
Princess Margaret Hospital
University of Toronto
Toronto, Ontario
Canada

Kenneth Hu, MD
Department of Radiation Oncology
Beth Israel Medical Center
New York, NY

Jessica Hunn, MD
Gynecologic Oncology Fellow
Division of Gynecologic Oncology
University of Chicago
Chicago, IL

Christian Hyde, MD
Cancer Treatment Centers of America
Southeastern Regional Medical Center
Newnan, GA

Salma K. Jabbour, MD
Assistant Professor of Radiation Oncology
Cancer Institute of New Jersey
New Brunswick, NJ

Sameer Keole, MD
Department of Radiation Oncology
Mayo Clinic
Phoenix, AZ

Deepak Khuntia, MD
Dorothy E. Schneider Cancer Center
San Mateo, CA

Christopher R. King, PhD, MD
Associate Professor
Department of Radiation Oncology
UCLA School of Medicine
Los Angeles, CA

Brian Robert Knab, MD
Medical Director
Elliot Regional Cancer Center at Londonderry
Londonderry, NH

Andrew B. Lassman, MD
Memorial Sloan-Kettering Cancer Center
New York, NY

Andrew K. Lee, MD, MPH
Associate Professor
Department of Radiation Oncology
The University of Texas MD Anderson
 Cancer Center
Houston, TX

Nancy Y. Lee, MD
Memorial Sloan-Kettering Cancer Center
New York, NY

Stanley L. Liauw, MD
Associate Professor of Radiation and
 Cellular Oncology
University of Chicago Medicine
Chicago, IL

Stephen T. Lutz, MD
Blanchard Valley Regional Health Center
Findlay, OH

Ronald C. McGarry, MD, PhD
Clinical Associate Professor and Vice Chairman
Department of Radiation Medicine
University of Kentucky
Lexington, KY

Minesh P. Mehta, MD
Professor of Radiation Oncology
Northwestern University, Feinberg School of
    Medicine
Chicago, IL

Loren Mell, MD
Associate Professor
Department of Radiation Oncology
University of California San Diego
Moores Cancer Center
La Jolla, CA

Najeeb Mohideen, MD
Radiation Oncology Associates
Northwest Community Hospital
Arlington Heights, IL

Alan T. Monroe, MD
Penrose Cancer Center
Colorado Springs, CO

Paul L. Nguyen, MD
Assistant Professor of Radiation Oncology
Director of Prostate Brachytherapy
Dana-Farber/Brigham and Women's
    Cancer Center
Harvard Medical School
Boston, MA

Michael A. Nichols, MD, PhD
Coastal Carolina Radiation Oncology
Wilmington, NC

Kenneth Olivier, MD
Mayo Clinic
Rochester, MN

Brian O'Sullivan, MB, BCh, BAO, FRCPC
Professor
Department of Radiation Oncology
Princess Margaret Hospital
University of Toronto
Toronto, Ontario
Canada

Catherine C. Park, MD
Associate Professor
Department of Radiation Oncology
Helen Diller Family Comprehensive Cancer Center
San Francisco, CA

James Piephoff, MD
Director of Radiation Oncology
Saint Anthony's Hospital
Alton, IL

Alan Pollack, MD, PhD
Professor and Chair of Radiation Oncology
Sylvester Comprehensive Cancer Center
University of Miami
Miami, FL

Shyam S. Rao, MD, PhD
Memorial Sloan-Kettering Cancer Center
New York, NY

William F. Regine, MD
Chair, Department of Radiation Oncology
University of Maryland Medical Center
Baltimore, MD

Stephen K. Ronson, MD
St. Joseph Hospital
Baltimore, MD

Devin D. Schellenberg, MD, FRCPC
Clinical Assistant Professor
Department of Radiation Oncology and
    Developmental Radiotherapeutics
British Columbia Cancer Agency
Surrey, British Columbia, Canada

Steven E. Schild, MD
Mayo Clinic
Scottsdale, AZ

Haider A. Shirazi, MD
Evergreen Park, IL

Ori Shokek, MD
York Cancer Center
York, PA

**William Small, Jr., MD, FACRO, FACR,
    FASTRO**
Professor and Vice Chairman
Department of Radiation Oncology
Associate Medical Director
Robert H. Lurie Comprehensive Cancer Center
Northwestern University Feinberg School of Medicine
Chicago, IL

Richard G. Stock, MD
Radiation Oncology Associates
New York, NY

Gray B. Swor, MD
21st Century Oncology
Sarasota, FL

Robert K. Takamiya, MD
Seattle Prostate Institute at Swedish
    Medical Center
Seattle, WA

Wade Thorstad, MD
Associate Professor
Department of Radiation Oncology
Washington University School of Medicine
Siteman Cancer Center
St. Louis, MO

Andrew Vassil, MD
Department of Radiation Oncology
Strongsville Family Health Center
Strongsville, OH

Gregory Videtic, MD, CM, FRCPC
Cleveland Clinic
Cleveland, OH

**John N. Waldron, MSc,
  MD, FRCPC**
Assistant Professor
Department of Radiation Oncology
Princess Margaret Hospital
University of Toronto
Toronto, Ontario
Canada

Tim R. Williams, MD, FACR, FASTRO
Medical Director
Department of Radiation Oncology
Lynn Cancer Institute
Boca Raton Regional Hospital
Boca Raton, FL

Julia S. Wong, MD
Assistant Professor
Department of Radiation Oncology
Harvard Medical School
Dana Farber Cancer Institute
Boston, MA

Catheryn Yashar, MD
Associate Professor
Department of Radiation Oncology
University of California San Diego
Moores Cancer Center
La Jolla, CA

Michael J. Zelefsky, MD
Professor of Radiation Oncology
Vice-Chair Clinical Research
Chief, Brachytherapy Service
Memorial Sloan-Kettering Cancer Center;
Professor of Radiation Oncology
Weill-Cornell Medical School
New York, NY

W. Ken Zhen, MD
Professor of Radiation Oncology
University of Nebraska Medical Center
Omaha, NE

Preface

The treatment of cancer patients continues to advance as new technologies emerge and ongoing studies come to fruition that help dictate our treatment approaches. However, as often noted in clinical practice, our patients frequently present with scenarios for which level I evidence is not available and a more individualized approach to each patient is warranted. It is in these scenarios that one must go beyond the pages of our textbooks and begin to practice the art of medicine. In these circumstances, treatment decisions are based on a combination of consensus opinion algorithms, expert opinions, and extrapolating from what limited data are available. The purpose of this book is to analyze common difficult clinical situations—much the same as the popular difficult case sessions at the annual ASTRO meeting. We choose to examine these difficult clinical situations from various vantage points. These various perspectives included the three editors of this book, one academic physician, one community-based physician and, at least during the editing of this book, a resident physician.

We asked experts in the field to compose example cases of commonly encountered clinical scenarios for which clear evidence-based randomized trials did not exist. The case examples were developed to guide discussions on treatment recommendations, with a review of current issues, and any potential data utilized to drive treatment decisions. The cases are organized into sections corresponding to the major treatment areas of radiation oncology: Breast, Gastrointestinal, Gynecology, Genitourinary, Head and Neck, Thorax, and Central Nervous System. Each of these sections has a section editor who also was asked to provide a treatment recommendation for each case. In addition to the expert opinion, each case example was reviewed by a second academic physician and by a practicing nonacademic community-based radiation oncologist. We hope the discussions that develop from the cases are thought provoking and continue outside the covers of this book.

An endeavor like this takes the help of a multitude of individuals without whom this book would not have been possible. We wish to thank all of the authors for sharing their experiences and expertise, as well as our patients for continuing to educate us on the art of medicine.

■ **INTRODUCTION** ■

Section Editor: Tim R. Williams

Clinical Judgment in the Era of "Evidence-Based Medicine"

Not everything that counts can be counted, and not everything that can be counted counts.
—Albert Einstein

INTRODUCTION

Fundamentally, the physician's role in the health care system is to solve clinical problems. Until relatively recently, the physician's judgment has been the final authority as to which treatment is most appropriate for a given individual's case. Much of medicine is discretionary, however, and there is a great variation in practice patterns across geographical areas [1]. Increasingly, "evidence-based medicine" is promoted as a method of developing rational, consistent, and effective treatment strategies. There should be no debate as to the value of a learned physician synthesizing and incorporating the body of medical knowledge into a logical plan of care for the patient. At another level, however, different stakeholders interpret the concept of "evidence-based medicine" in different ways. There is no universally accepted standard as to how much evidence is required to support a physician's opinion for a given clinical situation, and it has been suggested that only about 20% of current medical practice can be justified by evidence-based standards [2]. More often than these other stakeholders realize, the physician must develop a treatment plan on the basis of imperfect, ambiguous, and premature medical research. This chapter will review the meaning of "evidence" and discuss its value in supporting the decision-making process.

CLINICAL CASES

In the United States, over 1 million people a year receive radiation treatments, delivered by almost 5,000 Board-Certified radiation oncologists. Often, the "evidence" to support the oncologist's judgment is imperfect, premature, or nonexistent. All practicing radiation oncologists will be familiar with the following situations:

A 64-year-old female with metastatic small cell cancer who received a "good partial response" from chemotherapy presents with three brain metastases: 2.0, 1.8, and 1.5 cm in size. She tolerated her chemotherapy well, except for significant fatigue, from which she is now recovering. The medical oncologist is recommending second-line chemotherapy upon systemic progression, and she has considerable, but not overwhelming, disease with bilateral mediastinal lymphadenopathy and a solitary adrenal metastasis. Her Karnofsky Performance Status (KPS) is essentially 100, and she wants to travel across the country in a month to attend her grandson's bar mitzvah. Should she receive whole brain radiation, stereotactic radiosurgery, or both?

An 83-year-old male presents with an elevated PSA of 7.9 and a negative digital rectal exam (DRE). An ultrasound biopsy is positive for 3/12 cores with Gleason 3 + 3 = 6 disease. He has no other medical problems and takes only a daily aspirin and a statin. His family history is unavailable; his parents were killed in World War II. He says he will do "whatever the doctor recommends." Should he be treated?

A 78-year-old man on Sutent® with a history of metastatic renal cell carcinoma, presents with two enlarging lung nodules, one on each side, both biopsy proven, measuring 2.8 and 2.3 cm. His disease is otherwise stable. The patient is a retired executive with a KPS of 100. He "wants the doctors to be very aggressive with his case" as he "has always been a fighter." Should the lung lesions be treated with stereotactic body radiation therapy (SBRT)?

These are not hypothetical cases; each one of them is an actual case that came to my office for evaluation. Rendering an opinion as to the most appropriate treatment required much more than an assessment of the data and information available from the medical literature. In reality, the assessment involved more than the oncologic parameters of the case, complex as they were. A holistic approach was essential and required a more comprehensive review of the patient. This assessment and the cognitive formulation of the treatment plan can best be described using the term *judgment*. This judgment, arising as it does from the intimate doctor–patient relationship, is highly valued by our society. It should never be subordinate to collateral stakeholders, such as an insurance company, hospital administrator, negligence attorney, government bureaucracy, or any other third party peripherally connected to the case.

But how does the physician use data to develop this judgment? How should the available information in the medical literature be considered when developing an opinion? What tools are available to the physician?

THE HIERARCHY OF EVIDENCE

Evidence is the basis for the judgment of the appropriate use of interventions in clinical medicine. There have been many efforts to stratify the relative usefulness of evidence on the basis of the structure and statistical legitimacy of medical information. The concept of a "hierarchy," however, at least in terms of relative importance, is misguided [3]. Although the meta-analysis and the randomized controlled trial (RCT) are often referred to as the "gold standard" of medical data, they are not without limitations, and other types of clinical trials can provide much useful guidance. Even case reports and expert opinion, when taken in context, can assist the oncologist when making decisions. For example, it is very common for a physician to contact a recognized expert, or one of their previous professors, for advice on a particularly difficult case.

Randomized Controlled Trials

It must be recognized, though, that the RCT can provide great confidence in a particular therapy. The main advantage of an RCT is that it effectively eliminates selection bias. For many years, large cooperative groups, such as the Radiation Therapy Oncology Group (RTOG) and the National Surgical Adjuvant Breast and Bowel Project (NSABP), have been successfully organizing and executing RCTs.

Many legitimate clinical questions have been successfully resolved through the use of randomized controlled clinical trials. The value of postoperative radiation therapy after wide excision for breast cancer and the value of stereotactic radiosurgery for patients with solitary brain metastases are but two examples [4,5]. The confidence in these types of trials can be so compelling that one might be tempted to conclude that they are the only type of evidence that should be considered valid, and other "less rigorous" study methodologies are less reliable, less useful, or illegitimate. To some, the suggestion becomes self-evident, that only prospective, randomized, double-blind clinical trials are acceptable when determining the relative merit of various alternative treatments. The abstract idea that a particular treatment should only be justified when data from "Level 1 RCTs" are available exists only in the minds of nonclinical academicians, statisticians, insurance benefit managers, and administrative bureaucracies. In the three cases presented earlier, there are no prospective, randomized trials available to offer guidance. RCTs have limitations including appropriateness, generalizability, and cost.

Appropriateness

There are some treatments that have an effect so dramatic that the idea of validating it through a randomized clinical trial would be inappropriate. In these situations, the recognized benefit is realized from the application of straightforward medical principles. There is no usefulness of proving the benefit with an RCT. The classic example of such a dramatic effect is insulin therapy for diabetes. Other examples include blood transfusion for hemorrhagic shock or abscess drainage for pain relief [6]. In oncology, combination chemotherapy with cisplatin, vinblastine, and bleomycin for metastatic testicular cancer and radiation therapy for vocal cord cancer would be examples of treatments with effects so dramatic that selection bias can be eliminated as an explanation for the clinical effect.

In addition, a randomized trial may be inappropriate for ethical reasons. It would be inappropriate, for example, to perform a randomized trial in humans designed to assess the dose-response relationship for chemotherapy-induced hepatotoxicity. It would also be unethical to run a study in radiation oncology assessing the side-effect profiles in clinically localized prostate cancer of intensity-modulated treatment versus single AP:PA cobalt-60 radiation treatment at 80 centimeters source-to-skin distance (SSD) with compression cones and a single point-dose calculation (a treatment which was common in the 1970s).

This point illustrates what is probably the greatest limitation for the use of RCTs in radiation oncology, namely the dubious utility of an RCT when the endpoint is far in the future and the pace of technological innovation moves ahead of the trial itself, so that by the time the trial is completed, the treatments being evaluated are commonly regarded as obsolete. The innovation of intensity-modulation has revolutionized the treatment process in radiation oncology and it was incorporated into clinical practice quickly, on the basis of sound medical and physics principles, long before the time that would have been required for an RCT to evaluate it relative to more primitive treatment planning algorithms.

Generalizability

The conditions under which an RCT is performed are, by definition, controlled. Patient populations in these trials are reasonably homogeneous, treatment times well defined and limited, with collateral factors, which might influence the fidelity of the trial, minimized [7]. In clinical practice, patients are much more heterogeneous, they often have one or more comorbid conditions, and they are constrained by personal, logistical, and financial impediments.

In oncology, the most important question regarding generalizability is age. Most RCTs have age limits, generally in the mid-70s. There is a real question as to whether or not results from successful RCTs can be extrapolated to patients in their more senior years. Another issue is the presence of comorbid conditions, which can significantly limit a patient's ability to tolerate a treatment regime proven to be of benefit in an RCT. Other factors can include gender, ethnicity, socioeconomic status, and treatment-related factors including dose, timing, and duration of therapy [8].

Cost

RCTs are expensive. The average cost per patient included in an RCT has been estimated to be about $10,000 to 15,000, and the median cost to run a trial to be about $5,000,000 [3, pp. 18–19]. In radiation oncology, it goes without saying that it would be fiscally impossible to obtain Level 1 RCT data for even a minority of clinical situations. And even if it were possible, the pace of technological development and the length of time required to complete the trial would undermine the value of the outcome.

Observational Studies

Other studies, such as single-arm "Phase 2" trials, case control studies, case series, historical controlled trials, and others, are often considered inferior to RCTs. While it is true that RCTs are less vulnerable to selection bias than observational trials, a treatment protocol that has a significant benefit over traditional therapy may be deemed appropriate on the basis of an observational study alone [9]. Observational trials become much more controversial when the anticipated benefit is small. There is no standardized nomenclature to describe the various types of observational studies. The following are some of the types of observational studies.

Historical Controlled Trials

Historical controlled trials are best used when the likely benefits of a new treatment are generally accepted on the basis of the natural history of the condition being treated and the known limitations of current treatment techniques. Compared to RCTs, they are much easier and less expensive to run. In oncology, an example of the successful use of an historical controlled trial supporting a new therapy was imatinib for chronic myeloid leukemia (CML) [10]. Based on the known pharmacology of imatinib, as well as the natural history of CML, a prospective randomized trial was unnecessary, if not unethical, and based on a trial using historical controls imatinib was validated as the standard of care for CML.

The main criticism of historical controlled trials is selection bias in the control group. It is possible that a study design might allow patients with different or more advanced disease to corrupt the control group. It is also possible that supportive therapies might not have been as advanced in the older historical group, degrading the quality of the comparison. Authors of these trials must take great care to ensure that the natural history of this group accurately represents the known and accepted natural history of the disease being studied. Clearly defined selection criteria are critical, but these limitations should not be used to de-prioritize the potential value of historical controlled trials.

In 1990, a seminal article written by AIDS researchers was published describing the criteria under which historical controlled trials could be used to validate the value of certain AIDS therapies [11]. They reported five criteria:

1. There must be no appropriate control group.
2. There must be sufficient evidence to confirm that patients not receiving treatment have a universally poor prognosis.
3. The new therapy must not have a side-effect profile that would outweigh the potential benefit to the patient.
4. There must be a reasonable expectation that the potential benefit will be great enough to be unambiguous.
5. The scientific rationale for the treatment must be such that a positive result would be widely accepted.

There are many conditions in oncology, and many therapeutic interventions, which could quite reasonably fit these criteria, allowing historical controlled trials to have a legitimate place in a physician's decision-making process.

Case Controlled Studies

In a case controlled study, one group with a disease or condition is retrospectively identified and compared with a similar "control" group that does not have the condition. Case controlled studies are the mainstay of epidemiology. As such, they are "observational" in the sense that the subjects of the study are not randomized to one group or another; rather, they are "observed" to be in their particular group.

The main advantages of case controlled studies are that they are relatively inexpensive, simple to run, allow for the analysis of multiple risk factors, and provide results quickly. In some situations they can answer questions that cannot be answered by other types of investigational trials.

The disadvantages of case controlled studies are that they are subject to recall bias, to confounding variables, and may be compared to an inappropriately selected control group.

Case controlled studies have a place in oncology and often provide valuable insight and information to the treating physician. They have been used for many years to show the link between smoking and lung cancer [12,13].

Case Series

Case series, also variably called *retrospective analysis* or historical series, refer to the post hoc evaluation of a treatment technique over a period of time. Generally they are from a single institution, and sometimes reflect the long experience of a single investigator. They are common in radiation oncology, particularly in prostate cancer. They are considered inferior to RCTs because they lack a control group, are subject to selection bias, may include a more heterogeneous patient population, and may include patients treated with dissimilar techniques. Advantages of retrospective series include their substantially lower costs and simplicity. In some clinical situations they may be the only practical way to gather information on the clinical effectiveness of a particular treatment. A well-devised, properly conducted retrospective analysis can be very compelling evidence to support a treatment strategy.

SUMMARY OF SIGNIFICANCE FOR RADIATION ONCOLOGY

Radiation oncologists must make a determination as to what the most appropriate therapy is for a particular patient with a specific clinical situation. They do this by evaluating the available data. The most straightforward data come from RCTs, but most of the time RCTs for the patient's particular clinical situation are unavailable. When they are available, the results may not be generalizable to the given clinical situation. Alternatively, or in addition to RCTs, a historical controlled trial and/or a case series is available. The physician must evaluate these data with an eye on their limitations as well, such as whether or not the trial suffers from selection bias, or the patient population isn't consistent with the patient's clinical situation. The physician's own professional experience is also essential, and must be considered. It is the responsibility of the treating physician to aggregate this information and render a judgment as to the proper treatment.

EXAMPLES OF FLAWED DECISION PROCESSES IN ONCOLOGY

Two significant examples exist illustrating the pitfalls of the decision-making process in oncology. They are the rapid, premature acceptance of autologous stem cell rescue after high-dose chemotherapy for advanced breast cancer and the postulated value of hormone replacement therapy in postmenopausal women.

High-Dose Chemotherapy With Autologous Bone Marrow Transplant (HDC-ABMT)

In 1990, an article by William Peters reported the preliminary analysis of a phase 2 study in which patients with 10 or more positive lymph nodes who had received high-dose chemotherapy followed by an autologous stem cell rescue had a 3-year survival 40% better than historical controls that had received conventional chemotherapy [14].

Based predominantly on this trial, HDC-ABMT rapidly became widely accepted as the most appropriate choice for this high-risk population. Concerns were raised, however, about this and other preliminary phase 2 trials. One concern was that patients who were accepted for HDC-ABMT had already received a response to previous chemotherapy regimens, and these patients were known to have a better prognosis than nonresponders. A 1992 review also raised the issue of significant complications and side effects and noted that the responses generally lasted only a few months [15]. The problems with the available body of literature at the time were selection bias, short follow-up time, small sample size, lead-time bias, and publication bias in favor of positive results. There was still considerable interest in the technique, however, and a consensus emerged that RCTs were needed, but they probably would only confirm that which was generally already agreed upon, namely that HDC-ABMT was an important and valuable advance in clinical oncology.

The first report from a randomized trial became available in 1995. It came from a researcher in South Africa, and it was small, relatively short, and positive [16]. In 1996, the National Comprehensive Cancer Network considered the available evidence and concluded that HDC-ABMT should not be considered the primary treatment for high-risk breast cancer patients, and more study was needed. In their report, HDC-ABMT was still "controversial ... outside of the confines of a clinical trial" [17].

Subsequent trials were either equivocal or unequivocally negative, with one exception. A 1997 paper by William Peters reported a survival advantage in metastatic patients when compared to observation alone, but standard therapy was not used as an historical control group [18]. Three other trials showed unequivocally negative results [19–21]. A fourth study, which showed dramatically positive results, was discredited after it was discovered that the author had unethically forged the results and had committed gross scientific misconduct. Regrettably, it was the same author who published the initial randomized trial in 1995, which had generated so much initial enthusiasm [22]. The question of the usefulness of HDC-ABMT was finally adjudicated in 2000, some 10 years after the controversy began, with an article in the *New England Journal of Medicine* by Edward Stadtmauer and colleagues [23].

The history of the evolution of the medical literature regarding HDC-ABMT is instructive not only for the fact that a treatment paradigm that was initially thought to be effective on the basis of case control studies was later shown to be ineffective based on prospective, controlled, randomized trials. Clearly, a treatment as dramatic and potentially dangerous as high-dose systemic chemotherapy with bone marrow compromise and subsequent stem cell rescue requires clear and convincing evidence of its superiority over standard therapy. However, many thoughtful, intelligent, and well-meaning oncologists embraced the technology well before such data existed. In a survey of medical oncologists performed in 1989, just as the treatment was gaining acceptance, 79% thought that the treatment should be routinely offered to high-risk patients [24]. The overall consensus among practicing oncologists was that the treatment made logical sense on the basis of the recognized biology of breast cancer, their overall clinical experience, and the evolution of other aggressive treatment strategies that had preceded HDC-ABMT. Therefore, acceptance in mainstream clinical practice should occur contemporaneously with the accrual of randomized trials, if indeed randomized trials were needed at all [25]. Basically, the physicians were ahead of the data, and there existed an "acceptance bias" that compromised their judgment.

Beyond the medical and scientific issues, however, there were other social forces that were influencing the evaluation process. Political and legal pressure was being exerted on physicians, insurance companies, and government agencies. The treatment of breast cancer is supported by numerous advocacy groups. The National Alliance of Breast Cancer Organizations (NABCO), for example, represents under one umbrella over 400 support and advocacy organizations. The treatment of breast cancer has great public appeal and receives much media attention. There were many examples of the local and national media "exposing" the insurance industry's efforts to deny coverage for HDC-ABMT, and there were numerous lawsuits against insurance carriers for denial of coverage. Besides the physician's support, premature as it was, there was enormous social pressure to make HDC-ABMT standard treatment and to have it covered by insurance companies. Between 1990 and 1999, an estimated 42,680 transplants were performed at an estimated cost of $3.4 billion dollars. Ninety percent of the patients were treated offprotocol [26].

HDC-ABMT represented a significant dose escalation compared with prior therapy, which itself included some of the most aggressive therapeutic regimens in all of oncology. Aside from the various limitations and shortcomings of the individual studies and the time it took to reasonably evaluate the technology thoroughly, the evaluation process was flawed. Acceptance bias on the part of oncologists and pressure from social forces combined to corrupt the basic progress of science. The clinical judgment of the clinician, which is essential for patients to receive the appropriate treatment, was subverted and thousands of patients received treatment significantly more intense and yet no more effective than standard therapy.

The Long-Term Effects of Hormone Replacement Therapy

Great controversy has existed over the years concerning the potential benefits and possible risks of hormone replacement therapy in postmenopausal women. Initially used to prevent menopausal symptoms, some early case controlled studies suggested other possible benefits, such as a reduction in ischemic heart disease. The magnitude of this effect was thought to be as much as 50% [27]. Likewise, data from the Nurses Health Study, a prospective observational study of almost 120,000 nurses followed for over 20 years, also showed benefit [28]. In addition, based on case controlled studies, there was a suggestion that hormone replacement therapy might prevent or delay the onset of Alzheimer's disease [29]. There was also benefit suggested for osteoporosis [30] and colon cancer [31]. Based on these and numerous other individual, somewhat limited studies, a consensus emerged that the overall body of evidence supported the widespread use of hormone replacement therapy in postmenopausal women, and it was widely adopted.

In 2002, the results from the Women's Health Initiative, a very large, prospective, randomized trial were published. It included 16,000 women followed for 5 years. The trial showed a significant *increase* in cardiovascular disease, breast cancer, and strokes in patients being treated with hormone replacement therapy. Based on the data, the risks of hormone replacement significantly exceeded the benefits [32]. Many thousands of patients were summarily told to discontinue their hormone replacement. Many other studies, including some large, prospective, randomized trials, have subsequently become available. As these trials were published, it became clear that hormone replacement therapy in postmenopausal women is associated with an increased risk of breast cancer, coronary heart disease, stroke, and pulmonary embolus [33–36], and probably provides little, if any, protection against Alzheimer's disease [37]. It is protective for colorectal cancer and osteoporosis [38,39], and its effects on endometrial cancer remain controversial [40].

Hormone replacement therapy for postmenopausal women thus evolved from an initial acceptance on the basis of known concepts of physiology and early and encouraging case controlled studies. A large population of patients are potential candidates for the therapy, however, and estrogens are widely metabolized, and variably so, in each individual patient. As more studies were completed and large, prospective, randomized trials became available, previously unrecognized or minimized risks became evident. A 2004 meta-analysis of 30 previous prospective trials, including 26,708 postmenopausal patients with a mean follow-up of 4.5 years showed that, despite the risks, there was no increased mortality for patients taking hormone replacement [41].

So should a postmenopausal woman receive hormone replacement? Despite the availability of multiple "Level 1" clinical trials, including meta-analyses, prospective, double-blind, placebo-controlled randomized trials, and large prospective observational studies, the physician is still left with incomplete information with which to make a recommendation. Each patient must be evaluated independently and each will have a different risk–benefit profile. The data from the medical literature provide only the framework within which the physician works. The ultimate decision to treat will depend not only on this body of evidence, but most importantly on the physician's judgment based on a synthesis of the available information, comprehensive familiarity with the patient's clinical condition, and professional experience.

THE CONCEPT OF COMPARATIVE EFFECTIVENESS RESEARCH

While often promoted as a new way of assisting physicians in their decision-making process, the concept of "comparative effectiveness" is not new [42]. According to the Institute of Medicine, comparative effectiveness research (CER) is designed to "assist consumers, clinicians, purchasers, and policy makers to make informed decisions that will improve health care at both the individual and population levels" [43]. Fundamentally, CER is an attempt to more explicitly define the relative merit of alternative treatments in common clinical practice. CER differs from scientific research in three important respects:

1. It can compare, in a single analysis, any number of alternatives.
2. It generally focuses on "real-world" outcomes, as opposed to scientific outcomes.
3. It provides information to a wide range of stakeholders, who may interpret the results differently depending on their individual perspectives.

In addition, CER often will focus on simple endpoints, have a greater focus on patient satisfaction and quality of life, and, significantly, will commonly include an assessment of cost effectiveness.

Comparative effectiveness, therefore, potentially offers a mechanism not only to assist physicians in their decision-making process, but also government regulators, third-party payers, policy makers, and patients making choices about their health care as well. Many types of treatments and outcomes can be compared, whether they are procedures, devices, drugs, hospitals, programs, or even entire health care systems [44].

There is, however, an inherent ambiguity in CER. The main uncertainty is how much evidence is required to show difference or equivalence between alternatives. The interpretation of comparative effectiveness information will be different depending on the individual reviewers' interests and motivations, and will vary from stakeholder to stakeholder. For example, the CER standard that the FDA might use in approving a new device for clinical use might be completely different from the standard a third-party payer might use to determine coverage (coverage standards will likely also vary from payer to payer, and even within individual plans from the same payer). In addition, there will also be a third standard a physician might use to determine whether or not to offer such a new device to a particular patient and the patient him/herself might have his or her own standard for determining the relative merit of the new device over the previous one. Thus, CER will always have a hint of antagonism attached to it, until such time as all stakeholders can agree on a "standard" standard, or such an outcome emerges as the result of legislative fiat.

A significant example of the use of CER in radiation oncology is the Agency for Healthcare Research and Quality (AHRQ) report on comparative effectiveness in prostate cancer. As a comprehensive review of the available literature for the treatment of prostate cancer it is without peer, and even with the assessment of the "quality" of the evidence, the authors concluded that "No one therapy can be considered the most effective treatment for localized prostate cancer due to limitations in the body of evidence" [45].

SUMMARY OF THE MEDICAL DECISION-MAKING PROCESS FOR RADIATION ONCOLOGISTS

Unfortunately for policy makers and payers, no two clinical situations are exactly the same. Every day physicians offer opinions in their best efforts to help their patients. RCTs, historical controlled trials, case series, comparative effectiveness research, and decision analysis tools are available to the physician, and are very helpful. It is the physician's responsibility to evaluate the patient's clinical situation, use the information available from all relevant sources, and recommend a course of treatment. Ideally, this recommendation should be free from any outside influence, including the physician's own prejudices. All sources of information can be considered potentially relevant, and the concept of a "hierarchy" of evidence is out of place from this larger perspective. Ultimately, what the patient needs is for the physician to assimilate all of the available information, irrespective of its "relative merit," and place the treatment alternatives in appropriate context for the patient's clinical situation. We call this process *judgment*, and it is the physician's obligation and responsibility to act as the moral fiduciary of the patient. To use an often-quoted phrase "Evidence doesn't make decisions, people do."

REFERENCES

1. Mullan F. Wrestling with variation: An interview with Jack Wennberg. *Health Aff.* 2004. doi 10.1377/hlthaff.var.73

2. Peréz C, Brady LW, Becker A. *The Principles and Practice of Radiation Oncology*, 4th ed. Philadelphia, PA: Lippincott, Williams & Wilkins; 2004: 2452.

3. Rawlins, M. The Harveian Oration of 2008, Royal College of Physicians of London, Delivered October 16, 2008.

4. Fisher B, Anderson S, Bryant J, et al. Twenty-year follow-up of a randomized trial comparing total mastectomy, lumpectomy, and lumpectomy plus irradiation for the treatment of invasive breast cancer. *New Engl J Med.* 2002;347(16): 1232–1241.

5. Andrews DW, Scott CB, Sperduto PW, et al. Whole brain radiation with or without stereotactic radiation boost for patients with one to three brain metastases: Phase three results of the RTOG 9508 randomised trial. *Lancet.* 2004;363(9422):1665–1671.

6. Glasziou P, Chalmers I, Rawlins M, McCulloch P. When are randomized trials unnecessary? Picking signals from noise. *BMJ.* 2007;334:349–351.

7. Rothwell PM. External validity of randomized controlled trials: To whom do the benefits apply? *Lancet.* 2005;365:82–93.

8. Tunis S, Stryer DB, Clancy CM. Practical clinical trials: Increasing the value of clinical research for decision making in clinical and health policy. *JAMA.* 2003;290:1624–1632.

9. Rochon P, Gurwitz JH, Sykora K, et al. Reader's guide to critical appraisal of cohort studies: 1. Role and design. *BMJ.* 2005;330:895–897.

10. Garside R, Round A, Dalziel K, et al. The effectiveness and cost-effectiveness of imatinib in chronic myeloid leukemia. *Health Technol Assess.* 2005;9:25.

11. Byar D, Schoenfeld DA, Green SB, et al. Design considerations for AIDS trials. *New Engl J Med.* 1990;323:1343–1348.

12. Wynder EL, Graham EA. Tobacco smoking as a possible etiologic factor in bronchogenic carcinoma. *JAMA.* 1950;143:329–336.

13. Peto R, Darby S, Deo H, et al. Smoking, smoking cessation, and lung cancer in the UK since 1950: Combination of national statistics with two case-control studies. *BMJ.* 2000;321(7257):323–329.

14. Peters WP, et al. Adjuvant chemotherapy involving high-dose combination cyclophosphamide, Cis-platin, and carmustine and autologous bone marrow support for stage II/III breast cancer involving ten or more lymph nodes (CALGB 8782): A preliminary report. *Proceedings of the American Society of Clinical Oncology.* 1990;9:22.

15. Eddy DM. High-dose chemotherapy with autologous bone marrow transplantation for the treatment of metastatic breast cancer. *J Clin Oncol.* 1992;13(4):657–670.

16. Bezwoda WR, Seymour L, Dansey RD. High-dose chemotherapy with hematopoietic rescue as primary treatment for metastatic breast cancer: A randomized trial. *J Clin Oncol.* 1995;13(10):2483–2489.

17. National Comprehensive Cancer Network. NCCN breast cancer guidelines. *Oncology.* 1996;10(11S):47–75.

18. Peters WP, Jones RB, Vredenburgh J, et al. A large prospective randomized trial of high-dose combination alkylating agents (CPB) with autologous cellular support (ABMS) as consolidation for patients with metastatic breast cancer achieving complete remission after intensive doxorubicin-based induction therapy (AFM). *Proceedings of the American Society of Clinical Oncology.* 1996;15:149.

19. Rodenhuis S, Richel DJ, van der Wall E, et al. Randomized trial of high-dose chemotherapy and haemopoietic support on operable breast cancer with extensive axillary lymph node involvement. *Lancet.* 1998;352:515–521.

20. Hortobagyi GN, Buzdar AU, Champlin R, et al. Lack of efficacy of adjuvant high-dose tandem combination chemotherapy (CT) for high-risk primary breast cancer (HRPBC): A randomized trial. *Proceedings of the American Society of Clinical Oncology.* 1998;17:123a.

21. Peters WP et al. A prospective, randomized comparison of two doses of combination alkylating agents (AA) as consolidation after CAF in high-risk primary breast cancer involving ten or more axillary lymph nodes: Preliminary results of CALGB 980Z/SWOG 9114/ NCIC MA-13. *Proceedings of the American Society of Clinical Oncology.* 1990;18:2.

22. Bezwoda WR. Randomized, controlled trial of high-dose chemotherapy (HD-CNVp) versus standard dose (CAF) chemotherapy for high-risk, surgically treated, primary breast cancer. *Proceedings of the American Society of Clinical Oncology.* 1999;18:2a (abstract 4).

23. Stadtmauer EA, O'Neill A, Goldstein LJ, et al. Conventional high-dose chemotherapy compared with high-dose chemotherapy plus autologous hematopoietic stem-cell transplantation for metastatic breast cancer. *New Engl J Med.* 2000;342(15):1069–1076.

24. Belanger D, Moore M, Tannock I. How American oncologists treat breast cancer: An assessment of the influence of clinical trials. *J Clin Oncol.* 1991;9(1):7–16.

25. Rajagopal S, Goodman PJ, Tannock IF. Adjuvant chemotherapy for breast cancer: Discordance between physician's perception of benefit and the results of clinical trials. *J Clin Oncol.* 1994;12(6):1296–1304.

26. Mello M, Brennan T. The controversy over high-dose chemotherapy with autologous bone marrow transplant for breast cancer. *Health Aff.* 2010;20(5):101–117.

27. Grady D, Rubin SM, Petitti DB, et al. Hormone therapy to prevent disease and prolong life in postmenopausal women. *Ann Intern Med.* 1992;117:1016–1037.

28. Grodstein F, Manson J, Colditz GA, et al. A prospective, observational study of postmenopausal hormone therapy and primary prevention of cardiovascular disease. *Ann Intern Med.* 2000;133:933–941.

29. Paganini-Hill A, Henderson V. Estrogen deficiency and risk of Alzheimer's disease in women. *Am J Epidemiol.* 1994;140(3):256–261.

30. Michaëlsson K, Baron JA, Farahmand BY, et al. Hormone replacement therapy and risk of hip fracture: Population based case control study. *BMJ.* 1998;316:1858–1863.

31. Roussouw JE, Anderson GL, Prentice RL, et al. Risks and benefits of estrogen plus progestin in healthy postmenopausal women: Principal results from the women's health initiative randomized, controlled trial. *JAMA.* 2002;288(3):321–333.

32. Writing Group for the Women's Heath Initiative Investigators. Risks and benefits of estrogen plus progestin in healthy postmenopausal women: Principal results from the Women's Health Initiative randomized controlled trial. *JAMA.* 2002;288:321–333.

33. Vickers MR, Collins N. Progress on the WISDOM trial – Women's international study of long duration estrogen after menopause. *Climacteric.* 2002;5(Suppl 1):133–134.

34. Simon JA, Hsia J, Cauley JA, et al. Postmenopausal hormone therapy and the risk of stroke: The heart and estrogen-progestin replacement study (HERS). *Circulation.* 2001;103:638–642.

35. Høibraaten E, Qvigstad E, Arnesen, et al. Increased risk of recurrent venous thromboembolism during hormone replacement therapy: Results of the randomized, double-blind, placebo-controlled estrogen in venous thromboembolism trial (EVTET). *Thromb Haemost.* 2000;84:961–967.

36. Hully S, Grady D, Bush T, et al. Randomized trial of estrogen plus progestin for secondary prevention of coronary heart disease in postmenopausal Women. *JAMA.* 1998;280:605–613.

37. Zandi P, Carlson M, Plassman B, et al. Hormone replacement therapy and incidence of Alzheimer's disease in older women: The Cache County study. *JAMA.* 2002;288(17):2123–2129.

38. Wells G, Tugwell P, Shea B, et al. Meta-analysis of the efficacy of hormone replacement therapy in treating and preventing osteoporosis in postmenopausal women. *Endocr Rev.* 2002;23:529–539.

39. Grodstein F, Newcomb P, Stampfer M. Postmenopausal hormone therapy and the risk of colorectal cancer: A review and meta-analysis. *Am J Med.* 1999;106:574–582.

40. Karageorgi S, Hankinson S, Kraft P, De Vivo, I. Reproductive factors and postmenopausal hormone use in relation to endometrial cancer risk in the Nurses' Health Study Cohort 1976-2004. *Int J Cancer.* 2010;126(1): 208–216.

41. Salpeter S, Walsh J, Greyber E, et al. Mortality associated with hormone replacement therapy in younger and older women. *J Gen Intern Med.* 2004;19(7):791–804.

42. Jacobson G. *Comparative Clinical Effectiveness and Cost-Effectiveness Research: Background, History, and Overview.* Washington, DC: Congressional Research Service; October 17, 2007.

43. Institute of Medicine. *Initial National Priorities for Comparative Effectiveness Research.* Washington DC: National Academies Press; 2009, p. 41.

44. Garrison L Jr, Neumann P, Radensky P, Walcoff S. A flexible approach to evidentiary standards for comparative effectiveness research. *Health Aff.* 2010;29(10):1812–1817.

45. Wilt TJ, Shamliyan T, Taylor B, et al. *Comparative Effectiveness of Therapies for Clinically Localized Prostate Cancer.* Comparative Effectiveness Review Number 13. Rockville, MD: Agency for Healthcare Research and Quality; February 2008, p. 19.

▪ BREAST ▪

Section Editor: Eleanor E. R. Harris

■ CASE 1 ■

Postmastectomy Radiotherapy in Pathologic Stage IIB Breast Cancer

CLINICAL PROBLEM

The management decisions regarding adjuvant radiation treatment for women undergoing mastectomy for early stage breast cancer often revolve around the management of the axilla. In many cases, the presence of nodal disease is the primary or even the only indication for postmastectomy radiation. Despite the publication of multiple randomized trials showing both improved local-regional control and overall survival benefit for postmastectomy radiation, also corroborated by a large meta-analysis, controversy remains regarding its use in patients with only 1 or 2 positive axillary nodes who have undergone an adequate axillary dissection. As the majority of women have only 1 to 2 positive nodes, this is a common area of debate among surgeons and radiation oncologists.

CASE EXAMPLE

A 42-year-old premenopausal woman in her usual state of good health presents for a routine annual screening mammogram, on which a new cluster of calcifications is noted in the upper inner quadrant of the left breast, with no palpable abnormality appreciated. Ultrasound confirms a spiculated hypoechoic mass in the corresponding position measuring 2.9 cm. MRI confirms a corresponding area of abnormal enhancement and no other suspicious areas of enhancement or suspicious adenopathy. A core biopsy reveals intermediate grade invasive lobular cancer, ER+, PR+, Her2–. Axillary ultrasound reveals no suspicious lymph nodes. Metastatic work up with CT of the chest, abdomen, and pelvis and a bone scan are negative. The patient undergoes a mastectomy with tissue expander placement and sentinel lymph node biopsy. Pathology reveals a 3.2-cm grade 2 invasive lobular cancer, with negative excision margins (greater than 2 mm), the presence of lymphovascular space invasion, and

1 positive sentinel node with a 6-mm focus of metastasis out of 2 sentinel nodes recovered. A subsequent completion axillary dissection reveals an additional positive axillary node with a 4-mm focus of metastasis out of 9 nodes recovered, for a total of 2 of 11 positive nodes, final pathologic stage T2N1aM0. What is the optimal postoperative management with respect to systemic therapy and postmastectomy radiation therapy?

Management Decisions

- Was mastectomy required, or was the patient a possible candidate for breast conservation therapy (BCT)?
- Is postmastectomy radiation therapy (PMRT) indicated, and if so, what are the indications? What are the risks and benefits of PMRT?
- Was it appropriate to perform an immediate reconstruction? What, if any, are the implications of the presence of the tissue expander in the radiation therapy planning?

MAJOR OPINION

Eleanor E. R. Harris

Surgical Management of the Breast in Clinical Stage I–II Breast Cancer

The long-term equivalence of mastectomy and BCT has been summarized serially by the Early Breast Cancer Trialists' Group (EBCTG) overview meta-analyses [1]. These studies show that with follow-up of 20 years or more, mastectomy and BCT are associated with superimposable survival outcomes. Therefore, virtually any patient with clinical stage I and II breast cancer is a potential candidate for BCT. Classic contraindications to BCT are few, and include technical inability to

15

perform a lumpectomy with acceptable cosmesis, clinical evidence of diffuse or multicentric disease in the breast or inability to achieve negative margins of excision, and inability to undergo radiation. The main contraindication to breast irradiation is prior irradiation to the thorax, eg, Hodgkin's lymphoma, as well as some rare autoimmune disorders associated with increased radiosensitivity, such as scleroderma (rheumatoid arthritis and lupus are generally no longer felt to be contraindications to radiation treatment). Other conditions are sometimes perceived as contraindications to BCT but currently lack supporting medical evidence, including young age, *BRCa1-2* mutation carrier, positive family history, or more aggressive tumor subtypes [2].

BCT rates increased steadily until recent years. Now, increasingly more women with early stage disease are being treated with mastectomy, for reasons that are not clear. Both the use of mastectomy for breast cancer treatment [3] and rates of contralateral prophylactic mastectomy [4] are increasing, but prospective analyses of the rationale are lacking. At the same time, multiple alternatives to conventional whole breast radiation treatment (6 weeks of treatment to the whole breast and a tumor bed boost at 1.8–2 Gy per fraction) have been developed and studied in recent years, including various hypofractionation regimens and accelerated partial breast irradiation techniques. The question of the most appropriate surgical and radiation treatment has become a very complex issue and requires an integrated, multidisciplinary management approach. Ideally, all of the specialists who will be involved in the patient's care will consult with the patient and each other before starting any treatment so that a complete treatment plan, including the recommendations for type of surgery, systemic therapy, and radiation therapy are delivered in a coordinated fashion, so as to optimize outcomes and minimize toxicity.

The choice of mastectomy or BCT is one of patient preference. Physicians and medical staff advising patients should make every effort to provide thorough information about all of the treatment options and take great care not to influence the patient's decision with their own personal biases or preferences, unless there is a clear medical indication for a particular treatment approach. Prospective studies have shown that the surgeon's perceived preference or advice, as well as the patient's concerns about breast loss or tumor recurrence, influence the decision between mastectomy and BCT, while aversion to radiation was not a significant predictor of the choice [5,6]. Fear of cancer or recurrence is cited in these surveys, although patients may not appreciate the difference between local recurrence risks, which differ slightly between BCT and mastectomy, and overall survival, which are absolutely equivalent between these 2 treatment options.

In summary, this patient is a good candidate for BCT, assuming lumpectomy is technically feasible with respect to cosmetic outcome. She would expect an equivalent long-term survival with either mastectomy or BCT. The advantage of mastectomy is the potential to avoid irradiation. The advantage of BCT is the preservation of her natural breast with potentially improved body image and overall satisfaction.

The Use of Postmastectomy Radiation in Stage II Breast Cancer

The use of PMRT for stage II disease is highly controversial. Early studies and meta-analyses showed a consistent reduction in local-regional recurrence with PMRT, but no survival benefit, and an increase in noncancer related deaths with PMRT, especially cardiovascular events [7]. Older studies used radiation techniques that exposed much larger volumes of lung and heart to substantial radiation doses compared to contemporary techniques. More recent trials have shown a survival benefit associated with PMRT when more refined radiation techniques have been employed. In 1997 and 1999, 3 randomized trials for node-positive patients of mastectomy and adjuvant systemic therapy with or without PMRT were published, both showing improved local-regional control and overall survival benefit in the PMRT arms. The Danish Breast Cancer Cooperative Group (DBCG) conducted 2 parallel trials: 82b included 1,708 premenopausal women treated with mastectomy and adjuvant cyclophosphamide, methotrexate, and 5-fluorouracil (CMF) [8] and 82c included 1,375 postmenopausal women treated with mastectomy and tamoxifen [9]. The British Columbia randomized trial included 318 women treated with mastectomy and CMF [10]. These trials all demonstrated not only a significant improvement in local-regional control, but also a significant survival benefit with PMRT. Women with any number of positive nodes were eligible for these studies. Criticisms of the Danish trial focus on the suggestion that the surgical technique was suboptimal, with inadequate axillary dissections performed, and too few axillary nodes obtained, as well as the higher than expected recurrence rates in the no radiation groups and use of outdated chemotherapy. In an interesting analysis, the Danish group showed that PMRT changed the patterns of recurrence, with fewer local-regional recurrences resulting in fewer patients overall with distant metastases, suggesting that failure to control microscopic disease locally leads to increased distant metastases [11]. The Early Breast Cancer Trialists' Collaborative Group (EBCTCG) has performed a large meta-analysis of 78 randomized trials for early breast cancer and has examined the benefit of PMRT. In their latest update, the group reported a reduction in local recurrences from 6% to 2% with PMRT in node-negative women with no reduction in breast cancer mortality at 15 years [1]. In node-positive women, the local recurrence rate was reduced from 23% to 6% with PMRT, with an absolute reduction in 15 year breast cancer mortality of 5.4% (60% compared to 55%).

Although women with stage T1-2N1 disease, including those with 1 to 3 positive axillary nodes, were included in the trials described, the use of PMRT in this subgroup has remained controversial. The EBCTCG examined the effect of number of positive nodes in women treated with mastectomy and adriamycin-based chemotherapy, and noted an absolute reduction in local recurrence of 12% (16% without versus 4% with PMRT) in patients with 1 to 3 positive axillary nodes. The Danish group examined the impact of number of positive nodes in the 82b and 82c trials, limiting this analysis to 1,152 patients with 8 or more nodes dissected [12]. For women with 1 to 3 positive nodes, the 15 year local recurrence rate without PMRT was 27% compared to 4% with PMRT. The 15 year overall survival was significantly better with PMRT in this group as well (57% with PMRT versus 48% without PMRT). The British Columbia group reported 20 year outcomes by subgroups of number of nodes involved, and for women with 1 to 3 positive nodes noted improvements in event-free survival, breast cancer specific survival, local-regional control, and overall survival with PMRT, although not surprisingly none of these comparisons for interaction between subgroups reached statistical significance in this small trial [10]. In a review of PMRT, Buchholz et al. report the 10 year local-regional recurrence rates in women with stage II breast cancer with 1 to 3 positive nodes among several other studies in which patients received variable systemic therapy regimens and did not receive PMRT, with rates ranging from 6% to 16% [13]. In an analysis of the SEER registry of postmastectomy patients with T1-2 tumors and 1 to 3 positive nodes and no PMRT compared to similar stage patients treated with BCT including breast irradiation, Buchholz et al. reported that radiation use was independently associated with a survival benefit in this stage subgroup [14]. The International Breast Study Group analyzed risk factors for recurrence after mastectomy in its series of trials, which enrolled over 5,300 women who underwent mastectomy followed by different adjuvant therapies, with no radiotherapy used in any of the trials [15]. With a median follow-up range of 12 to 15 years, the authors reported cumulative incidence function estimates for local-regional failures in patients with 1 to 3 positive nodes of 19% to 34%, varying by tumor size (T1 or T2), presence or not of lymphovascular invasion (LVI), and tumor grade. These data in aggregate make a compelling case for the strong consideration of PMRT in the majority of stage II patients with 1 to 3 positive nodes, with consideration of specific risk factors and comorbidities.

Several studies have attempted to identify risk factors for local-regional recurrence in postmastectomy patients with 1 to 3 positive nodes in order to help guide further recommendations for PMRT. In its series of patients treated with mastectomy and doxorubicin-based chemotherapy with no PMRT, MD Anderson Cancer Center identified several factors associated with an increased risk of local-regional recurrence over 25% even with only 1 to 3 positive nodes, including extracapsular extension, tumor size greater than 4 cm, close or positive margins, lymphovascular space invasion, and skin or muscle invasion [16]. Truong et al. used data from 2 institutional studies to examine the impact of nodal ratio (number of positive nodes divided by number of nodes dissected) on local-regional recurrence risk [17]. A nodal ratio of 20 or greater was associated with a 10 year local-regional recurrence risk of 23% to 29%, thus warranting consideration of PMRT. A recent study of 1,065 patients treated at Guy's and St. Thomas Hospitals in London with 1 to 3 positive nodes examined risk factors for regional supraclavicular or infraclavicular nodal failure [18]. Regional failure was associated with high grade and number of positive nodes, experienced in 30% of those with high-grade tumors and 3 positive nodes. On univariate analysis, the following risk factors emerged: number of positive nodes and nodal ratio, size of nodal metastases, tumor grade, and no hormonal therapy. In addition, they noted a significant association between age under 50 and premenopausal status and chest wall recurrence. Mastectomy and breast conservation patients were not analyzed separately. A similar study that included mastectomy (none with PMRT) and BCT (none with nodal radiation) patients with 1 to 3 positive nodes noted supraclavicular nodal failure associated with LVI, number of positive axillary nodes, level of involved nodes, and extracapsular extension, with higher failure rates associated with 2 or more factors present [19].

In the era of molecular subtyping [20], studies regarding the relative local recurrence rates for different breast cancer subtypes are being performed. Most such studies use retrospective cohorts of patients to ensure adequate follow-up time to report local recurrence risks, so do not necessarily reflect current treatment standards, particularly regarding systemic therapy. Voduc et al. showed a higher risk of local recurrence after BCT in patients with Her2+ cancers, but used data prior to the introduction of trastuzumab [21]. They also showed a higher risk of local and regional recurrence in all nonluminal A subtypes after mastectomy, especially in the triple negative phenotype. Wang et al. reported local-regional recurrence rates among 835 node-positive postmastectomy patients; 21% of the stage II patients received PMRT [22]. Patients with triple negative and Her2+ had significantly higher 5 year local-regional relapse rates (12% for triple negative, 12–15% for Her2+, compared to 6% for ER+/Her2–). In a study of 582 stage II–III patients treated with mastectomy, chemotherapy, and PMRT, 5 year local-regional recurrence was 8.6% in ER compared to 4.4% in ER+, and 7.5% for Her2– compared to 1.7% for Her2+, 86% of whom received trastuzumab [23]. Overall recurrence rates for triple negative were 12% versus 4% for nontriple negative, despite the use of PMRT, suggesting that adjustments in therapy may be warranted in this subgroup, but clearly further data are required. Only 23% of patients in this series were stage IIB and their prognosis by molecular subtype was not examined separately. The DBCG performed an analysis of the impact of hormone receptor status and Her2 expression on local-regional recurrence in 1,000 patients from the 82b and 82c randomized trials [24]. At a median follow-up of 17 years, the molecular profile did seem to impact the recurrence risk. Patients with receptor positive, Her2– tumors had an improved overall survival and greater improvements in local-regional control with PMRT than those with receptor negative and Her2+ tumors, although local-regional control was higher with PMRT in all subtypes. The chemotherapy used in the premenopausal trial was CMF, and tamoxifen was used for only 1 year as only adjuvant therapy in the postmenopausal trial, and trastuzumab was not available. These results likely reflect the ineffectiveness of the systemic therapies in use in this era for the higher risk subtypes, so that PMRT had no impact on survival owing to uncontrolled micrometastatic disease. More data are required to assess the impact of molecular subtype on local-regional recurrence risk in 1 to 3 positive node patients [25].

The American Society of Clinical Oncology (ASCO) published PMRT guidelines in 2001 and found insufficient evidence at that time to routinely recommend PMRT for T1-2 tumors with 1 to 3 positive nodes. The Steering Committee on Clinical Practice Guidelines for the Care and Treatment of Breast Cancer was convened by Health Canada. They published PMRT guidelines in 2004, and stated that the role of PMRT for 1 to 3 positive nodes was "currently undefined" [26]. The most recent American College of Radiology Appropriateness Criteria Panel on PMRT from 2008 recommends treating a stage T1N1 case with 1 to 3 positive nodes. The National Comprehensive Cancer Network (NCCN) Clinical Practice Guidelines states that PMRT should be "strongly considered" for postmastectomy patients with 1 to 3 positive nodes (NCCN version 2.2011).

In summary, PMRT should be recommended for this patient. She has the following constellation of risk factors for local-regional recurrence: young age, premenopausal status, 2 positive nodes with macrometastases, nodal ratio approaching 20%, LVI, and a T2 tumor size. Level I randomized data have shown a survival benefit associated with PMRT for patients with this stage of disease.

Sequencing of Reconstruction and Postmastectomy Radiation

If a patient with early stage breast cancer chooses mastectomy, the decision regarding immediate or delayed reconstruction must be addressed preoperatively. A consultation with a plastic surgeon is required to discuss the numerous technical options for autologous tissue or implant reconstruction, as well as the optimal timing of reconstruction given the patient's disease status, comorbidities, and likelihood of requiring PMRT. Advantages of immediate reconstruction may include reducing the number of surgical procedures, and a possible psychological impact for the patient [27]. However, rates of overall complications may be higher for immediate versus delayed tissue expander/implant reconstructions, leading to higher reoperation rates [28,29]. Prospective studies have shown that with or without immediate reconstruction, women undergoing mastectomy experience negative feelings of body transformation, including mutilation and modified emotional, physical, and relational changes [30,31]. One study demonstrated that women seeking immediate reconstruction had more impairment in quality of life and poorer psychosocial functioning (more depression, affective distress, and poorer adjustment to their cancer diagnosis) compared to those who had delayed reconstructions [32]. Women having both immediate and delayed reconstructions experience improvements in body image after reconstruction [33]. The highest satisfaction rates are achieved by BCT compared to mastectomy with or without reconstruction [34–36]. The main advantage of delayed reconstruction compared to immediate is the ability to assess complete pathologic staging in order to determine the need for PMRT and the potential for reduced overall complications.

The treatment target volumes for PMRT are based on established patterns of local-regional recurrence without radiation and include the entire chest wall and mastectomy scar, and the regional axillary, infraclavicular and supraclavicular nodes, with or without the internal mammary nodes (IMNs). Typically, the undissected axilla superior to the axillary dissection bed will be contoured. However, under certain circumstances, the entire axilla may need to be included in the target volume, such as presence of bulky disease, extracapsular extension, inadequate axillary dissection (less than 6 nodes obtained), or use of sentinel node biopsy only. Bolus should typically be used on the chest wall even when a reconstruction has been performed, as the skin and scar are common sites of recurrence postmastectomy and are thus important target volumes. At the same time, the dose to the heart and lungs must be minimized to avoid long-term risks of radiation-related morbidity and mortality, in particular cardiovascular events. Immediate reconstruction can substantially affect the choice of radiation techniques, and is associated with increased morbidity with PMRT compared to delayed reconstruction, especially for tissue expander/implant reconstructions [37–40]. While a variety of radiation techniques exist to achieve the necessary target coverage, including electron beams, tangential 3D conformal, forward-planned and inverse-planned intensity modulated radiation therapy (IMRT), immediate reconstruction often interferes with the ability to achieve optimal dose–volume constraints, likely completely precluding the use of electrons, and potentially leading to increased heart and lung volumes irradiated. Prostheses used for reconstruction and their ports may contain higher atomic number (Z) materials than tissue, affecting the radiation dose distribution and increasing the dose at implant/tissue interfaces [41,42]. For these reasons, delayed reconstruction is preferred when PMRT is planned. An alternative approach has been reported by MD Anderson Cancer Center, called the *delayed-immediate reconstruction* [43]. In this technique, step 1 involves performing a skin-sparing mastectomy with placement of a tissue expander. In stage 2, after final pathologic assessment, patients not requiring PMRT had immediate reconstruction, while those requiring PMRT had delayed reconstruction. The tissue expander can be partially or fully deflated prior to radiation planning as needed to optimize the radiation dose distribution, with re-expansion prior to the permanent reconstruction.

Overall, there is a distinct lack of randomized or prospective data to guide the decisions regarding the timing of reconstruction when PMRT is indicated and whether reconstruction impairs the efficacy of PMRT. Conclusions from the available retrospective series are difficult to draw owing to differing patient selection, lack of uniform criteria for evaluation of outcomes, and lack of robust correlates between morbidity and patient satisfaction. This is evidenced by the huge range of rates for acceptable cosmesis reported among published series, ranging from 7% to 88% [44]. Overall postreconstruction complication rates are also affected by comorbidities, such as diabetes, obesity, and smoking habits. Certain techniques can decrease the risk of complications when reconstruction and PMRT are combined, including submuscular implant placement, use of textured implants, and possibly combining implant with autologous tissue. Meticulous radiation technique with optimization of homogeneity and minimal use of chest wall boost dose, unless strongly indicated, will also help reduce toxicity.

These decisions should be discussed thoroughly with individual patients by all members of the treatment team preoperatively, including the surgeon, plastic surgeon, and radiation oncologist, so that a personalized treatment plan accounting for the relevant medical and clinicopathologic factors, as well as patient preferences, is agreed upon. Clinical stage I patients may generally undergo immediate reconstruction. Clinical stage I and II patients may be staged preoperatively with axillary ultrasound and nodal biopsy as indicated to further assess the possible need for PMRT. Clinical stage II often presents the most controversial situation, because the indications for PMRT will be primarily dependent on the pathologic findings after mastectomy. In this group, potential indications for PMRT include young age or premenopausal status, T2 or T3 tumor size, high grade histology, gross multicentric disease, triple negative (ER−/PR−/Her2−) or Her2+ tumor, LVI, positive margins of excision, multiple positive nodes, extranodal extension, and the use of neoadjuvant chemotherapy [22,23,45,46]. Clinical stage III patients should not be offered immediate reconstruction owing to the requirement for PMRT.

In summary, for this case, the patient presented with clinical stage IIA disease, including clinically negative nodes, but with pathologic stage IIB disease. Her preoperative risk factors predictive of a recommendation for PMRT include young age, premenopausal status, and T2 tumor size. The choice of immediate reconstruction was reasonable, although delayed-immediate technique may have been advisable. She should have had a consultation with a radiation oncologist preoperatively to discuss her risk factors for possible PMRT and to counsel her regarding the pros and cons of immediate versus delayed reconstruction if PMRT were indicated, in order for her to make a fully informed decision about her treatment. The presence of positive sentinel nodes intraoperatively should be discussed with the patient as a potential reason to abort a planned immediate reconstruction, owing to the increased chance of PMRT being recommended. In women with known indications for PMRT, delayed reconstruction is strongly preferred in order to allow for optimal radiation treatment planning and to reduce long-term complications and cosmetic decrement.

ACADEMIC COMMENT

Catherine C. Park

The role of PMRT in stage II breast cancer has increased in recent years, given the results of the Danish trials and the Oxford overview, demonstrating not only a local-regional benefit, but also a survival benefit, with the use of PMRT. Patients with a very high risk for local-regional recurrence, that is 4 or more involved axillary nodes, or with T3 disease and any positive nodes, routinely receive PMRT [47]. However, patients with T1-2 tumors with 1 to 3 positive nodes fall into a controversial category because there is not as much evidence to uniformly recommend PMRT. Several studies have shown that aside from tumor size and nodal positivity, patient and tumor characteristics can substantially increase risk warranting PMRT. More often than not, PMRT is considered especially if high risk features are present, such as LVI, young age, grade III disease, extranodal extension, and close or positive margins. Extent of LVI may also be helpful, although data on this issue are scant. One study indicated that having 2 or more high risk features was associated with substantially increased local-regional recurrence risk in this group of patients [48]. The importance of biologic subtype remains unclear in this setting, and at present, data are lacking with regard to whether certain subtypes, such as triple-negative disease, are indications for PMRT.

The potential benefit of any patient who undergoes PMRT should be carefully weighed against the possible morbidities. Although delayed reconstruction is the preferred approach when PMRT is certain, many patients opt for immediate reconstruction, often with a tissue expander, if given the option. Thin patients with few autologous options also are more likely to undergo immediate reconstruction with a tissue expander, with further decisions made after the pathology from the mastectomy is available. Again, a detailed discussion with the plastic surgeon and patient is critical in order to achieve realistic expectations regarding complications. The technical challenges of treating a tissue expander include avoidance of the heart, minimizing lung volumes in the radiation field, and avoiding the contralateral breast (or reconstruction). If IMNs are to be treated, the presence of a reconstruction can make this more difficult. In some cases, it may be advisable to remove or deflate the tissue expander prior to completing radiation planning, if an acceptable beam geometry cannot be attained. In some cases, acellular dermal matrix is used to improve coverage of the lower pole of the tissue expander and help recreate a more natural-appearing inframammary fold. Whether this can improve outcomes in patients who need PMRT remains to be seen.

This is a young patient with +2/11 axillary lymph nodes and LVI. A detailed discussion of the risks and benefits of PMRT, as stated above, is crucial. Her risk of local-regional recurrence without PMRT is likely in the 10% to 15% range. Expecting an approximately 2/3 reduction in local regional recurrence, we would recommend PMRT for this patient. A small survival benefit is also likely, especially in younger patients who lack comorbidities, and who can be treated safely with precise RT techniques.

COMMUNITY PRACTITIONER COMMENT

Gray B. Swor

This particular patient scenario brings to light many issues that we struggle with in daily clinical practice. In regard to the surgical management of this patient, she may in fact be a candidate for BCT. There is no mention of breast size, but if the surgeon feels that she does not have ample breast tissue to undergo lumpectomy with acceptable cosmetic result, then neoadjuvant chemotherapy could be offered followed by lumpectomy if she has a favorable response. In randomized clinical trials, between 38% and 64% of women underwent breast conserving surgery in the neoadjuvant arms [49]. This patient chose to undergo reconstruction post mastectomy and a tissue expander was placed at the time of surgery. In patients who are not anticipated to need postoperative radiotherapy, immediate reconstruction with a permanent implant can be performed with a favorable cosmetic outcome [50]. If radiotherapy is a possibility, however, then placement of a tissue expander at the time of mastectomy is appropriate and should not impact the ability to administer radiotherapy. The tissue expander may need to be deflated prior to the initiation of radiotherapy to optimize treatment planning. The tissue expander preserves the skin chest wall envelope, allowing delayed/immediate reconstruction with a permanent implant or reconstruction with autologous tissue at a later time after

adjuvant treatment is completed. The toxicities associated with postmastectomy radiotherapy would include capsular contracture, implant malposition, and rupture, although these issues can be addressed at the time of final reconstruction with acceptable cosmesis in most cases.

The role of postmastectomy radiotherapy in patients with 1 to 3 positive axillary lymph nodes has been debated for decades. It has been well established that there is a benefit in terms of local and regional control with postmastectomy radiotherapy. Recent large randomized trials with relatively long follow-up have now shown an overall survival benefit when postmastectomy radiotherapy is offered to patients with less than 4 positive axillary lymph nodes. In fact, the absolute magnitude of the overall survival benefit afforded by postmastectomy radiotherapy is similar in patients with 1 to 3 positive lymph nodes, and those with 4 or more positive lymph nodes. Many of the studies performed have been criticized for quality of radiotherapy and extent of axillary surgery, however. There are other factors that may influence the magnitude of benefit of postmastectomy radiotherapy in patients with only 1 to 3 positive axillary lymph nodes. These factors include young age or premenopausal status, estrogen receptor negative status, the presence of LVI, the number of axillary lymph nodes, the size of the primary tumor (greater than 3 cm), medial tumor location, and percent nodal involvement (greater than 20%).

In this particular patient's scenario, postmastectomy radiotherapy should be strongly considered, although she has relatively low volume nodal disease. This is a premenopausal patient with a moderate-sized primary located in the upper inner quadrant. Therefore, there is concern for possible spread to the supraclavicular and internal mammary regions. I would counsel this patient about postmastectomy radiotherapy, which, on the basis of available data, would improve local-regional control and survival. The treatment area would include the left chest wall, level III axillary lymph nodes, supraclavicular lymph nodes, and internal mammary region because of the primary tumor location. If she had not undergone completion axillary lymph node dissection, then the level I and II axilla would be covered as well. I would recommend a dose of 50 to 50.4 Gy in 25 to 28 fractions to the chest wall with appropriate bolus and nodal regions. I would not recommend boost to the mastectomy scar in this particular patient, as there is no indication that this would improve her local control and could negatively impact her reconstruction outcome.

SECTION EDITOR'S NOTE

Eleanor E. R. Harris

Although the patient was a candidate for BCT, she opted for mastectomy, an increasingly common patient choice. While the reasons for the shift toward mastectomy for early stage disease in recent years are unclear, women may be motivated by the misconception that mastectomy provides better survival outcomes, by the desire to avoid radiation, or by improved access to plastic surgeons able to provide immediate reconstructions and increased use of skin-sparing mastectomy. The literature describing complications of postmastectomy radiation after immediate reconstruction are not particularly robust, but there appears to be an increased risk of complications that affect cosmesis compared to delayed reconstruction performed several months after PMRT. More importantly, the presence of a reconstructed breast or implant changes the anatomy in an unfavorable way in many patients, compromising the quality of the radiation dose plans, potentially leading to higher volumes of heart and lung irradiated, and virtually eliminating the ability to adequately boost the chest wall if needed (such as for a positive margin).

The case describes a common scenario, in which a patient with clinically node-negative cancer elects for mastectomy and immediate reconstruction only to find positive nodes on final pathology. This creates a dilemma for the surgeon—should the surgeon abort the immediate reconstruction given that the use of PMRT becomes much more likely? The case also creates a dilemma of radiation oncologist—should the implant be removed or deflated prior to simulation? Should the radiation be omitted owing to the increased risk of complications?

These scenarios should be discussed with the patient in advance of the surgery by the surgeon and radiation oncologist to review the alternative approach of breast conservation, the indications for postmastectomy radiation, and the pros and cons of the timing of reconstruction and the use of PMRT. Patient's fears regarding radiation therapy can be addressed proactively as well. Both, the surgeon and radiation oncologist should clearly describe the extensive body of randomized data and meta-analyses that show that long-term survival for stage I and II breast cancer is absolutely equivalent with the use of either mastectomy or BCT. Patients have fewer complications and better quality radiotherapy with lumpectomy and radiation than with mastectomy, immediate reconstruction, and PMRT, and should be aware of the implications of their choices. Omission of radiation in a premenopausal woman with multiple risk factors for local-regional recurrence potentially compromises her survival. Cosmetic or quality of life concerns should not take precedence over therapeutic procedures, unless this is the patient's express informed choice.

Assuming this patient had a clear understanding that radiation may still be recommended depending on final pathology, it was not unreasonable for her to have chosen immediate reconstruction in light of her negative lymph node staging. Unfortunately, she now finds herself in the proverbial "worst case scenario," requiring both, an axillary dissection and PMRT. I would definitely recommend PMRT, with target volumes to include the chest wall using bolus, undissected axilla, and supraclavicular nodes (I personally would not include the IMNs in this stage II left-sided patient with only 2 positive axillary nodes, but if included, heart dose constraints must be met). In such cases, I typically recommend that the tissue expander be deflated to flatten the chest wall contour (or if the permanent implant has been placed, to consider its removal). This will usually allow a significantly better dose distribution to be achieved. If the patient does not wish to manipulate the implant, then an acceptable treatment plan should be attempted, recognizing that inverse planned intensity modulated technique will likely provide the optimal target volume coverage while minimizing the dose to the heart. It is paramount to strictly adhere to guidelines for dose constraints on the cardiac structures, particularly in a young woman with an excellent prognosis. In my opinion, this patient would have been best treated with BCT. With a lumpectomy and sentinel node biopsy, she could have avoided the axillary dissection, as she meets the criteria for the ACOSOG Z011 trial, which is not applicable to mastectomy patients [51]. She would expect equivalent survival outcomes while undergoing fewer surgical procedures and with a lower risk of treatment-related toxicity.

REFERENCES

1. Clarke M, Collins R, Darby S, et al. Effects of radiotherapy and of differences in the extent of surgery for early breast cancer on local recurrence and 15-year survival: An overview of the randomised trials. *Lancet.* 2005;366(9503): 2087–2106.

2. Pierce LJ, Levin AM, Rebbeck TR, et al. Ten-year multi-institutional results of breast-conserving surgery and radiotherapy in BRCA1/ 2-associated stage I/II breast cancer. *J Clin Oncol.* 2006;24(16):2437–2443.

3. McGuire KP, Santillan AA, Kaur P, et al. Are mastectomies on the rise? A 13-year trend analysis of the selection of mastectomy versus breast conservation therapy in 5865 patients. *Ann Surg Oncol.* 2009;16(10):2682–2690.

4. Tuttle TM, Habermann EB, Grund EH, et al. Increasing use of contralateral prophylactic mastectomy for breast cancer patients: A trend toward more aggressive surgical treatment. *J Clin Oncol.* 2007;25(33):5203–5209.

5. Temple WJ, Russell ML, Parsons LL, et al. Conservation surgery for breast cancer as the preferred choice: A prospective analysis. *J Clin Oncol.* 2006;24(21):3367–3373.

6. Molenaar S, Oort F, Sprangers M, et al. Predictors of patients' choices for breast-conserving therapy or mastectomy: A prospective study. *Br J Cancer.* 2004;90(11):2123–2130.

7. Cuzick J, Stewart H, Peto R, et al. Overview of randomized trials of postoperative adjuvant radiotherapy in breast cancer. *Cancer Treat Rep.* 1987;71(1):15–29.

8. Overgaard M, Hansen PS, Overgaard J, et al. Postoperative radiotherapy in high-risk premenopausal women with breast cancer who receive adjuvant chemotherapy. Danish Breast Cancer Cooperative Group 82b Trial. *N Engl J Med.* 1997;337(14):949–955.

9. Overgaard M, Jensen MB, Overgaard J, et al. Postoperative radiotherapy in high-risk postmenopausal breast-cancer patients given adjuvant tamoxifen: Danish Breast Cancer Cooperative Group DBCG 82c randomised trial. *Lancet.* 1999;353(9165):1641–1648.

10. Ragaz J, Olivotto IA, Spinelli JJ, et al. Locoregional radiation therapy in patients with high-risk breast cancer receiving adjuvant chemotherapy: 20-year results of the British Columbia randomized trial. *J Natl Cancer Inst.* 2005;97(2): 116–126.

11. Nielsen HM, Overgaard M, Grau C, et al. Study of failure pattern among high-risk breast cancer patients with or without postmastectomy radiotherapy in addition to adjuvant systemic therapy: Long-term results from the Danish Breast Cancer Cooperative Group DBCG 82 b and c randomized studies. *J Clin Oncol.* 2006;24(15):2268–2275.

12. Overgaard M, Nielsen HM, Overgaard J. Is the benefit of postmastectomy irradiation limited to patients with four or more positive nodes, as recommended in international consensus reports? A subgroup analysis of the DBCG 82 b&c randomized trials. *Radiother Oncol.* 2007;82(3): 247–253.

13. Buchholz TA, Strom EA, Perkins GH, McNeese MD. Controversies regarding the use of radiation after mastectomy in breast cancer. *Oncologist.* 2002;7(6):539–546.

14. Buchholz TA, Woodward WA, Duan Z, et al. Radiation use and long-term survival in breast cancer patients with T1, T2 primary tumors and one to three positive axillary lymph nodes. *Int J Radiat Oncol Biol Phys.* 2008;71(4):1022–1027.

15. Wallgren A, Bonetti M, Gelber RD, et al. Risk factors for locoregional recurrence among breast cancer patients: Results from International Breast Cancer Study Group Trials I through VII. *J Clin Oncol.* 2003;21(7):1205–1213.

16. Katz A, Strom EA, Buchholz TA, et al. Locoregional recurrence patterns after mastectomy and doxorubicin-based chemotherapy: Implications for postoperative irradiation. *J Clin Oncol.* 2000;18(15):2817–2827.

17. Truong PT, Woodward WA, Thames HD, et al., The ratio of positive to excised nodes identifies high-risk subsets and reduces inter-institutional differences in locoregional recurrence risk estimates in breast cancer patients with 1-3 positive nodes: An analysis of prospective data from British Columbia and the M.D. Anderson Cancer Center. *Int J Radiat Oncol Biol Phys.* 2007;68(1):59–65.

18. Yates L, Kirby A, Crichton S, et al. Risk factors for regional nodal relapse in breast cancer patients with one to three positive axillary nodes. *Int J Radiat Oncol Biol Phys.* 2012;82(5):2093–2103.

19. Yu JI, Park W, Huh SJ, et al. Determining which patients require irradiation of the supraclavicular nodal area after surgery for N1 breast cancer. *Int J Radiat Oncol Biol Phys.* 2010;78(4):1135–1141.

20. Sørlie T, Perou CM, Tibshirani R, et al. Gene expression patterns of breast carcinomas distinguish tumor subclasses with clinical implications. *Proc Natl Acad Sci USA.* 2001;98(14):10869–10872.

21. Voduc KD, Cheang MC, Tyldesley S, et al. Breast cancer subtypes and the risk of local and regional relapse. *J Clin Oncol.* 2010;28(10): 1684–1691.

22. Wang SL, Li YX, Song YW, et al. Triple-negative or HER2-positive status predicts higher rates of locoregional recurrence in node-positive breast cancer patients after mastectomy. *Int J Radiat Oncol Biol Phys.* 2011;80(4):1095–1101.

23. Panoff JE, Hurley J, Takita C, et al. Risk of locoregional recurrence by receptor status in breast cancer patients receiving modern systemic therapy and post-mastectomy radiation. *Breast Cancer Res Treat.* 2011;128(3):899–906.

24. Kyndi M, Overgaard M, Nielsen HM, et al. High local recurrence risk is not associated with large survival reduction after postmastectomy radiotherapy in high-risk breast cancer: A sub-group analysis of DBCG 82 b&c. *Radiother Oncol.* 2009;90(1):74–79.

25. Recht A, Edge SB, Solin LJ, et al. Postmastectomy radiotherapy: Clinical practice guidelines of the American Society of Clinical Oncology. *J Clin Oncol.* 2001;19(5):1539–1569.

26. Truong PT, Olivotto IA, Whelan TJ, et al. Clinical practice guidelines for the care and treatment of breast cancer: 16. Locoregional post-mastectomy radiotherapy. *CMAJ.* 2004;170(8):1263–1273.

27. Fernández-Delgado J, López-Pedraza MJ, Blasco JA, et al. Satisfaction with and psychological impact of immediate and deferred breast recon-struction. *Ann Oncol.* 2008;19(8):1430–1434.

28. Hvilsom GB, Friis S, Frederiksen K, et al. The clinical course of immediate breast implant reconstruction after breast cancer. *Acta Oncol.* 2011;50(7):1045–1052.

29. Sullivan SR, Fletcher DR, Isom CD, Isik FF. True incidence of all complications following immediate and delayed breast reconstruction. *Plast Reconstr Surg.* 2008;122(1):19–28.

30. Piot-Ziegler C, Sassi ML, Raffoul W, Delaloye JF. Mastectomy, body deconstruction, and impact on identity: A qualitative study. *Br J Health Psychol.* 2009;15(Pt 3):479–510.

31. Harcourt DM, Rumsey NJ, Ambler NR, et al. The psychological effect of mastectomy with or without breast reconstruction: A prospective, multicenter study. *Plast Reconstr Surg.* 2003;111(3):1060–1068.

32. Roth RS, Lowery JC, Davis J, Wilkins EG. Quality of life and affective distress in women seeking immediate versus delayed breast reconstruction after mastectomy for breast cancer. *Plast Reconstr Surg.* 2005;116(4):993–1002; discussion 1003–1005.

33. Atisha D, Alderman AK, Lowery JC, et al. Prospective analysis of long-term psychosocial outcomes in breast reconstruction: Two-year postoperative results from the Michigan Breast Reconstruction Outcomes Study. *Ann Surg.* 2008;247(6):1019–1028.

34. Al-Ghazal SK, Fallowfield L, Blamey RW. Comparison of psychological aspects and patient satisfaction following breast conserving surgery, simple mastectomy and breast reconstruction. *Eur J Cancer.* 2000;36(15):1938–1943.

35. Figueiredo MI, Cullen J, Hwang YT, et al. Breast cancer treatment in older women: Does getting what you want improve your long-term body image and mental health? *J Clin Oncol.* 2004;22(19):4002–4009.

36. Janni W, Rjosk D, Dimpfl TH, et al. Quality of life influenced by primary surgical treatment for stage I-III breast cancer-long-term follow-up of a matched-pair analysis. *Ann Surg Oncol.* 2001;8(6):542–548.

37. Javaid M, Song F, Leinster S, et al. Radiation effects on the cosmetic outcomes of immediate and delayed autologous breast reconstruction: An argument about timing. *J Plast Reconstr Aesthet Surg.* 2006;59(1):16–26.

38. Kronowitz SJ, Robb GL. Radiation therapy and breast reconstruction: A critical review of the literature. *Plast Reconstr Surg.* 2009;124(2):395–408.

39. Chawla AK, Kachnic LA, Taghian AG, et al. Radiotherapy and breast reconstruction: Com-plications and cosmesis with TRAM versus tissue expander/implant. *Int J Radiat Oncol Biol Phys.* 2002;54(2):520–526.

40. Pinsolle V, Reau V, Pelissier P, et al. Soft-tissue reconstruction of the distal lower leg and foot: Are free flaps the only choice? Review of 215 cases. *J Plast Reconstr Aesthet Surg.* 2006;59(9):912–917; discussion 918.

41. Chu FC, Kaufmann TP, Dawson GA, et al. Radiation therapy of cancer in prosthetically augmented or reconstructed breasts. *Radiology.* 1992;185(2):429–433.

42. Klein EE, Kuske RR. Changes in photon dose distributions due to breast prostheses. *Int J Radiat Oncol Biol Phys.* 1993;25(3):541–549.

43. Kronowitz SJ, Hunt KK, Kuerer HM, et al. Delayed-immediate breast reconstruction. *Plast Reconstr Surg.* 2004;113(6):1617–1628.

44. Senkus-Konefka E, Wełnicka-Jaśkiewicz M, Jaśkiewicz J, Jassem J. Radiotherapy for breast cancer in patients undergoing breast recon-struction or augmentation. *Cancer Treat Rev.* 2004;30(8):671–682.

45. Yang PS, Chen CM, Liu MC, et al. Radiother-apy can decrease locoregional recurrence and increase survival in mastectomy patients with T1 to T2 breast cancer and one to three positive nodes with negative estrogen receptor and posi-tive lymphovascular invasion status. *Int J Radiat Oncol Biol Phys.* 2010;77(2):516–522.

46. McGuire SE, Gonzalez-Angulo AM, Huang EH, et al. Postmastectomy radiation improves the outcome of patients with locally advanced breast cancer who achieve a pathologic complete response to neoadjuvant chemotherapy. *Int J Radiat Oncol Biol Phys.* 2007;68(4):1004–1009.

47. Recht A, Gray R, Davidson NE, Fowble BL. Locoregional failure 10 years after mastectomy and adjuvant chemotherapy with or without tamoxifen without irradiation: Experience of the Eastern Cooperative Oncology Group. *J Clin Oncol.* 1999 Jun;17(6):1689–1700.

48. Truong PT, Olivotto IA, Kader HA, et al. Selecting breast cancer patients with T1-T2 tumors and one to three positive axillary nodes at high postmastectomy locoregional recurrence risk for adjuvant radiotherapy. *Int J Radiat Oncol Biol Phys.* 2005;61(5):1337–1347.

49. Moreno-Aspitia A. Neoadjuvant therapy in early stage breast cancer. *Crit Rev Oncol Hemat.* 2012;82:187–199.

50. Salgarello M, Barone-Adesi L, Terribile D, Masetti R. Update on one-stage immediate breast reconstruction with definitive prosthesis after sparing mastectomies. *Breast.* 2011;20:7–14.

51. Giuliano AE, Hunt KK, Ballman KV, et al. Axillary dissection vs no axillary dissection in women with invasive breast cancer and sentinel node metastases: A randomized clinical trial. *JAMA,* 2011;305(6):569–575.

■ CASE 2 ■

Indications for Radiation After Neoadjuvant Chemotherapy for Stage II–IIIA Breast Cancer

CLINICAL PROBLEM

Neoadjuvant chemotherapy (NAC), which was originally used to downstage locally advanced breast cancers in order to achieve operability, is increasingly being used in earlier clinical stage II and III patients. Goals of NAC in earlier stage patients include providing the benefit of systemic therapy to control micrometastatic disease earlier in the treatment course (although no evidence exists suggesting a survival benefit to NAC), gaining understanding in the responsiveness of the disease to treatment, and improving the rate of breast conservation therapy (BCT) in women who have slightly larger tumors and/or smaller breast size. Women undergoing NAC are clinically staged prior to chemotherapy, and are frequently downstaged pathologically at the time of postchemotherapy surgery. Controversy exists regarding the role of adjuvant radiation therapy to the nodal regions after NAC when lumpectomy is performed, and to the chest wall with or without regional nodes if mastectomy is performed. Traditional indications for adjuvant radiation, such as number of positive nodes and tumor size, may not be accurately known after downstaging, and prechemotherapy clinical staging information must be taken into account, as well as the postchemotherapy pathologic stage.

CASE EXAMPLE

A 38-year-old woman 10 months postpartum detects a tender mass in the upper outer right breast, which persists over 2 months without significant change, but without resolution. At 12 months postpartum, she discontinues breast-feeding and seeks the advice of her OB/GYN who also palpates a mobile mass in the breast without skin changes and no clinically apparent axillary adenopathy. Mammograms and ultrasound studies are obtained, which reveal a 4.5 cm solid mass with spiculated margins, BiRad category 5. Core biopsy shows high grade invasive ductal carcinoma (IDC), ER–/PR–/Her2–, with associated high grade ductal carcinoma in situ (DCIS). Axillary ultrasound reveals a 1.2 cm lymph node with no fatty hilum, which is positive for metastatic adenocarcinoma on fine needle aspiration (FNA). Breast MRI confirms the presence of a 4.7 cm enhancing mass with no satellite lesions and an enlarged enhancing axillary lymph node. There are no abnormalities in the left breast, no family history of breast cancer, and the patient has no other medical problems requiring intervention. Genetic testing is pending.

The patient is recommended to undergo NAC with dose dense Adriamycin and Cytoxan followed by Taxol. A clip is placed prechemotherapy in the primary tumor. At the completion of chemotherapy, she has no clinical evidence of palpable mass in the breast or axilla and postchemotherapy MRI shows complete resolution of previously noted abnormalities.

Management Decisions

- The patient desires to keep her breast. Is she a candidate for breast conservation surgery?
- If lumpectomy and axillary dissection is performed and there is a complete pathologic response, what radiation fields and doses would be required?
- Can she have a sentinel node biopsy, or is axillary dissection required?
- If the patient has mastectomy and has a complete pathologic response in the breast, and a negative axillary dissection with 0/12 lymph nodes (LN) removed, is postmastectomy radiation indicated? If so, what dose and fields would be treated?

- If the patient has a mastectomy and has 2 cm of residual disease in the breast with negative margins, and negative axillary node dissection (0/12 nodes removed), is postmastectomy radiation indicated?
- If the patient has mastectomy and sentinel lymph node biopsy (SLNB) 1 of 2 positive sentinel nodes (7 mm), and 2/12 additional positive axillary nodes, if postmastectomy radiation is indicated, what fields and dose would be treated?

MAJOR OPINION

Catherine C. Park

Use of BCT After NAC for Operable Breast Cancer

Several randomized clinical trials have reported comparable local regional recurrence (LRR) rates in patients undergoing breast-conserving surgery following NAC compared to those undergoing adjuvant chemotherapy [1–4]. In the National Surgical Adjuvant Breast and Bowel Project (NSABP) B-18 trial that randomized women to neoadjuvant or adjuvant chemotherapy, there was no difference in ipsilateral breast tumor recurrence among patients who received preoperative chemotherapy versus postoperative chemotherapy (13% of 506 patients vs. 10% of 450 patients, respectively, p = .21). Importantly, the cumulative incidences of all local recurrences, as well as distant recurrences, were not significantly different between the 2 groups (p = .08 and p = .22, respectively) [5]. Further evidence that comparable local–regional control rates could be achieved in patients receiving breast-conservation treatment in the neoadjuvant setting is reflected in a study from MD Anderson Cancer Center that included less than 38% with initial stage III disease. Local recurrence rates at 6.7 years follow-up were very low, 2.7%. Notably, in that study, surgeons did not routinely attempt to resect the original tumor volume and the 3 patients that recurred had small to moderate volumes of breast resected [3].

It should be noted, however, that when comparing patients in the NSABP B-18 study who were initially intended to undergo mastectomy but were converted to breast-conservation, the LRR rates appeared higher in the neoadjuvant group versus the adjuvant group, 15.7% versus 9.9%, respectively; p < .04 [5]. In addition, a meta-analysis of 11 trials performed during 1983–1999 of 3,946 patients show that the hazard rate for LRR was significantly increased after NAC (RR = 1.22, 95% CI = 1.04 to 1.43), compared with adjuvant therapy, especially when fewer NAC patients received adjuvant radiation (RR = 1.53, 95% CI = 1.11 to 2.10) [6,7]. In addition, patients with less than a pathologic complete response (pCR) have increased risk for LRR after breast-conserving therapy [4,8]. These data reflect the importance of the ability to adequately identify and resect residual disease and the importance of radiation therapy (RT), even in the setting of pCR and breast preservation.

"Triple negative subtype" (TNS) molecular subtype is measured by immunohistochemical analysis of ER/PR/ and Her-2 (including FISH). Patients with TNS have relatively increased rates of LRR after breast-conserving therapy following adjuvant chemotherapy [7,9–11]. Interestingly, limited date indicate that in the neoadjuvant setting, patients with TNS have higher rates of pCR, although it is unclear whether this translates into a better local–regional control rate [12]. It remains unclear why TNS is associated with higher LRR in the adjuvant setting; some possibilities include an earlier pattern of LRR (vs. total increase), more intrinsically aggressive disease, or relative radioresistance. Presently, TNS itself is not a contraindication to breast-conserving surgery and radiation.

Following successful lumpectomy and negative axillary node dissection, the patient should receive external beam photon radiotherapy to cover the entire breast to 45 to 50 Gy with a boost to the tumor bed to a dose of 10 to 16 Gy. If axillary dissection reveals a pathologic node-negative axilla, then it is reasonable to omit the regional nodal fields and treat the breast alone in most cases. However, some institutions have reported decreased numbers of axillary nodes retrieved following NAC [13], while others have not [14]. If the axillary node dissection is less than adequate (less than 10 nodes removed), there may be a risk for false-negative axilla, and regional nodal radiation may be considered on a case-by-case basis. In addition, other factors such as initial tumor size, grade, molecular subtype, presence and extent of lymphovascular invasion (LVI), the estimated number and size of involved lymph nodes on initial clinical staging, and patient age should be taken into account. A constellation of high-risk features create a more compelling case for treating the regional nodes even after a pCR.

In summary, if breast conserving surgery (BCS) is technically feasible, this patient is a candidate for partial mastectomy and postoperative breast irradiation followed by a tumor bed boost.

Management of the Axilla After NAC

NAC often results in pathologic downstaging of axillary nodes in a significant proportion of patients (30–40%) [8,12,15]. Several studies have shown the feasibility and accuracy of sentinel node mapping and biopsy in the postneoadjuvant setting. In the NSABP B-27 trial, 428 patients underwent sentinel lymph node (SLN) mapping and biopsy prior to axillary lymph node dissection (ALND). The success rate for identifying and removing the SLN was 84.8%, and was significantly higher when radiocolloid was used with or without Lymphazurin blue dye ($p < .03$) [16]. There was a 10.7% rate of false-negatives, which is consistent with the risk for false-negatives in the adjuvant setting. Seven other single institution studies report a success rate between 84.3% and 93.5%; however, the false-negative rates are quite variable ranging from 0% to 33% [16]. Interestingly, patients who achieved pCR had the lowest chance of having involved axillary nodes (15.5%) and, subsequently, a very low risk for a false-negative result (1.7%). Thus, at this time, retrospective studies indicate that the false-negative result would likely be low, however, axillary dissection would be a prudent choice to avoid this risk. A phase 2 trial, American College of Surgeons Oncology Group (ACOSOG) 1071, will evaluate the role for SLN surgery and axillary node dissection following neoadjuvant chemotherapy in patients with node-positive breast cancer.

In summary, the current standard of care is to perform axillary node dissection in patients who present with a biopsy-proven positive node. However, several studies have shown that SLN mapping and biopsy after NAC has a high success rate and low risk for false-negatives, and may be an acceptable alternative to axillary node dissection. The ACOSOG 1071 study is designed to directly address this issue.

The Role of Postmastectomy RT After NAC With or Without Complete Pathologic Response

There are no results from randomized studies to guide the use of postmastectomy radiation therapy (PMRT) following NAC. However, a number of single institution studies and results from the NSABP trials offer some guidance. The recommendation for PMRT follows an assessment of the initial stage, as well as the degree of response to NAC.

In patients who have had pCR, as the patient in the present case, the recommendation for PMRT may be on the basis of the stage of the presenting disease. For this patient, the initial presenting stage was a large stage IIB. In a series from MD Anderson, patients with stage IIIA or higher and pCR benefitted from PMRT after NAC (LRR rates 33% vs. 3%, $p < .006$) [15]. A subset analysis of 16 patients with stage IIB disease and pCR from the same series had 0% LRR. However, patients who presented with stage IIB who did not have pCR also benefitted from PMRT (26% vs. 11%, $p < .0001$). Data from St. Cloud France also shows that patients presenting with stage II or III disease who achieve ypN0 status have low rates of LRR (less than 3–9%), and derive no benefit from PMRT [17]. Thus, single institution series indicate that this patient would have a low risk of LRR after mastectomy on the basis of the presenting stage and pCR. However, such studies are limited by small numbers, heterogeneity in treatment approach, and variable follow-up times.

In addition, other factors may also influence the decision for PMRT. A subset analysis of very young patients, less than 35 years of age, indicates that LRR rates may be substantial (44% vs. 0% without and with PMRT, respectively, $p < .004$) in patients presenting with stage IIB or higher, especially if residual nodal disease is present [18]. They did not report on the very small subset of patients who achieved pCR. It is unclear whether this data directly applies to this case, although it is of concern.

The degree of residual disease burden has been strongly correlated with outcomes in the neoadjuvant setting. In the MD Anderson series, patients presenting with greater than stage IIB, or who had greater than 2 cm residual disease in the breast derived a significant benefit from PMRT ($p < .001$) [15]. This was also true for patients with 4 or more positive nodes. In patients with other adverse pathologic features such as LVI or extra-capsular extension (ECE), a subset analysis indicates that these patients may have higher LRR [19]. The indications for PMRT would not be significantly modified if the patient has an adequate negative axillary node dissection. Rather, the axillary nodes may be omitted in this situation, and the chest wall should be treated with tangential radiation to 50 Gy in 25 to 28 fractions. A case-by-case assessment should be made for including the supraclavicular field in this case.

If the axillary node involvement is found on the sentinel node biopsy, completion of the axillary dissection is clearly indicated. However, the role for PMRT is controversial in this situation. The NSABP studies indicate that patients with ypN1 disease who initially present with clinical T2N1 disease have approximately 17% risk for LRR without PMRT (unpublished); however, patients with ypN1 (1 to 3+ nodes) in the MD Anderson series have 5% LRR without PMRT. Subset analyses can be very unstable statistically; however, in the absence of data, these results indicate that the risk may be substantial in patients presenting with T2-T3 disease and ypN1 after NAC.

In summary, based on limited data, patients who present with stage IIB disease, but achieve pCR after NAC, generally have a low risk of LRR where PMRT may not be justified. However, one could potentially justify the use of PMRT in stage IIB disease and pCR on the basis of young age or other patient or tumor related factors that substantially increase risk. If a recommendation for PMRT is made, the entire chest wall should be treated to 45 to 50 Gy. Treatment of the axillary regional nodes in the setting of pCR would not likely add significant benefit. The decision to treat the supraclavicular nodal region should be made on an individualized basis after consideration of other tumor factors. For those patients who present with more advanced disease, or have residual disease in the breast and/or axilla after NAC, it is likely of benefit to give PMRT as it will decrease LRR risk. Young age and triple negative subtype are potential risk factors for LRR postmastectomy. This case involves a very young patient with a large T2, node-positive, triple negative cancer. She would likely benefit from PMRT regardless of her chemotherapy response.

ACADEMIC COMMENT

Julia S. Wong

As already stated, the potential goals of NAC for operable breast cancer are: (a) conversion of local therapy from mastectomy to BCT, if desired; (b) assessment of response to systemic therapy (typically on protocol); and (c) avoidance of delays in the initiation of systemic therapy in patients at high risk of distant failure. For this patient, NAC may have been necessary in order to offer BCT, rather than mastectomy. Whether upfront BCS is an option partly depends on the size of the tumor

in relation to the breast, and the tumor's location. Contraindications include gross multicentric disease and extensive suspicious calcifications that cannot be encompassed with BCS. Given the results of NSABP B-18 showing a slightly higher local recurrence rate in patients receiving NAC compared to traditional adjuvant systemic therapy, although not statistically significant, it seems prudent to have clearly negative margins if BCT is being considered after NAC, in particular, for young patients and those with triple negative disease in whom higher local recurrence rates, in general, are a concern. Clips need to be placed at the time of the initial core biopsy, to help guide the surgeon, as some patients may have a radiographic complete response.

The optimal management of the clinically-negative axilla in the setting of NAC continues to evolve. We know that SLN after NAC is feasible and accurate, but the interpretation of these results in relation to initial stage and subsequent local–regional therapy recommendations is not always straightforward. Ideally, patients undergo imaging of the axilla as part of the initial diagnostic work-up, and any suspicious axillary nodes identified on CT, MRI, or ultrasound are evaluated at that time with an FNA. Patients with known axillary involvement at diagnosis are candidates for completion axillary dissection (not solely SNB) after NAC until further data become available regarding outcomes of SNB alone after NAC in this population.

In the setting of a positive axillary FNA followed by NAC, and then completion axillary dissection, the patient would typically receive 44 to 50 Gy to the whole breast followed by a boost to the tumor bed. If there were multiple suspicious lymph nodes at diagnosis, the addition of a regional nodal field to treat the undissected nodes (Level III/supraclavicular) may be considered. Whether this is necessary is not clear.

No firm guidelines exist at present for the use of PMRT after NAC. The "rules" for its use have been based on pathology obtained at diagnosis. How best to interpret post-NAC pathology, with respect to the use of PMRT and the fields to be treated, is not well defined. In this case, we would consider initial clinical stage; given that this is a large T2 tumor with at least 1 involved axillary node in a young patient, PMRT would likely be offered. The chest wall would be treated to about 50 Gy, with or without a scar boost. Inclusion of the supraclavicular nodes may be considered, but the main benefit is from the treatment of the chest wall. After an adequate, negative axillary dissection, the axilla should not be irradiated as there is little benefit, and such treatment increases the risk of lymphedema.

If residual axillary disease is identified on axillary dissection after NAC, the extent of the RT fields would depend on the initial stage, the number of lymph nodes involved, the extent of the dissection, and the volume of nodal disease. Supraclavicular radiation should be strongly considered, however, as the accurate initial number of positive nodes cannot be definitively known for risk stratification purposes.

How to optimize the combination of PMRT and breast reconstruction is a topic of ongoing debate. There is much controversy and not enough data to provide clear guidelines on the best approach. The treatment policies, therefore, tend to vary by institution with no clear "right" or "wrong." For patients who we already know will need PMRT, our preference is to recommend delaying reconstruction until all adjuvant therapy is complete. This allows us to optimize radiation planning techniques to avoid lung and heart, but commits the patient to autologous flap reconstruction, as an implant alone is usually not possible after chest wall RT. For patients in whom the need for PMRT is unclear, patients who are unwilling to accept delayed reconstruction, or patients in whom delayed reconstruction is not a viable option, we will consider placement of a tissue expander at the time of mastectomy. This decision is usually accompanied by a detailed discussion with the patient regarding the pros and cons with respect to the effect of a tissue expander on radiation planning and the potential complications to the reconstruction, which are increased by the use of RT.

COMMUNITY PRACTITIONER COMMENT

Gray B. Swor

NAC in this situation has several advantages. It allows early systemic intervention in a high-risk patient, assessment of the response to chemotherapy, and increases the rate of BCT (approximately 20–30%). Fortunately, in this case example, the patient had an excellent clinical and radiographic response to NAC. She would, therefore, be a candidate for BCS. This would include lumpectomy and axillary staging, either ALND or SLNB. Since she was found to have a positive axillary lymph node at the time of diagnosis, axillary staging cannot be avoided following neoadjuvant treatment. If her SLN is positive, then axillary node dissection usually follows although further axillary surgery is unlikely to change her management. Currently, there is not sufficient data to support omitting completion axillary node dissection after NAC. In the American College of Surgeons Oncology Group Z0011 trial [20] comparing SLNB alone with ALND in patients with a positive SLN, patients who received NAC were excluded from the study. Therefore, it is difficult to draw any conclusion regarding the safety of omitting ALND in the neoadjuvant setting. Likewise, if she undergoes mastectomy, she will require axillary staging as above.

If mastectomy is planned and the patient desires reconstruction, she would be a candidate for immediate–delayed reconstruction with a tissue expander placed at the time of mastectomy or delayed reconstruction using autologous tissue at a later time following adjuvant therapy (usually a year). If immediate–delayed reconstruction is performed, the tissue expander may need to be deflated prior to RT to optimize treatment planning and delivery. After completion of adjuvant radiotherapy, the expander can be re-expanded to the desired volume. The expander can be swapped out for the permanent implant later (usually 8–12 months to allow for healing time).

If this patient undergoes lumpectomy or mastectomy and is found to have residual disease in the breast or lymph nodes, then subsequent recommendations for systemic therapy are usually in the context of a clinical trial. Since she is ER negative, she is not a candidate for antiestrogen therapy, nor is she a candidate for Herceptin as she is Her-2 neu negative.

The decision regarding adjuvant RT should be based on pretreatment clinical staging. In this current scenario, we have a patient with a very large clinical T2 lesion (the distinction between 4.7 cm and 5 cm being arbitrary) and at least 1 positive axillary lymph node. She also has several poor-risk features including premenopausal status, negative receptor status, and a high-grade lesion. For these reasons, comprehensive RT is recommended. So if she has BCS, the whole breast and regional lymph nodes, including the Level III axilla and supraclavicular nodes, would be treated to a dose of approximately 50 Gy in 28 fractions. If no axillary node dissection is performed, then the Level I and II axillary nodes would be included in the treatment area. If, however, she undergoes

ALND, the dissected axilla would be avoided. In the situation of BCS, a boost to the lumpectomy bed would be recommended to a dose of 10.8 Gy in 6 fractions. Likewise, if she has a mastectomy, the chest wall would be treated with appropriate bolus, including the Level III axilla, and supraclavicular regions if ALND is performed—the Level I and II axilla would be included only if SLNB alone is performed. As with upfront mastectomy, certain pathologic features may warrant targeting the full axilla, including bulky nodal disease, ECE, inadequate axillary dissection (less than 6 nodes obtained) or use of sentinel node biopsy only. The chest wall and lymphatic dose should be approximately 50.5 Gy in 28 fractions. A boost to the mastectomy scar would also be recommended for an additional 10 to 10.8 Gy in 5 to 6 fractions.

SECTION EDITOR'S NOTE

Eleanor E. R. Harris

The majority of randomized clinical trials for both BCT and mastectomy have been performed in the setting of adjuvant chemotherapy. Results for the use of NAC have been studied in a small number of randomized trials and reported by several institutions, notably in large series from the MD Anderson Cancer Center. These studies have not asked questions about the use of radiation, which has usually been at the treating physician's discretion in mastectomy patients, or forbidden as in the NSABP B18 and B27 trials. Classic indications for radiation, especially after mastectomy, have been based on pathologic surgical staging prior to chemotherapy. The likelihood of downstaging in the breast and nodes after NAC raises some questions about the indications for radiation. An area of increasing interest and study is the use of NAC for marginally operable cancers to improve the rate of BCS. The randomized trials of chemotherapy sequencing have shown no survival difference by the timing of chemotherapy and surgery, and have also shown that a pCR is a positive prognostic factor regardless of surgical management.

In this case of a young woman with a large clinical stage T2N1 cancer initially and an excellent clinical response to NAC, she fits this latter category and is a reasonable candidate for BCS. In fact, this approach may be preferable. She likely requires an axillary dissection, given the presence of clinically positive and pathologically confirmed axillary nodes at diagnosis. She also requires

radiation to the breast or chest wall and regional nodes regardless of what surgical management of the breast is used, because of the presence of several risk factors, including pathologically positive nodes prechemotherapy, large tumor size, and triple negative histology.

I would recommend postlumpectomy radiation to the breast and regional nodes to a conventional dose of 46 to 50 Gy in 2 Gy per fraction, assuming good dose homogeneity (if greater than 7%, consider using 1.8 Gy per fraction), and a tumor bed boost of 10 to 16 Gy for total tumor bed dose of 60 to 66 Gy. I tend to prescribe a total dose of 66 Gy for young women and for triple negative cancers, on the basis of the limited data. The optimal boost dose after pCR is not known. Although some would omit a boost after whole breast radiation in this scenario, I would still provide it given her high-risk histology.

If this patient were to undergo mastectomy, even in the setting of a pCR, I would still recommend postmastectomy radiation to the chest wall and remaining regional nodes on the basis of her prechemotherapy staging. While this is more controversial, there are emerging data that premenopausal women with stage II triple negative cancers have a higher rate of LRR after mastectomy if radiation is omitted than after BCT [21]. These trends have not been sufficiently evaluated in the setting of NAC use, and the impact of pCR on these trends is not well understood. Therefore, I would not recommend omission of PMRT given its proven survival benefit in node-positive disease.

REFERENCES

1. Cance WG, Carey LA, Calvo BF, et al. Long-term outcome of neoadjuvant therapy for locally advanced breast carcinoma: Effective clinical downstaging allows breast preservation and predicts outstanding local control and survival. *Ann Surg.* 2002;236(3):295–302. Discussion 302–303.

2. Fisher B, Brown A, Mamounas E, et al. Effect of preoperative chemotherapy on local-regional disease in women with operable breast cancer: Findings from National Surgical Adjuvant Breast and Bowel Project B-18. *J Clin Oncol.* 1997;15(7):2483–2493.

3. Peintinger F, Symmans WF, Gonzalez-Angulo AM, et al. The safety of breast-conserving surgery in patients who achieve a complete pathologic response after neoadjuvant chemotherapy. *Cancer.* 2006;107(6):1248–1254.

4. Chen AM, Meric-Bernstam F, Hunt KK, et al. Breast conservation after neoadjuvant chemotherapy: The MD Anderson Cancer Center experience. *J Clin Oncol.* 2004;22(12):2303–2312.

5. Boehmler JH 4th, Butler CE, Ensor J, Kronowitz SJ. Outcomes of various techniques of abdominal fascia closure after TRAM flap breast reconstruction. *Plast Reconstr Surg.* 2009;123(3):773–781.

6. Jackson WB, Goldson AL, Staud C. Postoperative irradiation following immediate breast reconstruction using a temporary tissue expander. *J Natl Med Assoc.* 1994;86(7):538–542.

7. Nguyen PL, Taghian AG, Katz MS, et al. Breast cancer subtype approximated by estrogen receptor, progesterone receptor, and HER-2 is associated with local and distant recurrence after breast-conserving therapy. *J Clin Oncol.* 2008;26(14):2373–2378.

8. Wolmark N, Wang J, Mamounas E, et al. Preoperative chemotherapy in patients with operable breast cancer: Nine-year results from National Surgical Adjuvant Breast and Bowel Project B-18. *J Natl Cancer Inst Monogr.* 2001;(30):96–102.

9. Voduc KD, Cheang MC, Tyldesley S, et al. Breast cancer subtypes and the risk of local and regional relapse. *J Clin Oncol.* 2010;28(10):1684–1691.

10. Millar EK, Graham PH, O'Toole Sa, et al. Prediction of local recurrence, distant metastases, and death after breast-conserving therapy in early-stage invasive breast cancer using a five-biomarker panel. *J Clin Oncol.* 2009;27(28):4701–4708.

11. Straver ME, Rutgers EJ, Rodenhuis S, et al. The relevance of breast cancer subtypes in the outcome of neoadjuvant chemotherapy. *Ann Surg Oncol.* 2010;17(9):2411–2418.

12. Rastogi P, Anderson SJ, Bear HD, et al. Preoperative chemotherapy: Updates of National Surgical Adjuvant Breast and Bowel Project Protocols B-18 and B-27. *J Clin Oncol.* 2008;26(5):778–785.

13. Neuman H, Carey LA, Ollila DW, et al. Axillary lymph node count is lower after neoadjuvant chemotherapy. *Am J Surg.* 2006;191(6):827–829.

14. Boughey JC, Peintinger F, Meric-Bernstam F, et al. Impact of preoperative versus postoperative chemotherapy on the extent and number of surgical procedures in patients treated in randomized clinical trials for breast cancer. *Ann Surg.* 2006;244(3):464–470.

15. Huang EH, Tucker SL, Strom EA, et al. Postmastectomy radiation improves local-regional control and survival for selected patients with locally advanced breast cancer treated with neoadjuvant chemotherapy and mastectomy. *J Clin Oncol.* 2004;22(23):4691–4699.

16. Mamounas EP, Brown A, Anderson S, et al. Sentinel node biopsy after neoadjuvant chemotherapy in breast cancer: Results from National Surgical Adjuvant Breast and Bowel Project Protocol B-27. *J Clin Oncol.* 2005;23(12):2694–2702.

17. Le Scodan R, Selz J, Stevens D, et al. Radiotherapy for stage II and stage III breast cancer patients with negative lymph nodes after preoperative chemotherapy and mastectomy. *Intl J Radiat Oncol Biol Phys.* 2012;82(1):e1–e7.

18. Garg AK, Oh JL, Oswald MJ, et al. Effect of postmastectomy radiotherapy in patients <35 years old with stage II-III breast cancer treated with doxorubicin-based neoadjuvant chemotherapy and mastectomy. *Intl J Radiat Oncol Biol Phys.* 2007;69(5):1478–1483.

19. Huang EH, Tucker SL, Strom EA, et al. Predictors of locoregional recurrence in patients with locally advanced breast cancer treated with neoadjuvant chemotherapy, mastectomy, and radiotherapy. *Intl J Radiat Oncol Biol Phys.* 2005;62(2):351–357.

20. Giuliano AE, Hunt KK, Ballman KV, et al. Axillary dissection vs no axillary dissection in women with invasive breast cancer and sentinel node metastases: A randomized clinical trial. *JAMA,* 2011;305(6):569–575.

21. Abdulkarim BS, Cuartero J, Hanson J, et al. Increased risk of locoregional recurrence for women with T1-2N0 triple-negative cancer treated with modified radical mastectomy without adjuvant radiation therapy compared with breast conserving therapy. *J Clin Oncol.* 2011;29(21):2852–2858.

Management of Elderly Patients With Early Stage Breast Cancer

CLINICAL PROBLEM

The optimal management of elderly women with early stage breast cancer is controversial. Most clinical trials have excluded women over the age of 70, so information on outcome benefit in this age group is lacking for both systemic and radiation therapy (RT). A recent randomized trial in women over age 70 with stage T1N0 ER+ breast cancer of postlumpectomy tamoxifen with or without whole breast radiation showed a statistically significantly reduction in local recurrence in the radiation arm with no survival difference. Other epidemiologic studies show that undertreatment of older women with breast cancer is common and associated with a higher risk of dying from breast cancer. Older women are more likely to have comorbidities, but when physiologic age and comorbidity status are accounted for, they are likely to tolerate standard therapy well.

CASE EXAMPLE

A 72-year-old woman with osteoarthritis, hyperlipidemia, and hypertension has a new abnormal density in the upper inner quadrant of the right breast on routine screening mammogram measuring 8 mm, corresponding to a hypoechoic mass on ultrasound. Physical exam by her primary physician confirms a 10 mm firm mass and no axillary adenopathy. Core biopsy shows an intermediate-grade invasive ductal carcinoma (IDC), ER+ (85%), PR+ (5%), and Her2 2+ by immunohistochemistry (IHC) with a fluorescent in situ hybridization (FISH) score of 1.5. The patient undergoes lumpectomy with sentinel lymph node biopsy. Pathology reveals a 9 mm intermediate-grade IDC with focal lymphovascular space invasion, closest margin width of 1 mm superiorly, and a micrometastasis measuring 0.8 mm in 1 of 2 sentinel lymph nodes (SLNs). She has an Oncotype Dx Recurrence Score of 19.

Management Decisions

• Does the patient require a completion axillary dissection? A re-excision of the lumpectomy bed?
• Is postlumpectomy radiation indicated? If so, what options for dose fractionation and radiation field arrangements could be considered?
• Is systemic therapy indicated? If so, which agents?

MAJOR OPINION

Julia S. Wong

Breast Conservation Options in Elderly Patients With Early Stage Breast Cancer

Management of the Axilla and Margins When Using Breast Conservation Therapy

Sentinel node biopsy is the standard of care for patients with an invasive disease who are clinically node-negative and who require surgical evaluation of the axilla. Until recently, completion axillary dissection was the recommended course of action for a positive sentinel node, if the metastatic deposit was a micrometastasis or larger. A meta-analysis of 8,059 patients, 96% of whom had successful sentinel node mapping, found a 42% rate of lymph node involvement; among patients with a positive sentinel node, 53% had additional positive nodes at completion axillary dissection [1]. The issue of which patients require completion dissection is a source of ongoing debate. The Memorial Sloan-Kettering nomogram was developed to estimate the risk of additional positive nodes in the setting of a positive sentinel node, using pathologic size, tumor type and nuclear grade, lymphovascular invasion, multifocality, estrogen receptor status, method of detection of sentinel node metastases, number of positive sentinel nodes, and number of negative sentinel nodes [2]. The receiver operating characteristic (ROC) was 0.76 in a retrospective population and 0.77 in a prospective group. Other groups have tested the nomogram with varying results in terms of reliability [3,4].

The significance of the presence of only micrometastatic disease in a sentinel node, both with respect to prognosis and how this should affect management decisions, remains unclear, especially as there is considerable variability regarding how it is detected. Until recently, the standard of care was to recommend completion axillary dissection for patients with micrometastatic (or larger) disease in a sentinel node. The American College of Surgeons Oncology Group (ACOSOG) Z0011 trial is a prospective study randomizing patients with clinical stage T1-T2, N0 breast cancer with 1 to 2 positive sentinel nodes, who underwent lumpectomy and tangential breast RT, to either completion axillary dissection versus no further axillary treatment [5,6]. Although the trial closed early because of slow accrual and lower-than-anticipated recurrence rates, there were 856 evaluable patients with a median follow-up of 6.3 years. The local regional recurrence rate was 3.4% overall; 1.8% in the sentinel node biopsy-only group and 3.6% in the axillary dissection group. Twenty-seven percent of the patients in the axillary dissection group had additional positive nodes in the completion dissection. Of note, the radiation doses and the extent of the superior field border were not described. These details are of interest as it is established that the superior portion of the tangential fields includes some of the Level I and II axillary nodes [7,8] and almost certainly contributed to regional control.

Criteria for breast-conserving surgery include negative margins (with the possible exception of the posterior/deep margin and the superficial/skin margin if the margin is at the limit of the anatomic extent of the breast tissue). In some settings, a focally positive margin is considered acceptable, especially if systemic therapy will be given, as local control remains excellent (7% at 8 years in 1 retrospective study) [9]. The definition of what constitutes an adequate margin varies according to variables such as extent of disease in the breast, extent of resection, patient age, and the extent of disease near the margin. Cosmetic issues can also affect whether a re-excision is feasible. As a result, situations involving close margins (less than 1 or 2 mm) in patients interested in

breast-conserving surgery need to be evaluated on an individual basis. Of note, modern series show excellent local control with breast-conserving surgery plus radiation, likely reflecting the impact of improved imaging, attention to margins, and the use of systemic therapy. In a retrospective study of 793 patients who underwent breast conservation therapy (BCT), at a median follow-up time of 70 months, the overall 5-year cumulative incidence of local recurrence was 1.8%, and when analyzed by receptor status as a surrogate for subtype, all groups had a local recurrence rate under 10% [10]. The vast majority of this patient population had negative margins and received adjuvant systemic therapy.

In summary, given the available information and the very low rate of regional recurrence observed in the ACOSOG trial, it is reasonable to offer this approach to selected patients who meet the entry criteria and omit completion axillary dissection in this patient. Patients with high-risk features, who may not have been well represented in the trial population, may be considered for completion dissection. As for breast re-excision, this patient is older and has a small, ER-positive cancer. If the margin in question is focally close, re-excision may reasonably be omitted, especially if she is planning to receive RT ($\pm$ endocrine therapy). If the margin is close along a broad front, especially if there is the presence of an extensive intraductal component, re-excision is recommended. The radiation oncologist and surgeon should review the extent of disease at the or near the margin with the pathologist.

Role of RT in Elderly Women Treated With Breast Conservation

RT consistently reduces the local recurrence by about two-thirds after lumpectomy. Efforts to select "favorable" subgroups which do not benefit from breast irradiation have been unsuccessful. However, the absolute benefit of RT is smaller in patients who are at lower baseline risk of local recurrence, and there has been interest in whether RT may be omitted in selected older patients. The Cancer and Leukemia Group B (CALGB) C9343 trial included 636 women aged 70 or older, who had clinical stage I, ER-positive breast cancer and who underwent lumpectomy and received tamoxifen, randomizing them to RT or no RT [11,12]. Surgical evaluation of the axilla was not required. Patients had negative margins, defined as no tumor on ink. No survival difference was seen. At a median follow-up of 10.5 years, ipsilateral breast recurrence was 8% in the no RT arm and 2% in the RT arm. Forty-three percent of the participants had died, but only 7% were due to breast cancer. Compliance with endocrine therapy is variable, and some patients ultimately discontinue it. Patients with long life expectancies may feel that a reduction in local recurrence is a worthy endpoint, even if breast cancer-specific survival in unaffected. It is worthwhile to critically assess comorbidities in this patient population when making recommendations for RT [13]. Radiation techniques have improved over the past 1 to 2 decades, especially with respect to reduced heart and lung doses and improved homogeneity, lessening the acute and long-term morbidity of RT.

The use of hypofractionation, typically defined as dose per fraction larger than 2 Gy per day with reduced number of total fractions, has been studied in several trials of early stage breast cancer. Data from Canada on the use of hypofractionated RT, showing that 42.5 Gy given in 16 treatments to the whole breast, without a boost, results in equivalent local control and cosmetic results at 10 years compared to standard fractionation, provides another option for patients who otherwise would not consider RT [14,15]. Patients in this study had T1 or T2 tumors, a negative Level I/II axillary dissection, negative margins (no invasive or intraductal carcinoma at ink), and the maximum width of breast tissue was limited to 25 cm. The START trials in England, which compared 5 to 0 Gy in 25 fractions to several hypofractionation regimens (39 Gy in 13 fractions, 41.6 Gy in 13 fractions, or 42.9 Gy in 13 fractions) similarly showed no significant differences in local control or late normal tissue effects among the different fractionation regimens [16,17].

The European Organisation for Research and Treatment of Cancer (EORTC) evaluated the impact of a boost to the tumor bed in addition to whole breast irradiation in a randomized trial [18,19]. More than 5,000 patients were randomized to receive 50 Gy to the whole breast, with or without a 16 Gy boost. Although the proportional benefit of a boost for local control was consistent, the absolute benefit of a boost in this age group was small. Patients older than 60 years who did not receive a boost had a 10-year local recurrence rate of 7.3%, compared to 3.8% for patients who received a boost. In a subgroup analysis, there was no significant effect of margin status on local recurrence at 10 years. In a multivariate analysis, a high grade was associated with an increase in local recurrence (reduced with the use of a boost), as was young age (age less than 50 years).

In summary, based on the findings of the CALGB trial, it is reasonable to discuss the option of omitting RT in this older patient, who would have been eligible for this trial, if she agrees to take a full course of endocrine therapy. This trial did not require surgical staging of the axillary nodes, and two-thirds of patients in the trial did not have an axillary dissection or sentinel node biopsy, so some enrolled would have had microscopically positive nodes. A positive axillary node is associated with an increased risk of local regional recurrence, so warrants consideration of the use of breast irradiation. In particular, if the tolerability of endocrine therapy is in question, and given in addition the presence of a close margin, tangential RT to the whole breast and including the lower axillary nodes is likely the preferred option. Standard fractionation of 45 to 50 Gy over 4 to 5 weeks with or without a boost may be offered. Hypofractionated whole-breast RT without a boost to 42.56 Gy in 3 weeks is a good alternative, if acceptable dose homogeneity can be achieved.

Use of Accelerated Partial Breast Irradiation

Accelerated partial breast irradiation (APBI) has become increasingly popular given its premise, namely, to treat only the area at highest risk of recurrence, the lumpectomy cavity, because that is where most local recurrences are seen, and treat in a shorter timeframe (usually twice a day over 4–5 days) rather than a multiple-week course of standard external beam RT. Various techniques are available: interstitial (which has the longest follow-up in published studies, but is the most labor intensive), balloon catheter (such as MammoSite; easier technically than the interstitial technique), intraoperative RT (requires specialized equipment), or 3-dimensional conformal beam arrangements using a standard linear accelerator (often utilizing noncoplanar beams). Depending on the institution, one of these approaches may bc favored. Studies of 3-D conformal techniques have the shortest follow-up, but data continue to mature. Four-year data from William Beaumont Hospital on 94 patients treated with 3-D conformal approaches shows a 1.1% local recurrence rate, 4% grade 3 toxicity

(1 transient breast pain and 3 fibrosis), and an 89% good/excellent rating for cosmesis [20].

The selection of patients suitable for APBI remains controversial. The ongoing National Surgical Adjuvant Breast and Bowel Project (NSABP)-39 randomized study comparing whole-breast RT to APBI will help in this regard. At institutions not participating in this or another APBI trial, the American Society for Radiation Oncology (ASTRO) has published consensus guidelines to help determine which patients can be safely treated with APBI off protocol [21]. Three categories were defined: suitable, cautionary, and unsuitable. This patient falls into the "unsuitable" category given the micrometastasis in a sentinel node, presence of lymphovascular invasion (LVI), and a margin of less than 2 mm, the latter 2 characteristics being in the "cautionary" category. The Groupe Européen de Curiethérapie-European Society for Therapeutic Radiology and Oncology (GEC-ESTRO) has published APBI guidelines as well [22]. The 3 categories defined were low, intermediate, and high risk. This patient has 2 intermediate risk features (margin less than 2 mm and pN1mi nodal status) and 1 high risk feature (LVI).

In summary, APBI is increasingly widely used in early stage cancer. The criteria for its use continue to evolve as more long-term data become available, and is particularly attractive to older patients because of concerns about length of treatment and toxicity. Until more mature randomized trial data are available, published guidelines for patient selection for APBI should be utilized, such as the ASTRO consensus guidelines. This particular patient does not meet the published ASTRO criteria of suitability, and therefore is not an optimal candidate for APBI.

Adjuvant Systemic Therapy Use in Elderly Patients With Early Stage I–II Breast Cancer

Patients with hormone-sensitive cancers are candidates for adjuvant endocrine therapy. The relative benefit of chemotherapy in this clinical situation is quite low, and the mainstay of systemic therapy is endocrine therapy, especially given the differential in toxicity profile between chemotherapy and endocrine therapy, which is a concern in an older patient with multiple comorbidities. The advent of genomic analysis (Oncotype DX, MammaPrint) now allows clinicians to define more specific benefits of the addition of chemotherapy to endocrine therapy for the individual patient. The Oncotype DX assay consists of a 21-gene panel, is performed on paraffin-embedded tissue, and derives a recurrence score (low, intermediate, or high) that corresponds to a risk of recurrence at 10 years, for ER-positive, node-negative patients who take tamoxifen for 5 years. The test is both prognostic and predictive [23,24]. Patients with a low recurrence score derive little benefit from the addition of chemotherapy, whereas those with a high recurrence score derive substantial benefit. While developed for node-negative patients, there are data supporting its use in node-positive patients [25]. The MammaPrint assay utilizes 70 genes and has been shown to independently predict disease outcome and survival [26], but requires fresh frozen tissue, thus limiting its clinical use.

Tamoxifen has been shown to reduce recurrence rates about 50% in patients aged 70 or older [27]. Alternatively, aromatase inhibitors (AIs) may be considered instead of, or combined sequentially with, tamoxifen. Several trials have been designed to assess this issue, including the ATAC, BIG 1-98, IES, and MA-17 trials [28–33]. There is currently no consensus on the optimal regimen, but many would strive to include an AI, either after tamoxifen, or as the sole endocrine therapy, if feasible. The toxicity profile of tamoxifen versus an AI must be considered.

In summary, for this patient with a strongly ER-positive, stage I breast cancer, endocrine therapy, without chemotherapy, is appropriate. If chemotherapy is being considered, an Oncotype DX test may be obtained to ascertain the patient's risk of distant failure at 10 years if on tamoxifen. Depending on the risk category, the medical oncologist may feel that a discussion about the risks and benefits of adding chemotherapy to endocrine therapy may be warranted. In this patient with osteoarthritis, depending on the severity of her joint symptoms and her other comorbidities, the medical oncologist may consider tamoxifen more appropriate. Compliance in this age group can also present challenges.

ACADEMIC COMMENT

Eleanor E. R. Harris

The definition of *elderly* is a controversial subject and should not be solely based on chronological age. Clinical trials, by necessity, incorporate discrete eligibility criteria and often use specific age cutoffs that are, in truth, somewhat arbitrary, yet become adopted in practice. Physiologic age, comorbidities, performance status, patient preference, and life expectancy are critically important parameters in the medical decision-making process that are seldom used as eligibility criteria for clinical trials. Many of the randomized trials for early stage breast cancer excluded women above a certain age cutoff, particularly for systemic therapy questions, resulting in a relative paucity of data in older age groups. There also appears to exist clinician biases that older women will not tolerate standard treatment as well as younger patients, which is not borne out of data, particularly when comorbidities are accounted for. Older women in good health tolerate standard breast irradiation quite well [13,34]. Compliance with a full 5-year course of endocrine therapy, however, has been reported to be relatively low in studies of the general population (as opposed to clinical trial participants), with up to one-quarter of women no longer filling their prescriptions at 1 year, dropping off to only 50% at 4 years [35]. There are studies that show higher rates of death from breast cancer in older populations when undertreated [36].

These complex issues are important to consider when choosing the optimal therapy for an elderly patient. Although the trial reported by Hughes shows no survival benefit for the addition of breast irradiation to tamoxifen in women over 70 years of age, it was not powered to demonstrate this difference [12]. The power calculations for this study were based on time to local or regional recurrence. For the locoregional recurrence endpoint, at 8 years there was a statistically significant benefit to the use of radiation, which lowered the locoregional recurrence rate from 9% to 2% ($p = .015$). This outcome depends on completion of a full 5-year course of endocrine therapy. Whether such a local control benefit is clinically meaningful is for the individual patient and her physician to determine.

Elderly patients in good health with limited comorbidities should be treated similarly as other groups of low-risk breast conservation patients. It should also be recognized that not all elderly patients in fact present with low-risk disease. Standard therapies with proven local–regional and survival benefit should not be avoided simply because of the patient's chronological age. If the patient is deemed physiologically able to tolerate standard radiation and systemic therapies, they should be offered.

COMMUNITY PRACTITIONER COMMENT

Gray B. Swor

This patient is a reasonably healthy 72-year-old with a pT1b N1(mic) M0 intermediate-grade infiltrating ductal carcinoma, ER positive, PR positive, and negative HER-2 by FISH. The main issues in the surgical management of this patient include the close margin and axillary staging. Pathologically, she is found to have a 1 mm surgical margin superiorly. This is technically a negative margin. There is no universally agreed upon definition of a negative margin; however, the definition used in most trials is no tumor at the inked surgical margin. Successful BCT is precedent on margins free of invasive and in situ disease with acceptable cosmesis. I do not believe that this particular patient requires re-excision. This close margin could be addressed with an additional boost dose of RT if there is concern.

In regard to her axillary nodal staging, axillary lymph node dissection (ALND) has been the standard approach for patients with a positive SLN, although the management of patients with low volume disease in the SLN has been controversial. In light of the ACOSOG Z0011 Phase 3 Trial, patients who underwent sentinel lymph node dissection (SLND) alone compared with those who underwent completion ALND for a positive SLN experienced no detriment in terms of overall survival or disease-free survival in patients with T1 and T2 breast cancers. Axillary recurrence rates were similar in both groups. Therefore, I believe that ALND could be safely omitted in this individual assuming she will undergo adjuvant breast and Level I and II axillary radiotherapy. Omitting the ALND would reduce the potential toxicities of further axillary surgery, including postoperative seroma formation, arm and breast lymphedema, paresthesias, and numbness in the underarm area.

Medical management of this patient is controversial. Even though she has a small intermediate-grade tumor and is strongly ER+, she does have a positive SLN and is found to be in a low/intermediate risk category on Oncotype DX testing, with a recurrence score of 19 translating into a systemic risk of recurrence of 12%. I think that chemotherapy should be considered, perhaps with regimens such as cyclophosphamide, methotrexate, and 5-fluorouracil (CMF), in an effort to minimize toxicities. Her expected survival benefit with adjuvant chemotherapy would perhaps be approximately 5%

to 7%. Antiestrogen therapy with an AI would be recommended for 5 years unless she has a contraindication, such as severe osteoporosis, in which case tamoxifen could be recommended.

There is current debate regarding post-lumpectomy radiotherapy recommendations in elderly women with favorable disease breast cancer. Some have concluded that radiotherapy can safely be omitted in this group of women who are ER-positive and on antiestrogen therapy as there is no survival benefit and the improvement in local control is small. In this sample patient, RT would be indicated after lumpectomy because she has several intermediate-risk features, including a positive SLN, intermediate-grade tumor, close surgical margin, and focal lymphovascular invasion. Treatment would include the whole breast and Level I and II axillary lymph nodes, if only sentinel lymph node biopsy is performed. If, however, completion ALND is performed, then the dissected axilla would be omitted from the treatment field. If this particular patient had a more generous surgical margin, was N0 with a low-grade tumor, and was on antiestrogen therapy, then perhaps omitting radiotherapy could be considered, although in large studies of women over 70 years there is consistently a reduction in local recurrence with adjuvant radiotherapy.

This particular patient has inquired about the use of accelerated partial breast radiotherapy. Patients must be carefully selected for this more limited treatment on the basis of the ASTRO consensus statement on APBI. This patient would be unsuitable because of her positive lymph node status. Even if her SLNs were negative, she would be considered cautionary as she had a less than 2 mm margin and focal LVI.

Although this patient is 72 years old, she does seem to be in good clinical condition. The ability to tolerate RT should not be a limiting factor in making treatment recommendations in elderly breast cancer patients as there is no evidence to suggest that they experience greater morbidity from treatment. In reviewing 2010 actuary data, her life expectancy would be approximately 87 years of age, therefore, a path of undertreatment should be avoided.

SECTION EDITOR'S NOTE

Eleanor E. R. Harris

Although showing a statistically significant benefit for the primary endpoint of local–regional control in the radiation arm, the results of the CALGB C9343 trial have been interpreted by many as being clinically insignificant, leading to advocacy for observing women over age 70 postlumpectomy who have T1N0, ER+ cancer. The study has several limitations, including small sample size and lack of data on both tolerance and compliance with the endocrine therapy required in both arms. Other studies have revealed problems with compliance with AIs, especially in the elderly population for whom musculoskeletal comorbidities are often preexisting. Population data that show that elderly women who are undertreated have a higher risk of dying of breast cancer raise concerns about the omission of radiation. These women are good candidates for hypofractionation regimens, or often meet the ASTRO "suitability" criteria for APBI, making the radiotherapy much more convenient with reduced risk of toxicity. Recent reports have shown little shift in clinical practice after the publication of the initial results of C9343 in 2004. Rather, the consensus seems to be that recommendations for breast irradiation should be individualized with consideration of the patient's performance status, comorbidities, and informed preferences. In my own experience, while I typically discuss the results of the C9343 trial with women who fit its eligibility criteria, the vast majority prefer to have radiation.

The C9343 study, which was conducted between 1994 and 1999, defined negative margins as "no tumor on ink." Also, the study did not require any axillary surgery if the patient was clinically node negative; over one-third of patients had no axillary dissection and the study predated the sentinel node era. It is highly unlikely that a micrometastasis would have been detected in that era in the women who underwent axillary dissection, so some percentage of enrolled patients would have had undetected micrometastases in their nodes, yet classified as N0, thus eligible to be randomized to no radiation. Subsequently, the ACOSOG Z011 trial has shown no benefit to completion axillary dissection in women undergoing lumpectomy and breast irradiation who have 1 or 2 positive sentinel nodes.

In light of these considerations, for this woman in her early 70s with limited comorbidities and early stage, relatively favorable cancer, I would not recommend completion axillary dissection. She has a focally close margin, which meets the definition of negative margin in C9343 and numerous NSABP studies. Several series have shown that the risk of residual disease on re-excision in this setting is low.

I personally review the margin in question with the pathologist to assess the focality of disease near the margin, but typically do not recommend re-excision. I would recommend postlumpectomy breast irradiation. This patient is a good candidate for either hypofractionation (such as 42.56 in 16 fractions) to the whole breast or some type of APBI. I lean toward the former, given the presence of N1mic disease, but would be comfortable with APBI if the patient had a strong preference and/or access issues. I would counsel the patient that she technically falls into the ASTRO Consensus Statement's "unsuitable" category because of N1mic pathology, although this statement does not specifically comment upon the categorization of micrometastatic nodal disease only. If the patient prefers, she could also have conventionally fractionated whole breast irradiation, although as demonstrated in the Canadian and START trials, there is no benefit to the longer course of treatment. With either fractionation scheme, I would omit the tumor bed boost, given the results of the EORTC boost trial, showing little benefit to additional boost in women over age 60, but increased fibrosis in the boost arm. The patient would likely be recommended to take 5 years of an AI, with tamoxifen as an alternative if she does not tolerate the AI.

REFERENCES

1. Kim T, Giuliano RE, Lyman GH. Lymphatic mapping and sentinel node biopsy in early-stage breast carcinoma: A metaanalysis. *Cancer*. 2006 Jan 1;106(1):4–16.
2. Van Zee K, Manasseh DM, Bevilacqua JL, et al. A nomogram for predicting the likelihood of additional nodal metastases in breast cancer patients with a positive sentinel node biopsy. *Ann Surg Oncol*. 2003 Dec;10(10):1140–1151.
3. Cserni G. Comparison of different validation studies on the use of the Memorial Sloan-Kettering Cancer Center nomogram predicting nonsentinel node involvement in sentinel node-positive breast cancer patients. *Am J Surg*. 2007;194:699–700.
4. Klar M, Jochmann A, Foeldi M, et al. The MSKCC nomogram for prediction the likelihood of non-sentinel node involvement in a German breast cancer population. *Breast Cancer Res Treat*. 2008 Dec;112(3):523–531.
5. Giuliano AE, McCall L, Beitsch P, et al. Locoregional recurrence after sentinel lymph node dissection with or without axillary dissection in patients with sentinel lymph node metastases. The American College of Surgeons Oncology Group Z0011 randomized trial. *Ann Surg*. 2010;252:426–433.
6. Giuliano AE, Hunt KK, Ballman KV, et al. Axillary dissection vs. no axillary dissection in women with invasive breast cancer and sentinel node metastasis. *JAMA*. 2011;305(6):569–575.
7. Schlembach PJ, Buchholz TA, Ross MI, et al. Relationship of sentinel and axillary level I-II lymph nodes to tangential fields used in breast irradiation. *Int J Radiat Oncol Biol Phys*. 2001;51:671–678.
8. Aristei C, Chionne F, Marsella AR, et al. Evaluation of level I and II axillary nodes included in the standard breast tangential fields and calculation of the administered dose: Results of a prospective study. *Int J Radiat Oncol Biol Phys*. 2001;51;69–73.
9. Park CC, Mitsumori M, Nixon A, et al. Outcome at 8 years after breast-conserving surgery and radiation therapy for invasive breast cancer: Influence of margin status and systemic therapy on local recurrence. *J Clin Oncol*. 2000;18:1668–1675.
10. Peintinger F, Symmans WF, Gonzalez-Angulo AM, et al. The safety of breast-conserving surgery in patients who achieve a complete pathologic response after neoadjuvant chemotherapy. *Cancer*. 2006;107(6):1248–1254.
11. Hughes KS, Schnaper LA, Berry D, et al. Lumpectomy plus tamoxifen with or without irradiation in women 70 years of age or older with early breast cancer. *N Engl J Med*. 2004 Sep 2;351(10):971–977.
12. Hughes KS, Schnaper LA, Cirrincione C, et al. Lumpectomy plus tamoxifen with or without irradiation in women age 70 or older with early breast cancer. *J Clin Oncol*. 2010;28:15s (Abstr 507).
13. Harris EE, Hwang WT, Urtishak SL, et al. The impact of comorbidities on outcomes for elderly women treated with breast-conservation treatment for early-stage breast cancer. *Int J Radiat Oncol Biol Phys*. 2008 Apr 1;70(5):1453–1459.
14. Whelan T, MacKenzie R, Julian J, et al. Randomized trial of breast irradiation schedules after lumpectomy for women with lymph node-negative breast cancer. *J Natl Cancer Inst*. 2002 Aug 7;94(15):1143–1150.
15. Whelan TJ, Pignol JP, Levine MN, et al. Long-term results of hypofractionated radiation therapy for breast cancer. *N Engl J Med*. 2010 Feb 11;362(6):513–520.
16. Owen JR, Ashton J, Bliss JM, et al. Effect of radiotherapy fraction size on tumor control in patients with early-stage breast cancer after local tumor excision: Long-term results of a randomized trial. *Lancet Oncol*. 2006;7:467–471.

17. START Trialist's Group. The UK Standardisation of Breast Radiotherapy (START) Trial A of radiotherapy hypofractionation for treatment of early breast cancer: A randomized trial. *Lancet Oncol.* 2008;9:331–341.

18. Bartelink H, Horiot JC, Poortmans PM, et al. Impact of a higher radiation dose on local control and survival in breast-conserving therapy of early breast cancer: 10-year results of the randomized boost versus no boost EORTC 22881-10882 trial. *J Clin Oncol.* 2007 Aug 1;25(22):3259–3265.

19. Jones HA, Antonini N, Hart AA, et al. Impact of pathological characteristics on local relapse after breast-conserving therapy: A subgroup analysis of the EORTC boost versus no boost trial. *J Clin Oncol.* 2009 Oct 20;27(30):4939–4947.

20. Chen PY, Wallace M, Mitchell C, et al. Four-year efficacy, cosmesis, and toxicity using three-dimensional conformal external beam radiation therapy to deliver accelerated partial breast irradiation. *Intl J Radiat Oncol Biol Phys.* 2010 Mar 15;76(4):991–997.

21. Smith BD, Arthur DW, Buchholz TA, et al. Accelerated partial breast irradiation consensus statement from the American Society for Radiation Oncology (ASTRO). *Intl J Radiat Oncol Biol Phys.* 2009 Jul 15;74(4):987–1001.

22. Polgár C, Van Limbergen E, Pötter R, et al. Patient selection for accelerated partial-breast irradiation (APBI) after breast-conserving surgery: Recommendations of the Groupe Européen de Curiethérapie-European Society for Therapeutic Radiology and Oncology (GEC-ESTRO) breast cancer working group based on clinical evidence (2009). *Radiother Oncol.* 2010 Mar;94(3):264–273.

23. Paik S, Shak S, Tang G, et al. A multigene assay to predict recurrence in tamoxifen-treated, node-negative breast cancer. *N Engl J Med.* 2004 Dec 30;351(27):2817–2826.

24. Paik S, Tang G, Shak S, et al. Gene expression and benefit of chemotherapy in women with node-negative, estrogen receptor-positive breast cancer. *J Clin Oncol.* 2006 Aug 10;24(23):3726–3734.

25. Albain K, Barlow W, Shak S, et al. Prognostic and predictive value of the 21-gene recurrence score assay in postmenopausal, node-positive, ER-positive breast cancer (S8814, INT0100). *Breast Cancer Res Treat* 2007;106(Suppl 1): #10.

26. van de Vijver MJ, He YD, van't Veer LJ, et al. A gene expression signature as a predictor of survival in breast cancer. *N Engl J Med.* 2002 Dec 19;347(25):1999–2009.

27. Early Breast Cancer Trialists' Collaborative Group. Effects of chemotherapy and hormonal therapy for early breast cancer on recurrence and 15-year survival: An overview of the randomised trials. *Lancet.* 2005;365(9472):1687–1717.

28. Arimidex, Tamoxifen, Alone or in Combination (ATAC) Trialists' Group, Forbes JF, Cuzick J, et al. Effect of anastrozole and tamoxifen as adjuvant treatment for early-stage breast cancer: 100 month analysis of the ATAC trial. *Lancet Oncol.* 2008;9(1):45–53.

29. Coates AS, Keshaviah A, Thürlimann B, et al. Five years of letrozole compared with tamoxifen as initial adjuvant therapy for postmenopausal women with endocrine-responsive early breast cancer: Update of study BIG 1-98. *J Clin Oncol.* 2007;25(5):486–492.

30. Coombes RC, Hall E, Gibson LJ, et al. A randomized trial of exemestane after two to three years of tamoxifen therapy in postmenopausal women with primary breast cancer. *N Engl J Med.* 2004;350(11):1081–1092.

31. Coombes RC, Kilburn LS, Snowdon CF, et al. Survival and safety of exemestane versus tamoxifen after 2-3 years' tamoxifen treatment (Intergroup Exemestane Study): A randomised controlled trial. *Lancet.* 2007;369(9561):559–570.

32. Goss PE, Ingle JN, Martino S, et al. Randomized trial of letrozole following tamoxifen as extended adjuvant therapy in receptor-positive breast cancer: Updated findings from NCIC CTG MA.17. *J Natl Cancer Inst.* 2005;97(17):1262–1271.

33. Ingle JN, Tu D, Pater JL, et al. Duration of letrozole treatment and outcomes in the placebo-controlled NCIC CTG MA.17 extended adjuvant therapy trial. *Breast Cancer Res Treat.* 2006;99(3):295–300.

34. Smith BD, Gross CP, Smith GL, et al. Effectiveness of radiation therapy for older women with early breast cancer. *J Natl Cancer Inst.* 2006;98(10):681–690.

35. Lin NU, Winer EP. Advances in adjuvant endocrine therapy for postmenopausal women. *J Clin Oncol.* 2008;26(5):798–805.

36. Dragun AE, Huang B, Tucker TC, Spanos WJ. Disparities in the application of adjuvant radiotherapy after breast-conserving surgery for early stage breast cancer: Impact on overall survival. *Cancer.* 2011;117(12):2590–2598.

■ **GASTROINTESTINAL** ■

Section Editor: Joseph M. Herman

■ CASE 1 ■

Pancreatic Cancer

CLINICAL PROBLEM

Patients with resected pancreatic cancer are at risk of both local and systemic recurrences. While it is clear that adjuvant chemotherapy is better than surgery alone, there is intense controversy regarding the role and timing of adjuvant radiation therapy (RT). In the United States and certain regions of Europe, if patients undergo a microscopic (R1) or macroscopic positive resection (R2), they receive either upfront chemoradiation (CRT) or CRT after 1 or 2 cycles of chemotherapy per the Radiation Therapy Oncology Group (RTOG) 9704 trial [1,2]. When resection margins are negative, patients often receive 2 to 6 cycles of chemotherapy followed by CRT. In Europe, CRT is either delayed until after 2 to 6 cycles of chemotherapy, or excluded.

CASE EXAMPLE

A 75-year-old Caucasian male with a history significant for prostate cancer, status post a radical prostatectomy, presents with painless jaundice, dark urine, clay-colored stool, midepigastric pain, and a 15-pound weight loss over the past 3 months. He is seen in the emergency room and found to have a direct bilirubin of 10 mg/dL and elevated liver function tests. Abdominal ultrasound demonstrates dilated bile ducts and a CT scan of the chest, abdomen, and pelvis with IV/oral contrast revealed a 3.0 cm lesion in the head of the pancreas with no evidence of venous or arterial involvement (Figures 3.1.1A,B), and a CA 19-9 of 121 U/mL. For comparison, see images of an unresectable pancreatic cancer due to encasement of arterial vessels (Figures 3.1.2A,B). After

a multidisciplinary evaluation, it is recommended that the patient undergoes surgical resection. He undergoes a pancreaticoduodenectomy, and final pathology reveals a 3.5-cm pancreatic head adenocarcinoma, 1 of 22 lymph nodes positive, superior mesenteric artery (SMA) margin microscopically positive (R1), with perineural and perivascular involvement (Figures 3.1.3 and 3.1.4). The patient is seen 5 weeks postoperatively. Restaging CT scan shows no evidence of recurrence and a repeat CA 19-9 is 39 U/mL. His incision is well healed and his Karnofsky performance status (KPS) score is 90.

Management Decisions

- What are the common prognostic factors for pancreatic cancer? What is the significance of lymph node ratio and postoperative CA 19-9 levels?
- Should patients receive gemcitabine or 5-fluorouracil (5-FU)-based adjuvant CRT?
- What dose of chemotherapy and radiation is optimal in the adjuvant setting?
- Are there any novel chemotherapeutic and/or targeted approaches?
- If pathology revealed an R0 resection, would adjuvant radiation still be necessary?
- If the decision is to use adjuvant CRT, when should it be timed in relationship to chemotherapy?
- What are the dose-limiting structures for radiation and what is the role of intensity modulated radiation therapy (IMRT)?
- Are there any established biomarkers to predict which patients may benefit from chemotherapy versus CRT in the adjuvant setting?
- Which patients should optimally receive neoadjuvant therapy as opposed to upfront surgery?

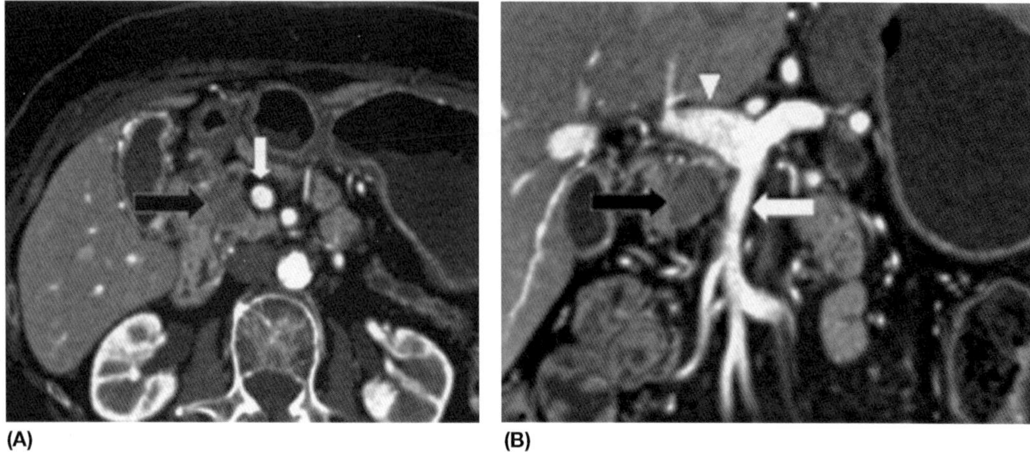

(A) **(B)**

FIGURE 3.1.1A,B ▪ Pancreas protocol CT scan displaying a resectable pancreatic tumor based on National Comprehensive Cancer Network (NCCN) criteria.

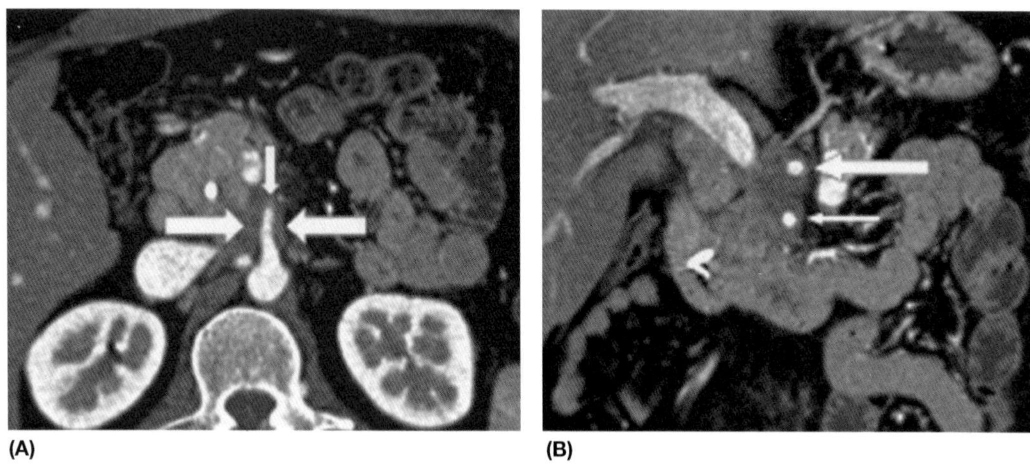

(A) **(B)**

FIGURE 3.1.2A,B ▪ Pancreas protocol CT scan displaying a uresectable pancreatic tumor based on NCCN criteria.

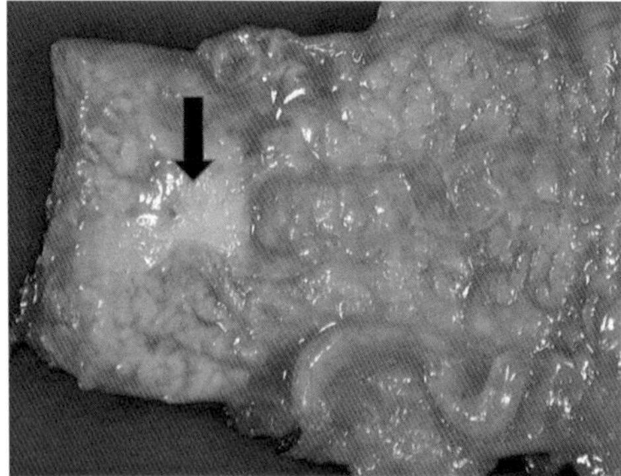

FIGURE 3.1.3 ▪ Gross picture showing a pancreatic tumor obstructing the pancreatic duct. (Compliments of Ralph Hruban).

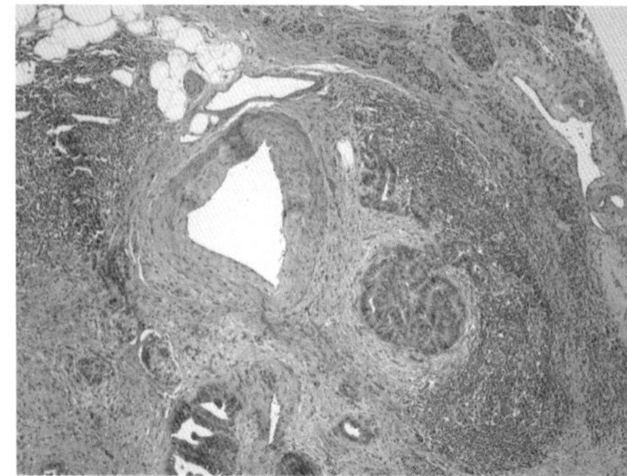

FIGURE 3.1.4 ▪ Histological section of a pancreatic adenocarcinoma showing the typical appearance of irregular malignant glands with perineural invasion. (Compliments of Ralph Hruban).

MAJOR OPINION

Joseph M. Herman

What Are Common Prognostic Factors for Pancreatic Cancer? How Do They Influence Treatment Management Decisions?

A few of the most published prognostic factors for adjuvant pancreatic cancer include margin status (R0 vs. R1/R2), tumor stage (T3/T4), grade (1 or 2 vs. 3), CA 19-9 level (higher than 90 U/mL), node status (positive vs. negative), number of lymph nodes positive, number of lymph nodes excised, percentage of lymph nodes positive versus number of lymph nodes excised, perineural/perivascular invasion, and family history of pancreatic cancer [3–5]. Studies suggest that patients with any of the high-risk prognostic factors should receive adjuvant therapy. If the disease is thought to be localized (known R1/R2 disease), then upfront CRT may be preferred. Having a high CA 19-9 (higher than 90 U/mL) postoperatively correlates with poor prognosis and suggests residual disease [6]. If a patient has an elevated CA 19-9 with an R0 resection, there may be metastatic disease outside of the tumor bed. Thus, these patients may be better treated with chemotherapy first, followed by CRT. Nomograms are being developed to help determine which patients are more at risk of local versus systemic recurrence [7,8].

Should Patients Receive Gemcitabine or 5-FU-Based Adjuvant Chemotherapy and Radiotherapy? What Dose of Chemotherapy Is Optimal? Are There Any Novel Chemotherapeutic and/or Targeted Approaches?

The benefit of 5-FU-based CRT was first seen in a small randomized trial performed by the Gastrointestinal Tumor Study Group (GITSG) [9], and supported by a subsequent European Organisation for Research and Treatment of Cancer (EORTC) trial and retrospective series [10–14]. However, the comparative benefit of chemotherapy and CRT was challenged by the European Study Group for

Pancreatic Cancer (ESPAC)-1 study, which showed a detriment in survival with CRT [15]. This study, however, was criticized for its lack of radiation delivery standardization. For example, the trial allowed "background" therapy, where patients could receive treatments other than those to which they had been randomized at the discretion of the treating physician. The trial's 2 × 2 design, which is intended for the simultaneous analysis of 2 independent effects within the framework of a single study, is not ideal for interpreting the results of this trial because administration of the first therapy could have influenced the second therapy. Moreover, there was a great deal of patient nonadherence within this trial, with only 70% of patients randomized to receive CRT receiving the prescribed dose of radiation (50% of nonadherence due to patient's decision to not receive assigned treatment) and only 50% of patients randomized to receive chemotherapy receiving the full course (33% of nonadherence due to patient's decision to not receive assigned treatment). In accordance with previous trials, a split-course radiation regimen was utilized; however, quality assurance for the RT was lacking because of no centralized review of the radiation fields. Finally, it is worth nothing that while patients in the CRT arm received only 2 cycles of 5-FU during radiation, patients in the chemotherapy and CRT followed by chemotherapy arms received more than 6 cycles of 5-FU. Despite these shortcomings, the ESPAC-1 trial does highlight the important benefit of adjuvant 5-FU chemotherapy.

The European Charité Onkologie (CONKO)-1 trial and ESPAC-3 trial also reported improved overall survival and disease-free survival with either 5-FU or gemcitabine when compared to observation alone [16,17]. Despite showing an early benefit of gemcitabine before and after 5-FU-based CRT, the results of RTOG 9704 were no longer significantly different with further follow-up [1,2]. So far, an optimal standard adjuvant treatment approach for patients with fully resected disease has not yet been determined. Likewise, for patients for whom radiation is excluded, the optimal chemotherapy regimen is debatable. Six months of 5-FU has been shown by studies to be equivalent to gemcitabine; however, these studies gave bolus 5-FU, which is rarely used in the United States where continuous infusion 5-FU is considered standard with radiation despite requiring a port and infusional pump. While oral capecitabine and CI 5-FU have been shown to be comparable when given concurrently with radiation, neither is established as a standard replacement if given in isolation for 6 months. Thus, if the decision is to exclude RT, most patients receive gemcitabine alone for 6 months. The optimal dose of chemotherapy with radiation is not clear. Full dose gemcitabine with either an attenuated dose of RT (36 Gy) [18,19] or conformal full dose RT (50–54 Gy) [20,21] have been shown to be tolerable and to have comparable survival. Biweekly low dose [22] or an attenuated dose (300–600 mg/m^2) of gemcitabine are also acceptable options [23]. For example, patients in ESPAC-3 received 5-FU plus folinic acid (folinic acid, 20 mg/m^2, intravenous bolus injection, followed by 5-FU, 425 mg/m^2 intravenous bolus injection given on days 1–5 every 28 days) [17]. Notable targeted therapies in the adjuvant setting include erlotinib with [24] and without [25] RT. The efficacy of this combination is currently being evaluated in the ongoing RTOG/Intergroup study. While other agents are being considered, these studies are small and efficacy data are limited.

If the Decision Is to Use Adjuvant Radiation, When Should It Be Timed in Relation to Chemotherapy?

Despite our collective best efforts to improve systemic therapy and optimize integration of the major cancer treatment modalities in the adjuvant therapy for pancreatic cancer, over 70% of patients develop systemic disease as a major mode of treatment failure. Internationally, there is now a trend to delay RT until an "adequate" amount of chemotherapy has been delivered to prevent systemic spread. Therefore, only those patients who are diseasefree after 4 to 6 months of systemic therapy have an opportunity to receive CRT. In a study by Desai et al., patients received 4 cycles of gemcitabine with cisplatin or capecitabine followed by capecitabine and conformal radiation. The median survival of 43 treated patients was an impressive 45.9 months [21]. Another study by Van Laethem et al. evaluated adjuvant gemcitabine alone versus gemcitabine-based CRT after curative resection for pancreatic cancer (EORTC-40013-22012/FFCD-9203/GERCOR phase 2 study) [23]. The addition of CRT resulted in improved local control over gemcitabine alone, but no improvement in survival. The approach of chemotherapy alone followed by CRT is also being tested in the international intergroup phase 3 trial where patients are receiving gemcitabine and erlotinib followed by capecitabine-based CRT. While integration of RT in this manner may be adequate for R0 resections, some question if systemic therapy alone optimally prevent local recurrence, particularly among patients with R1 resections.

Other chemotherapy combinations that have been explored in the metastatic setting are being considered in the adjuvant setting. For example, Abraxane is a nanoparticle albumin-bound form of paclitaxel (nab-paclitaxel). Abraxane was recently combined with gemcitabine in a phase 1/2 trial for patients with metastatic disease. Von Hoff et al. reported excellent outcomes with a median overall survival (OS) of 12 months, objective response rate of 48%, and progression-free survival (PFS) of 7.9 months [26]. Results of the phase 3 MPACT trial comparing gemcitabine and Abraxane to gemcitabine alone has resulted in a two month survival benefit with the addition of Abraxane. Similarly good results were seen in the randomized phase 3 trial by Conroy et al. who compared FOLFIRINOX (5-FU, leucovorin, irinotecan, and oxaliplatin) to single-agent gemcitabine in patients with metastatic pancreatic adenocarcinoma. FORFIRINOX led to an improvement in median OS (11.1 months vs. 6.8 months; HR 0.57, $p <$ .001), objective response rate (31.6% vs. 9.4%, $p <$ .001), and progression-free survival (6.4 months vs. 3.3 months; HR 0.47, $p <$ .001). Importantly, toxicities associated with the FOLFIRINOX regimen were not insignificant. Rates of grade 3–4 neutropenia (45.7% vs. 21%, $p <$ .001) and febrile neutropenia (5.4% vs. 1.2%, $p =$ .03) were more frequent in the combination arm and required the application of granulocyte colony stimulating factor (G-CSF) in 42.5% vs. 5.3% ($p <$ .001). Despite these toxicities, patient-reported quality of life was improved in the FOLFIRINOX arm when compared to gemcitabine alone. Still, FOLFIRINOX is an aggressive regimen with significant dose-limiting toxicities. Therefore, it is challenging to combine it with standard RT or new therapeutic agents. Alternate modalities such as immunotherapy may be easier to combine with FOLFIRINOX and/or radiation owing to its favorable toxicity profile [27]. In an attempt to improve the toxicity profile and efficacy of FOLFIRONOX alone, investigators are exploring fractionated stereotactic body radiation therapy (SBRT) as opposed to standard CRT.

If the Pathology Revealed an R0 Resection, Would Adjuvant Radiation Still Be Necessary?

Patients most likely to benefit from adjuvant RT have undergone an R0 resection and received adequate adjuvant chemotherapy. Unfortunately, the proportion of patients undergoing R1 resections remains high even in modern reports (range 19–45%) [1,10]. Patients who undergo R1 resections with or without adjuvant therapy have inferior median survival compared to those with R0 resections (range 8–18 vs. 20–25 months). It is therefore imperative that surgeons and multidisciplinary teams rely on improved CT/MRI imaging and functional imaging (PET/CT) to properly select those patients who should undergo neoadjuvant therapy as opposed to upfront surgery [28].

The majority of resected pancreatic cancer patients die from metastatic disease to the liver (70%). However, local and regional recurrence can also be fatal. Up to 40% of patients with R0 resections still develop local recurrences. In addition to the tumor bed, patients are also at risk of recurrences to regional lymph nodes, which can manifest with peritoneal nodular studding and result in malignant ascites. RT is thought to primarily prevent local recurrence in the retroperitoneal margin, otherwise known as the SMA margin. However, it is hypothesized that irradiation of the regional lymph node regions may also result in improved systemic control, although this is difficult to confirm [29]. One can, however, extrapolate from neoadjuvant therapy for resectable or borderline resectable disease where preoperative CRT results in improved margin and node-negative resections [30]. Therefore, even following an R0 resection, radiation should still be considered, especially if patients have other high-risk features.

What Are the Dose Limiting Structures With Adjuvant RT and What Is the Role of IMRT?

Elective nodal irradiation (ENI) is commonly used for adjuvant cases but is controversial for unresectable, neoadjuvant, or borderline resectable cases [31]. Conformal, IMRT, and breath hold/gating techniques can result in improved planning target volume (PTV) coverage with decreased dose to organs at risk (OARs) [32,33]. OARs include the kidneys, liver, small bowel, and spinal cord. If small margin expansions are used for clinical target volume (CTV) and PTV, breathing motion and set-up error should be evaluated or controlled per the American Association of Physicists in Medicine (AAPM) task group 76 guidelines (eg, active breathing control, 4D-CT scan) [34]. In general, IMRT should be used if normal tissue constraints cannot be met with conformal RT, the total dose is greater than 54 Gy, and/or full dose gemcitabine chemotherapy is given concurrently with RT. Otherwise, 3-D conformal RT is considered standard.

Are There Any Established Imaging Modalities or Biomarkers to Predict Which Patients May Benefit From Chemotherapy Versus CRT?

The benefit of evolving RT strategies now and into the future will likely be associated with the greatest impact in the setting of R0 resections and truly effective systemic therapy. We need to routinely integrate novel functional imaging (eg, PET), which can be used to better stage patients, assist with treatment planning, and assess treatment response [35–37]. In order to learn more about the natural history of this disease, it is imperative that we study novel blood, urine, and stool biomarkers and preoperative biopsies (DPC4) to better individualize treatment as opposed to relying on current conventional staging methods (CA 19-9) [38–40].

Which Patients Should Optimally Receive Neoadjuvant Therapy as Opposed to Upfront Surgery?

Staging is optimally determined with modern contrast-enhanced CT and/or MRI imaging with thin cuts through the pancreas along with endoscopic ultrasound (EUS). Patients are typically separated into 5 clinical scenarios: (a) neoadjuvant/resectable, (b) borderline resectable, (c) locally advanced/unresectable, (d) adjuvant/resectable, and (e) palliative [41,42]. Several studies have demonstrated higher likelihoods of downstaging and subsequent R0 resections following neoadjuvant therapy in patients with borderline resectable disease [43,44]. In cases where tumors are borderline resectable, surgeons should give strong consideration to an approach utilizing neoadjuvant therapy. Although such discussions may be challenging and require timely

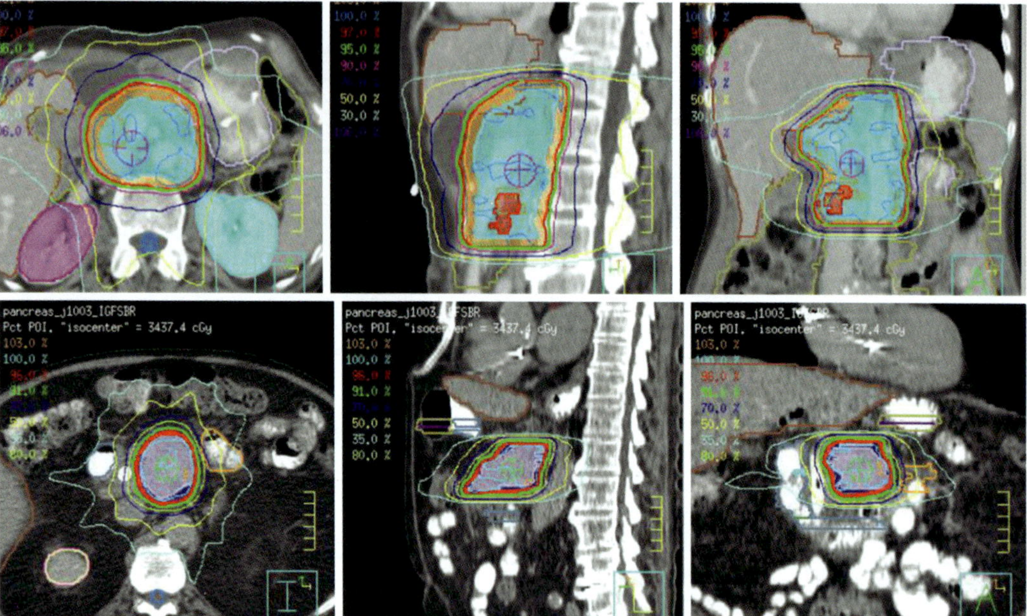

FIGURE 3.1.5 ■ Comparison of adjuvant IMRT treatment plan (1.8 to 50.4) as compared to a fractionated SBRT plan (6.6 Gy × 5).

consideration, a multidisciplinary forum is more likely to facilitate such discussions and be associated with the potential for improved outcome for pancreatic cancer patients [45].

No current standard exists for neoadjuvant treatment, although we use similar paradigms as for locally advanced unresectable disease [43,46,47]. Options include RT 45 to 54 Gy in 1.8 to 2.5 Gy fractions or 36 Gy in 2.4 Gy fractions [18]. Ideally, surgical resection should be attempted 6 to 8 weeks following CRT. Surgery can be performed more than 8 weeks following CRT; however, radiation induced fibrosis may potentially make surgery more difficult and increase the length of stay [48].

Final Recommendation

Every attempt should be made to enroll patients on a clinical trial if available. In this specific case (given the R1 resection), I would recommend upfront 5-FU (capecitabine)-based CRT as per RTOG 9704. RT is to be delivered with a dose of 45 to 46 Gy in 1.8 to 2 Gy fractions to the tumor bed, anastomoses, and adjacent lymph node regions followed by an additional 5 to 9 Gy to the tumor bed (required) and anastomoses (optional) [10]. The final boost dose is to be determined by the amount of small bowel in the radiation field. I would use IMRT to limit dose to OARs. Four to 6 weeks following CRT, patients would receive 4

additional months of infusional gemcitabine (1000 mg/m²/wk) [1]. Although eliminating or delaying RT may decrease the risk of metastatic disease, it may also increase the risk of local recurrence, which can cause extensive morbidity (pain and obstruction) and result in death [49]. As the most common site of a localized recurrence following surgical resection is the tumor bed or SMA margin, it may be ideal to use stereotactic body radiation therapy (SBRT) to sterilize the margin [50]. Fractionated SBRT uses a smaller radiation field (Figure 3.1.5), can be given in only 5 days, may (a) result in less toxicity, (b) allow for more aggressive chemotherapy such as FOLFIRINOX, and (c) improve quality of life when compared to CRT. However, additional prospective studies are needed to determine if SBRT is efficacious in the treatment of pancreatic cancer [51].

ACADEMIC COMMENT

William F. Regine

A discussion of the use of adjuvant therapy in the management of pancreatic cancer brings forward philosophies of therapeutic nihilism versus great hope for improvement. Our hope is to improve upon our historical results among patients who are actually able to undergo resection (10–15% of all pancreatic cancer patients). I focus my perspective on the patients who are able to undergo resection and the opportunity for improvement of outcome in this patient population. Although the advances of systemic therapy have been modest and surgical and radiation techniques/approaches have evolved significantly in the last decade, the 5-year survival for these patients remains "stuck" at approximately 15% to 20%. These survival numbers, or higher (up to 35%), are generally reserved for those patients who are able to undergo an R0 resection. Unfortunately, the likelihood of achieving an R0 resection in previously untreated patients at initial presentation is less than 5% to 10%.

The case here represents the typical presentation of a patient with a potentially resectable (and therefore curable) adenocarcinoma of the pancreatic head. All such patients are presented and managed by our multidisciplinary GI oncology team, which includes surgeons, medical oncologists, radiation oncologists, radiologists, and gastroenterologists. Such a patient, on presentation, would be required to undergo a "pancreatic-protocol CT," which involves thin sliced, high contrast-resolution CT scanning specifically done to evaluate resectability of the primary lesion in relation to surrounding organs and major vessels. Once such imaging confirms the patient to be "clearly" resectable (ie, no abutment or involvement of any major vessels such as the superior mesenteric artery/vein [SMA/SMV] or hepatic artery [HA]), the patient would currently undergo a Whipple procedure (often pylorus preserving, if the tumor was not invading the duodenum). When possible, we simulate the patient in the treatment planning position prior to surgery to allow for fusion with the postoperative scan allowing clear delineation of the preoperative tumor bed. If postoperative imaging confirms no evidence of interval development of disease, and postoperative CA 19-9 is lower than 180 U/mL in this setting of an R1 resection, our general approach is to first offer the patient participation in the Intergroup/RTOG 0848 phase 3 trial. If the patient declines protocol participation, off-protocol therapy in this setting is as per the previously discussed RTOG 9704 study with a single upfront cycle of gemcitabine followed by 5-FU-based CRT followed by an additional 3 cycles of gemcitabine [2].

The rationale for using RT early in the postoperative adjuvant treatment approach for patients having undergone an R1 resection relates to the observations and principles used in the management of locally advanced pancreatic adenocarcinoma. In general, it has clearly been demonstrated that patients who undergo an R1 resection have median and overall survivals very similar to those of patients with locally advanced and unresectable pancreatic adenocarcinoma. Thus, our rationale for inclusion of RT early in the postoperative adjuvant treatment course of R1 resection patients is, in part, based on the findings in the locally advanced setting where median and overall survival are improved by integration of concurrent CRT as compared to use of chemotherapy alone [52]. In addition, if the margin is clearly localizable (pancreatic remnant/anastomosis or clipped paravascular retroperitoneal area) with the help of the surgeon, this area would be boosted to a cumulative dose of 57 to 59.4 Gy, all at 1.8 Gy fraction. This would be done provided the dose constraints for bowel, stomach, and other surrounding organs could be met as similarly defined within the current Intergroup/RTOG 0848 protocol. All patients are currently treated with IMRT on the basis of our recently published institutional experience [33] and, when possible, patients are simulated prior to surgery and images are fused to the postoperative simulation to better localize the tumor bed. Following completion of CRT, the patient would undergo a follow-up staging examination within 3 to 4 weeks and continue with 3 additional cycles of gemcitabine as per RTOG 9704. The patient would receive this therapy even if there is interval development of tumor progression, if not a candidate for another trial (for patients with progression). After completion of all therapy, the patient would continue close follow-up with CT imaging every 3 to 4 months for at least 2 years.

Our off-protocol approach varies in similar patients according to initial postoperative margin status and CA 19-9 findings. If a patient undergoes an R0 resection, or has persistently elevated (higher than 180 U/mL) CA 19-9, systemic therapy with gemcitabine would be the primary emphasis. Therapy would then involve 5 cycles of gemcitabine (as per the Intergroup/RTOG 0848 trial) followed by restaging/imaging and CA 19-9 evaluation. If there are no signs of progression, the patient would undergo a sixth cycle of gemcitabine followed by 5-FU-based CRT, as previously described.

Having presented our current institutional philosophy/approach of the use of adjuvant therapy in the postoperative setting, our programmatic focus has been to acknowledge that the fundamental roles of surgery, chemotherapy, and radiotherapy should be viewed as "complementary" rather than "competing." I expect the latter to be the case in many tumor boards in which readers may find themselves participating. Our focus has been to evolve our treatment modalities toward the "best integrated approach" in the context of the findings from patient imaging/workup. Our threshold for utilizing neoadjuvant CRT has been lowered and it has become more routinely used in all patients with "borderline" resectable disease (as typically defined by any abutment of adjacent SMA/HA or involvement of a short segment of SMV), as well as increasing consideration for use in patients with markedly elevated CA 19-9 levels (currently defined as higher than 500 U/mL). The rationale for such a neoadjuvant approach has been well described [18,43,53]. It is clear that this evolving rationale, coupled with data suggesting more thorough pathologic examination, further increases the "true" R1 resection rate up to 85% [54,55]; as well, growing surgeon comfort with "operating" after neoadjuvant therapy will lead to increasing consideration for more routine use of neoadjuvant therapy even in the "clearly" resectable setting. Parallel to this development, our group is evolving its "complementary-integrated" CRT strategy toward smaller volume (gross disease only), short-course RT (≤3 weeks) with concurrent full-dose systemic therapy. We feel this combined modality evolution, coupled with improved understanding of the natural history of disease, and improved biomolecular markers and staging, offers great hope for improvement of future pancreatic cancer patient outcome.

COMMUNITY PRACTITIONER COMMENT

Ori Shokek

In regard to this case of a 75-year-old with a KPS score of 90 postoperatively with an R1 resection of a pancreatic head tumor (3 cm) and a single positive node, I would strongly recommend radiotherapy with concurrent 5-FU (CRT) as part of total adjuvant therapy along RTOG 9704 principles (ie, sequenced with gemcitabine as systemic therapy). Given the R1 resection, perhaps there is impetus to give CRT somewhat earlier in the course of total adjuvant therapy rather than after many cycles of gemcitabine. If I were faced with an R0 resection, there would still be an indication for radiotherapy, but this would be more controversial and there would be impetus to give a greater number of cycles of gemcitabine first. My use of vague terms (eg, "somewhat earlier") is intentional, and the optimal number of cycles is not known, in general or by resection margin status.

In considering this case, the data I consider mainly come from 4 significant studies. The utility of adjuvant chemotherapy in resected pancreatic head adenocarcinoma is firmly validated by the CONKO-01 and ESPAC trials [16,56,57]. Considerations regarding locoregional radiotherapy are more intricate. A survival advantage was suggested by the older GITSG and EORTC trials which tested adjuvant CRT versus no adjuvant therapy. But the ESPAC-1 trial was a multiarm study that tested CRT and suggested no benefit (and, furthermore, even a detriment) to radiotherapy. This has formed the basis of a current controversy. However, ESPAC-1 is problematic, flawed by the use of split-course, low total-dose radiotherapy, and by the permission of "background" therapy that was given to nearly half of all patients (per first report in *Lancet* in 2001), which was not mentioned in the second report. Furthermore, despite the majority (82%) of patients having R0 resections, the trial's pattern of failure data shows that nearly two-thirds had local recurrence alone (35%) or concurrent local recurrences with distant failure (27%). Thus, the notion that locoregional failure is an issue in pancreatic cancer is supported even by ESPAC-1. The trial's suggestion of lack of benefit to local radiotherapy is surprising but perhaps explained by ESPAC-1's flaws as described above and possibly also by the lack of effective systemic therapy prior to the CRT phase of total adjuvant therapy. It is possible that good radiotherapy (with modern techniques and doses), which comes after several cycles of full-dose gemcitabine, does have good utility, as supported by the recent study by Abrams et al. [58]. The current RTOG 0848 trial seeks to definitively confirm or refute this hypothesis.

It is difficult to judge where the balance lies between the need for early local therapy (CRT) and the need for early systemic therapy on the basis of a higher lymph node positive ratio, because a high lymph node ratio is concerning both ways—possibly suggesting additional adenopathy remaining postoperatively, as well as a higher chance of systemic dissemination. The pre- versus postoperative CA 19-9 change is likewise a difficult marker in trying to determine which is more immediately important—local or systemic therapy—as a persistently elevated CA 19-9 postoperatively may be explained by either unresected involved nodal disease or subclinical distant disease. Whether residual local disease in the R1 setting can explain a persistently elevated CA 19-9 is difficult to say. Given the available patterns of failure data as discussed, I do generally see a need to improve locoregional control and, accordingly, recommend radiotherapy routinely as part of total adjuvant therapy, unless there are case-specific reasons otherwise.

SECTION EDITOR'S NOTE

Joseph M. Herman

Given the controversy surrounding pancreatic cancer management, patients should ideally be discussed in a multidisciplinary setting after a pancreatic protocol CT scan and be considered for clinical trials. Outside the scope of a clinical trial, the minimum standard of care option is 6 months of adjuvant 5-FU or gemcitabine chemotherapy. In select cases (T1N0 margins negative), patients can be observed; however, even patients with early stage disease can have a recurrence locally and distantly. There is evidence that CRT in the adjuvant setting provides increased rates of local–regional control and overall survival, and will continue to play an important role in this disease. Advances in RT technology such as IMRT and SBRT hold the promise of improved locoregional control with decreased toxicity and morbidity. However, better identification of patients at risk of early local failure is needed. In the face of the high rate of distant metastasis in pancreatic cancer, it remains difficult for improved local control to have a dramatic impact on overall survival. It is clear that better systemic treatments such as FOL-FIRINOX and Abraxane are needed. Identification of molecular biomarkers and novel targeted therapies hold the potential to provide "personalized" treatment regimens optimized for an individual's cancer. This may finally lead to improvements in outcome that have been so elusive for this disease.

REFERENCES

1. Regine WF, Winter KA, Abrams RA, et al. Fluorouracil vs gemcitabine chemotherapy before and after fluorouracil-based chemoradiation following resection of pancreatic adenocarcinoma: A randomized controlled trial. *JAMA*. 2008 Mar 5;299(9):1019–1026.

2. Regine WF, Winter KA, Abrams R, et al. Fluorouracil-based chemoradiation with either gemcitabine or fluorouracil chemotherapy after resection of pancreatic adenocarcinoma: 5-year analysis of the U.S. Intergroup/RTOG 9704 Phase III Trial. *Ann Surg Oncol*. 2011;18(5):1319–1326.

3. Showalter TN, Winter KA, Berger AC, et al. The influence of total nodes examined, number of positive nodes, and lymph node ratio on survival after surgical resection and adjuvant chemoradiation for pancreatic cancer: A secondary analysis of RTOG 9704. *Int J Radiat Oncol Biol Phys*. 2011 Dec 1;81(5):1328–1335.

4. Klein AP, Brune KA, Petersen GM, et al. Prospective risk of pancreatic cancer in familial pancreatic cancer kindreds. *Cancer Res*. 2004;64(7):2634–2638.

5. Wang L, Brune KA, Visvanathan K, et al. Elevated cancer mortality in the relatives of patients with pancreatic cancer. *Cancer Epidemiol Biomarkers Prev*. 2009;18(11):2829–2834.

6. Berger AC, Garcia M Jr, Hoffman JP, et al. Postresection CA 19-9 predicts overall survival in patients with pancreatic cancer treated with adjuvant chemoradiation: A prospective validation by RTOG 9704. *J Clin Oncol*. 2008;26(36):5918–5922.

7. Brennan MF. Adjuvant therapy following resection for pancreatic adenocarcinoma. *Surg Oncol Clin N Am*. 2004;13(4):555–566, vii.

8. Hsu CC, Wolfgang CL, Laheru DA, et al. Early mortality risk score: Identification of poor outcomes following upfront surgery for resectable pancreatic cancer. *J Gastrointest Surg*. 2012 Apr;16(4):753–761. doi: 10.1007/s11605-011-1811-4. Epub 2012 Feb 7.

9. Further evidence of effective adjuvant combined radiation and chemotherapy following curative resection of pancreatic cancer. Gastrointestinal Tumor Study Group. *Cancer*. 1987;59(12):2006–2010.

10. Herman JM, Swartz MJ, Hsu CC, et al. Analysis of fluorouracil-based adjuvant chemotherapy and radiation after pancreaticoduodenectomy for ductal adenocarcinoma of the pancreas: Results of a large, prospectively collected database at the Johns Hopkins Hospital. *J Clin Oncol*. 2008;26(21):3503–3510.

11. Corsini MM, Miller RC, Haddock MG, et al. Adjuvant radiotherapy and chemotherapy for pancreatic carcinoma: The Mayo Clinic experience (1975-2005). *J Clin Oncol*. 2008;26(21):3511–3516.

12. Klinkenbijl JH, Jeekel J, Sahmoud T, et al. Adjuvant radiotherapy and 5-fluorouracil after curative resection of cancer of the pancreas and periampullary region: Phase III trial of the EORTC gastrointestinal tract cancer cooperative group. *Ann Surg*. 1999;230(6):776–782; discussion 782–784.

13. Hsu CC, Herman JM, Corsini MM, et al. Adjuvant chemoradiation for pancreatic adenocarcinoma: The Johns Hopkins Hospital-Mayo Clinic collaborative study. *Ann Surg Oncol.* 2010;17(4):981–990.

14. Hattangadi JA, Hong TS, Yeap BY, Mamon HJ. Results and patterns of failure in patients treated with adjuvant combined chemoradiation therapy for resected pancreatic adenocarcinoma. *Cancer.* 2009 Aug 15;115(16):3640–3650.

15. Neoptolemos JP, Stocken DD, Friess H, et al. A randomized trial of chemoradiotherapy and chemotherapy after resection of pancreatic cancer. *N Eng J Med.* 2004 Mar 18;350(12):1200–1210.

16. Oettle H, Neuhaus P. Adjuvant therapy in pancreatic cancer: A critical appraisal. *Drugs.* 2007;67(16):2293–2310.

17. Neoptolemos J, Büchler M, Stocken DD, et al. ESPAC-3(v2): A multicenter, international, open-label, randomized, controlled phase III trial of adjuvant 5-fluorouracil/folinic acid (5-FU/FA) versus gemcitabine (GEM) in patients with resected pancreatic ductal adenocarcinoma. *J Clin Oncol.* 2009;27(18s):abstr LBA4505).

18. Talamonti MS, Small W Jr, Mulcahy MF, et al. A multi-institutional phase II trial of preoperative full-dose gemcitabine and concurrent radiation for patients with potentially resectable pancreatic carcinoma. *Ann Surg Oncol.* 2006;13(2):150–158.

19. Allen AM, Zalupski MM, Robertson JM, et al. Adjuvant therapy in pancreatic cancer: Phase I trial of radiation dose escalation with concurrent full-dose gemcitabine. *Int J Radiat Oncol Biol Phys.* 2004;59(5):1461–1467.

20. Desai SP, Ben-Josef E, Normolle DP, et al. Phase I study of oxaliplatin, full-dose gemcitabine, and concurrent radiation therapy in pancreatic cancer. *J Clin Oncol.* 2007;25(29):4587–4592.

21. Desai S, Ben-Josef E, Griffith KA, et al. Gemcitabine-based combination chemotherapy followed by radiation with capecitabine as adjuvant therapy for resected pancreas cancer. *Int J Radiat Oncol Biol Phys.* 2009;75(5):1450–1455.

22. Blackstock AW, Mornex F, Partensky C, et al. Adjuvant gemcitabine and concurrent radiation for patients with resected pancreatic cancer: A phase II study. *Br J Cancer.* 2006;95(3):260–265.

23. Van Laethem JL, Hammel P, Mornex F, et al. Adjuvant gemcitabine alone versus gemcitabine-based chemoradiotherapy after curative resection for pancreatic cancer: A randomized EORTC-40013-22012/FFCD-9203/GERCOR phase II study. *J Clin Oncol.* 2010;28(29):4450–4456.

24. Ma WW, Herman JM, Jimeno A, et al. A tolerability and pharmacokinetic study of adjuvant erlotinib and capecitabine with concurrent radiation in resected pancreatic cancer. *Transl Oncol.* 2010;3(6):373–379.

25. Bao PQ, Ramanathan RK, Krasinkas A, et al. Phase II study of gemcitabine and erlotinib as adjuvant therapy for patients with resected pancreatic cancer. *Ann Surg Oncol.* 2011;18(4):1122–1129.

26. Von Hoff DD, Ramanathan RK, Borad MJ, et al. Gemcitabine plus nab-paclitaxel is an active regimen in patients with advanced pancreatic cancer: A phase I/II trial. *J Clin Oncol.* 2011 Dec 1;29(34):4548–4554.

27. Lutz E, Yeo CJ, Lillemoe KD, et al. A lethally irradiated allogeneic granulocyte-macrophage colony stimulating factor-secreting tumor vaccine for pancreatic adenocarcinoma. A Phase II trial of safety, efficacy, and immune activation. *Ann Surg.* 2011 Feb;253(2):328–335.

28. Abrams RA, Lowy AM, O'Reilly EM, et al. Combined modality treatment of resectable and borderline resectable pancreas cancer: Expert consensus statement. *Ann Surg Oncol.* 2009;16(7):1751–1756.

29. Asiyanbola B, Gleisner A, Herman JM, et al. Determining pattern of recurrence following pancreaticoduodenectomy and adjuvant 5-fluoro-uracil-based chemoradiation therapy: Effect of number of metastatic lymph nodes and lymph node ratio. *J Gastroint Surg.* 2009;13(4):752–759.

30. Katz MH, Fleming JB, Bhosale P, et al. Response of borderline resectable pancreatic cancer to neoadjuvant therapy is not reflected by radiographic indicators. *Cancer.* 2012 Dec 1;118(23):5749–5756. Epub 2012 May 17.

31. Murphy JD, Adusumilli S, Griffith KA, et al. Full-dose gemcitabine and concurrent radiotherapy for unresectable pancreatic cancer. *Int J Radiat Oncol Biol Phys.* 2007;68(3):801–808.

32. Spalding AC, Jee KW, Vineberg K, et al. Potential for dose-escalation and reduction of risk in pancreatic cancer using IMRT optimization with lexicographic ordering and gEUD-based cost functions. *Med Phys.* 2007;34(2):521–529.

33. Yovino S, Poppe M, Jabbour S, et al. Intensity-modulated radiation therapy significantly improves acute gastrointestinal toxicity in pancreatic and ampullary cancers. *Int J Radiat Oncol Biol Phys.* 2011;79(1):158–162.

34. Keall PJ, Mageras GS, Balter JM, et al. The management of respiratory motion in radiation oncology report of AAPM Task Group 76. *Med Phys.* 2006;33(10):3874–3900.

35. Chang DT, Schellenberg D, Shen J, et al. Stereotactic radiotherapy for unresectable adenocarcinoma of the pancreas. *Cancer.* 2009;115(3):665–672.

36. Ford EC, Herman J, Yorke E, Wahl RL. 18F-FDG PET/CT for image-guided and intensity-modulated radiotherapy. *J Nucl Med.* 2009;50(10):1655–1665.

37. Wahl RL, Herman JM, Ford E. The promise and pitfalls of positron emission tomography and single-photon emission computed tomography molecular imaging-guided radiation therapy. *Semin Radiat Oncol.* 2011;21(2):88–100.

38. Hoimes CJ, Moyer MT, Saif MW. Biomarkers for early detection and screening in pancreatic cancer. Highlights from the 45th ASCO annual meeting. Orlando, FL, USA. May 29–June 2, 2009. *JOP.* 2009;10(4):352–356.

39. Yachida S, White CM, Naito Y, et al. Clinical significance of the genetic landscape of pancreatic cancer and implications for identification of potential long-term survivors. *Clin Cancer Res.* 2012 Nov 15;18(22):6339–6347. doi: 10.1158/1078-0432.CCR-12-1215. Epub 2012 Sep 18.

40. Blackford A, Serrano OK, Wolfgang CL,et al. SMAD4 gene mutations are associated with poor prognosis in pancreatic cancer. *Clin Cancer Res.* 2009 Jul 15;15(14):4674–4679. Epub 2009 Jul 7.

41. Callery MP, Chang KJ, Fishman EK, et al. Pretreatment assessment of resectable and borderline resectable pancreatic cancer: Expert consensus statement. *Ann Surg Oncol.* 2009;16(7):1727–1733.

42. Tempero MA, Arnoletti JP, Behrman SW, et al. Pancreatic adenocarcinoma, version 2.2012: Featured updates to the NCCN Guidelines. *J Natl Compr Canc Netw.* 2012 Jun 1;10(6):703–713.

43. Evans DB, Varadhachary GR, Crane CH, et al. Preoperative gemcitabine-based chemoradiation for patients with resectable adenocarcinoma of the pancreatic head. *J Clin Oncol.* 2008;26(21):3496–3502.

44. Varadhachary GR, Wolff RA, Crane CH, et al. Preoperative gemcitabine and cisplatin followed by gemcitabine-based chemoradiation for resectable adenocarcinoma of the pancreatic head. *J Clin Oncol.* 2008;26(21):3487–3495.

45. Pawlik TM, Laheru D, Hruban RH, et al. Evaluating the impact of a single-day multidisciplinary clinic on the management of pancreatic cancer. *Ann Surg Oncol.* 2008;15(8):2081–2088.

46. White RR, Hurwitz HI, Morse MA, et al. Neoadjuvant chemoradiation for localized adenocarcinoma of the pancreas. *Ann Surg Oncol.* 2001;8(10):758–765.

47. Le Scodan R, Mornex F, Girard N, et al. Preoperative chemoradiation in potentially resectable pancreatic adenocarcinoma: Feasibility, treatment effect evaluation and prognostic factors, analysis of the SFRO-FFCD 9704 trial and literature review. *Ann Oncol.* 2009;20(8):1387–1396.

48. Gupta PK, Turaga KK, Miller WJ, et al. Determinants of outcomes in pancreatic surgery and use of hospital resources. *J Surg Oncol.* 2011 Nov 1;104(6):634–640.

49. Tepper J, Nardi G, Sutt H. Carcinoma of the pancreas: Review of MGH experience from 1963 to 1973. Analysis of surgical failure and implications for radiation therapy. *Cancer.* 1976 Mar;37(3):1519–1524.

50. Rwigema JC, Heron DE, Parikh SD, et al. Adjuvant stereotactic body radiotherapy for resected pancreatic adenocarcinoma with close or positive margins. *J Gastrointest Cancer.* 2012 Mar;43(1):70–76.

51. Timmerman R, Bastasch M, Saha D, et al. Optimizing dose and fractionation for stereotactic body radiation therapy. Normal tissue and tumor control effects with large dose per fraction. *Front Radiat Ther Oncol.* 2007;40:352–365

52. Loehrer PJ, Powell ME, Cardenes HR, et al. A randomized phase III study of gemcitabine in combination with radiation therapy versus gemcitabine alone in patients with localized, unresectable pancreatic cancer: E4201. *J Clin Oncol.* 2008;26(May 20 suppl):abst. 4506.

53. Small W, Jr, Berlin J, Freedman GM, et al. Full-dose gemcitabine with concurrent radiation therapy in patients with nonmetastatic pancreatic cancer: A multicenter phase II trial. *J Clin Oncol.* 2008;26(6):942–947.

54. Menon KV, Gomez D, Smith AM, et al. Impact of margin status on survival following pancreatoduodenectomy for cancer: The Leeds Pathology Protocol (LEEPP). *HPB.* 2009;11(1):18–24.

55. Esposito I, Kleeff J, Bergmann F, et al. Most pancreatic cancer resections are R1 resections. *Ann Surg Oncol.* 2008;15(6):1651–1660.

56. Evans DB, Hess KR, Pisters PW. ESPAC-1 trial of adjuvant therapy for resectable adenocarcinoma of the pancreas. *Ann Surg.* 2002;236(5):694; author reply 694–696.

57. Neoptolemos JP, Moore MJ, Cox TF, et al. Effect of adjuvant chemotherapy with fluorouracil plus folinic acid or gemcitabine vs observation on survival in patients with resected periampullary adenocarcinoma: The ESPAC-3 periampullary cancer randomized trial. *JAMA.* 2012 Jul 11;308(2):147–156. Erratum in: *JAMA.* 2012 Nov 14;308(18):1861.

58. Abrams RA, Winter KA, Regine WF, et al. Failure to adhere to protocol specified radiation therapy guidelines was associated with decreased survival in RTOG 9704-A phase III trial of adjuvant chemotherapy and chemoradiotherapy for patients with resected adenocarcinoma of the pancreas. *Int J Radiat Oncol Biol Phys.* 201 Feb 1;82(2):809–816.

■ **CASE 2** ■

Rectal Cancer

CLINICAL PROBLEM

For localized rectal cancer, the standard of care is neoadjuvant chemoradiation (CRT) followed by a low anterior resection (LAR) or abdomino-perineal resection (APR). These procedures, however, carry a higher risk of morbidity and mortality that may not be warranted for early T1-T2 distal lesions that have a lower rate of lymph node positivity. For distal, well-lateralized T2 lesions, local excision (LE) alone, with or without CRT (adjuvant/neoadjuvant), may result in higher local and distant recurrence rates, and is therefore controversial.

CASE EXAMPLE

A 55-year-old female presents with rectal bleeding. Subsequent colonoscopy, MRI (Figure 3.2.1), and endorectal ultrasound (ERUS) (Figure 3.2.2) reveal a 3-cm rectal lesion, freely mobile, located approximately 3 cm from the anal verge, and clinically staged with ERUS as uT2N0. Tumor biopsy is positive for moderately differentiated adenocarcinoma without lymphovascular space invasion (LVSI). Carcinoembryonic antigen (CEA) is 2.8 ng/mL.

Management Decisions

- Should a staging PET/CT be ordered?
- Which clinical characteristics make uT2 rectal cancer patients optimal candidates for LE?
- Which surgical techniques are ideal for LE of a T2 lesion?
- What data exist for neoadjuvant versus adjuvant CRT for uT2 lesions?
- If neoadjuvant therapy is given, what is the optimal time interval between completion of therapy and surgery?
- In the neoadjuvant setting, what chemotherapy should be given concurrently with radiation?
- In select cases, is it reasonable to exclude surgery after CRT?

MAJOR OPINION

Devin D. Schellenberg

Should a Staging PET/CT Be Ordered?

In this clinical scenario, the patient has already undergone the widely recommended staging exams, including contrast CT, ERUS, and pelvic MRI. For early rectal cancer, PET/CT is not recommended by the National Comprehensive Cancer Network (NCCN) guidelines, but considered potentially appropriate by the American College of Radiology (ACR) guidelines [1,2]. Specifically, PET/CT has shown to be less accurate than ERUS or pelvic MRI with endorectal coil in evaluating the T and N stages for early stage rectal cancer [3,4]. PET/CT does not adequately differentiate T2 versus T3 lesions and, in general, cannot characterize lymph nodes under 8 to 10 mm in size. PET/CT was not used in the 2 prospective trials evaluating LE [5,6].

Although PET/CT has been found to be more accurate in the staging of distant disease in more advanced colorectal cancers (altering stage in up to 30% of advanced colorectal cases) [7], currently there is no published evidence of its utility in local rectal cancer where distant metastases would be uncommon. Therefore, PET/CT should not be used as a replacement for MRI or ERUS. It may be used in conjunction with contrast CT chest, abdomen, and pelvis for distant staging, but the expected yield in this clinical scenario would be low.

54

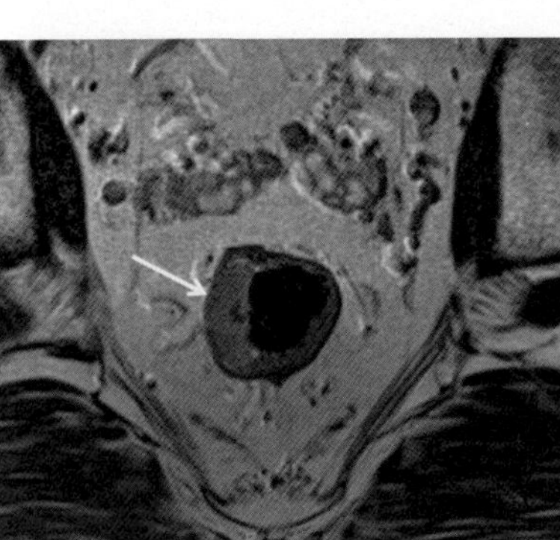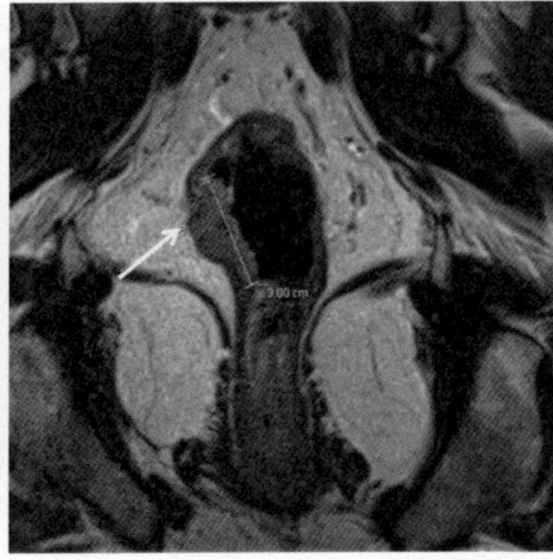

FIGURE 3.2.1 ■ Axial and coronal high resolution T2-weighted MRI. Tumor involves the mucosa, submucosa, and extends into the deep layer of the lamina muscularis propria with no extension beyond the muscularis propria.

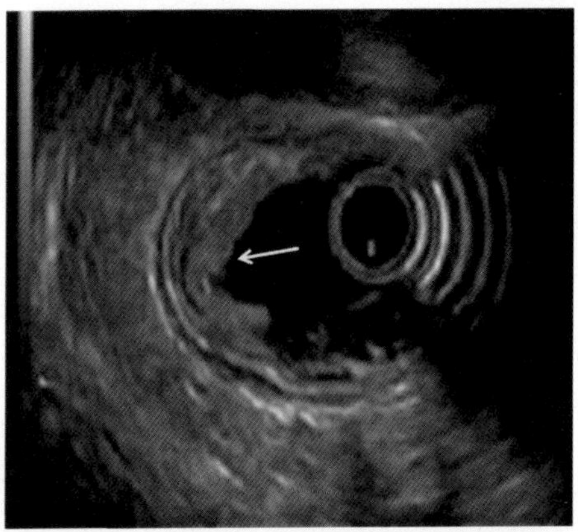

FIGURE 3.2.2 ■ Staging pull-through EUS examination is shown. Radial imaging at 7.5 MHz shows a rectal wall abnormality invading the muscularis propria and a thickened submucosal space suggesting tumor involvement. The tumor appears to extend into but not through the muscularis propria, shown here at the 9 o'clock position.

Which Clinical Characteristics Make uT2 Rectal Cancer Patients Optimal Candidates for LE?

In order for patients to be considered for LE, their tumors must be small, amenable to a transanal approach, and have a low risk of harboring clinically undetectable lymph nodes. LE was developed for early rectal cancer and though there are insufficient data to justify a clear size limitation, most institutions, cooperative trials, and guidelines state that LE should not be performed for lesions of greater than 3 to 4 cm in size, nor for circumferential lesions [1,2,6]. Although there are no strict distance guidelines, the proximal aspect of tumors was no further than 3 to 8 cm from the anal verge in most institutional series and prospective studies [5,6,8]. Achieving an accepted 1-cm tumor margin is difficult if tumors extend farther than 6 to 8 cm from the anal verge, though newer surgical techniques and the use of transanal endoscopic microsurgery (TEM) may expand the distance from the anal verge in the future.

Furthermore, as LE does not evaluate lymph node status, high-risk lesions based on poor differentiation (grade 3) or LVSI are poor candidates for LE. In almost all institutional series, lymphovascular invasion and high grade have correlated with increased rates of node-positive disease or local recurrence [1,9–12]. Institutional data have demonstrated high-grade tumors to result in lymph node positivity in 27% of cases versus only 4% in low-grade tumors [13]. While recurrence rates have been as high as 50% in resected pT2 tumors with either high grade and/or LVSI [10,14], tumors with myxoid differentiation and increased depth of invasion have correlated with poorer outcomes in some but not all series [10]. Though T1 versus T2 status certainly alters the local recurrence rates, the depth of invasion within T2 tumors has not been widely prognostic of lymph node positive disease or recurrence [15]. Therefore, LE consideration should be more directed by tumor grade and LVSI rather than tumor depth for T2 tumors of the distal anal canal.

Importantly, if a positive margin or T3 status is noted after LE, medically fit patients should proceed to APR or LAR surgery [1,2,16]. Positive margins have been associated with increased local recurrences on institutional multivariate analyses, and have been found to be the most predictive factor of local recurrence on systemic review [17,18]. Duek et al. found a 40% rate of residual tumor on immediate APR pathology after LE [19]. In addition, in the setting of T3 disease recurrences are often as high as 50% [20,21], with some series suggesting up to a 70% rate of lymph node metastases with T3 tumors [22] and Tsai et al. reporting a recurrence rate of 100% [23]. In the absence of significant comorbidities, patients with T3 or margin-positive LE should proceed with wider surgery as adjuvant therapy is highly unlikely to fully reduce the risk of local recurrence.

Which Surgical Techniques Are Ideal for LE of a T2 Lesion?

The 3 main operative approaches for LE are transanal, posterior trans-sphincteric (York Mason procedure), and posterior proctotomy (Kraske procedure). The posterior trans-sphincteric and posterior proctotomy approaches are less commonly used and involve posterior approaches with dissection above or below the levator ani to the rectum. Transanal excision (TAE) and TEM are the most common approaches and use either direct or endoscopic viewing of the rectal lesion. The aim is to excise the lesion down to the perirectal fat with a 1 cm margin. The mural defect is then closed or left to heal by secondary intention in certain larger lesions. All procedures described here involve removal of the lesion alone. Lymph node sampling is not performed.

In summary, TEM has been shown to be safe following CRT and is becoming the most commonly used surgical technique for LE. TEM appears to be more effective in achieving a negative margin compared to TAE, though this did not translate to a significant difference in patient outcomes on multivariate analysis retrospective studies [1,7,24].

What Data Exist for Neoadjuvant Versus Adjuvant CRT for uT2 Lesions?

There are no randomized, prospective trials evaluating neoadjuvant versus adjuvant CRT for uT2 tumors. Also, there are no randomized, prospective trials of LE alone versus LE plus CRT. As a result, the data supporting both neoadjuvant and adjuvant treatment are based on the high local recurrence rates for T2 tumors treated without adjuvant therapy and comparisons between institutional studies where adjuvant treatment was or was not used.

Though a direct comparison of local recurrence rates between institutions is not scientifically sound, local recurrence rates have regularly been greater in trials with LE alone. In 9 institutional series, local recurrence in uT2 lesions have varied between 3% and 50%, with only 1 trial reporting a recurrence rate under 10% [14,19,20,21,23,25,26]. Whereas, with the use of neoadjuvant therapy, local recurrence rates have varied between 4% and 11% in 4 trials with only 1 trial reporting a local recurrence rate above 10% [5,16,27,28]. The most convincing evidence for an effect of adjuvant treatment came from Duek et al. demonstrating local recurrence rates of 50% with LE alone and 0% with adjuvant radiation in a small institutional series [19]. Review of the LE trials demonstrates neoadjuvant treatment followed by LE to be safe and effective, though it may be associated with greater rates of wound breakdown [29].

A recommendation regarding neoadjuvant versus adjuvant CRT cannot be made at this time, though it appears that T2 tumors treated with LE alone have higher rates of recurrence than those treated with either neoadjuvant or adjuvant therapy. The most frequently reported treatment of uT2 is neoadjuvant CRT with 5-fluorouracil (5-FU)-based chemotherapy and radiation of 45 to 54 Gy in standard fractionations.

If Neoadjuvant Therapy Is Given, What Is the Optimal Time Interval Between Completion of Therapy and Surgery?

Similar to the setting of locally advanced rectal cancers, the optimal time interval between neoadjuvant therapy and surgery in early stage rectal cancer is set to facilitate both downstaging of the tumor as well as normal tissue healing from radiation. The interval has been 4 to 8 weeks in most studies [30,31]. In the prospective ACOSOG study, the recommended interval is 4 to 6 weeks [6].

Note: It is important that the location of the tumor be marked (usually by tattoo) prior to neoadjuvant therapy as the complete response rates to neoadjuvant therapy have been 33% to 61% in published trials [6,16,30].

In the Neoadjuvant Setting, What Chemotherapy Should Be Given Concurrently With Radiation?

Standard neoadjuvant CRT should include either a continuous IV infusion of 5-FU or oral capecitabine. The American College of Surgeons Oncology Group (ACOSOG) trial found excessive toxicity with preoperative treatment with capecitabine 850 mg/m² BID Monday to Friday and oxaliplatin 50 mg/m² IV, on days 1, 8, 22, and 29, such that a radiation dose reduction was required [6]. Multiagent chemotherapy with radiation continues to be evaluated in more advanced rectal cancer trials and in the early rectal cancer ACOSOG trial. However, without a demonstrable benefit in local control or clear evidence of improved survival in a randomized study, the standard of care should remain 5-FU or capecitabine-based chemotherapy as given for locally advanced cancers.

In Select Cases, Is It Reasonable to Exclude Surgery After CRT?

It appears that tumors that have poor responses to neoadjuvant treatment have higher local recurrence rates. All patients with recurrence in the Lezoche et al. series had ypT2 disease at resection, demonstrating limited response to neoadjuvant treatment [5], while Meadows et al. suggested those patients without a complete clinical response (cCR) should have an APR rather than LE because of elevated recurrence risks [32].

Conversely, patients with excellent tumor response or downstaging have improved prognoses in institutional studies and in a systemic review [32–34]. Smith et al. found nodal disease to be less than 5% in ypT0 patients [33] and institutions have examined observation in complete responders achieving very strict endoscopic criteria 8 weeks post neoadjuvant CRT [31,35]. However, outside of a clinical trial, surgery is recommended for all patients. Furthermore, altering surgical treatment (eg, TEM for patients with proven downstaging response and APR for nonresponders) is also experimental at present [34].

Final Recommendation

When evaluating patients with uT2N0, I first ensure the staging is as accurate as possible. This sometimes means referrals to centers with more expertise in transrectal ultrasound and/or review of the MRI (which sometimes has not been done with gadolinium or an endorectal coil). Most often, the referring surgeon has discussed management options, yet a lengthy and detailed review regarding the controversies involved and possible treatment outcomes occurs. I inform patients that if they are treated with APR (or LAR) and the final pathology is indeed pT2N0 (with negative margins), they will not require chemotherapy or radiation. This has been the standard treatment for decades. Furthermore, if they choose to undergo a LE, recurrence rates may be higher even with postoperative CRT. Though the practice is changing, preoperative treatment is currently not standard at my center. Those that receive it are forewarned that despite CRT, downstaging will not occur in all patients and a small minority of patients may have to undergo an APR (or LAR) for T3 disease or positive margins. If patients desire a LE, the surgery is performed by a small, specialized group of surgeons at my center. This allows a unified message regarding LE to be given by both the surgeon and the oncologist. I believe this in turn helps to facilitate informed and realistic decisions by patients regarding LE.

ACADEMIC COMMENT

William Blackstock

There is considerable desire to use LE as a definitive treatment for stage T1-T2 rectal cancer. In a 2009 Surveillance Epidemiology and End Results (SEER) analysis of 4320 patients with T1-T2 rectal cancers, 20% underwent either LE alone (13%) or LE plus adjuvant radiation therapy (7%) [36]. In an analysis of 25,825 patients using data from the National Cancer Data Base, the rates of LE increased between 1999 and 2001, with 46% of patients with T1 and 17% of patients with T2 lesions managed surgically with a LE [37]. Whether done using a conventional TAE, posterior trans-sphincteric (York Mason procedure), or posterior proctotomy (Kraske procedure), the operation has very low morbidity. When performed properly, there is no need for permanent or even temporary colostomy, the recovery is rapid, and long-term bowel function is excellent.

The work-up for this patient should include a baseline CT of the chest/abdomen/pelvis, routine laboratory tests, including a hemoglobin to discern potential bleeding. The utility of positron emission tomography utilizing fluorodeoxyglucose (FDG-PET) for the staging of patients with rectal cancer is uncertain. When possible, all patients should be evaluated by a colorectal surgeon who performs a rigid proctoscopy or sigmoidoscopy and endoscopic ultrasound (EUS) to evaluate the stage of the lesion and to discern any perirectal lymphadenopathy in order to further refine our clinical staging of the patient. It should be noted that EUS accurately provides T-stage in 70% of patients and less so for nodal staging. The accuracy of CT for predicting nodal involvement ranges from 22% to 73%. MRI has overall accuracies for T-staging of 65% to 86%. MRI is very accurate for identifying large T3 and T4 tumors, with sensitivities for prediction of T3 of 80% to 86% and specificity of 71% to 76% [38]. However, challenges still exist in the accurate detection of metastatic lymph nodes [39].

Tumor assessment, either at the time of the initial biopsy or following resection, is critical in patient selection. In general, the best candidates for LE include small (smaller than 4 cm), low-lying tumors confined to the muscularis propria. Patients with adverse pathologic features (signet ring histology, piece-meal resection, poor differentiation, LVSI, unclear margins) or whose tumors occupy more than 40% of the rectum are at high risk for local recurrence, and LE is generally not recommended [1]. There are limited data available for the use of neoadjuvant CRT for patients with T2N0 tumors prior to LE. ACOSOG recently completed a phase 2 (Z6041) study of 90 patients with T2N0 disease receiving preoperative radiation of 50.4 Gy with concurrent capecitabine/oxaliplatin chemotherapy [40]. Patients were required to have T2N0 disease confirmed with either EUS or endorectal MRI. The tumors could not exceed 4 cm and were within 8 cm from the anal verge. Forty-four percent of patients at the time of the LE were found to have a pathologic complete response and 64% of patients were downstaged. We await long-term follow-up of this study to discern if local control is compromised by utilizing this strategy. Despite these findings, preoperative CRT prior to LE is not standard of care for patients with T2N0 rectal cancer and it should be restricted to select patients or be conducted on clinical trial.

The data for postoperative CRT following LE is more robust. The Cancer and Leukemia Group B completed a phase 2 study in which 51 patients with T2N0 lesions received 50.4 Gy with concurrent 5-FU chemotherapy [41]. With a median follow-up of over 7 years, the local recurrence rates for patients with T2 disease was 18%. It should be noted that despite intense staging, 32% of the 51 patients were excluded from the study when they were found to have tumors that were either larger than 4 cm in diameter or the size was unclear. Twenty-five percent of patients were found to have higher than T2 disease and in 39% of excluded patients, the margin status was unclear.

In general, LEs are optimally performed utilizing the TEM approach. TEM is a minimally invasive surgical procedure that allows for LE of rectal lesions that are difficult to directly visualize. The TEM operating system includes a specialized magnifying resectoscope and ports for carbon dioxide gas insufflation and irrigation, and allows the passage of dissecting instruments.

Our approach to patients with pT2N0 disease following TEM is to assess the patient 4 to 6 weeks following resection. Patients with optimal histologic characteristics (as outlined earlier) receive postoperative radiation to a dose of 50.4 Gy in 1.8 Gy daily fractions. This is delivered with concurrent 5-FU or capecitabine chemotherapy. The external beam radiation therapy is delivered with megavoltage linear accelerators ($\geq$6 MV) using a 3 to 4 field pelvis technique following CT-based simulation and computer-assisted treatment planning. The superior border of the target volume is placed at or above the second sacral segment, but not more cephalad than the interspace between the fifth lumbar vertebra and the first sacral segment. The inferior border is intended to exclude perineal skin except in circumstances when transcoccygeal or trans-sacral excision was employed or the surgical incision extended caudally to include a portion of the anal canal. Bolus material is applied to surgical skin incisions. For the opposed lateral fields, the posterior border is placed 1.5 cm posterior to the sacral edge. The inguinal nodes are included in the initial target volume for patients with low-lying primary cancers below 4 cm from the anal verge or patients with cancers involving the anal canal.

Routine follow-up would include pelvic imaging, CEA assessment, and physical examination every 3 to 4 months the first year. If the patient remains without evidence of disease, this interval is increased to every 4 to 6 months for 2 additional years and then yearly for 2 additional years.

COMMUNITY PRACTITIONER COMMENT

Stephen K. Ronson

The treatment of a low-lying stage I adenocarcinoma of the rectum presents a potentially complex set of treatment decisions. These treatment decisions become more complicated when the patient is clinically staged as uT2N0, group stage I. Workup in this case should include full colonoscopy, CT of the chest/abdomen/pelvis, as well as EUS for accurate tumor staging and perirectal nodal evaluation with the addition of a PET/CT or MRI for further nodal evaluation if any questionable lymph nodes are found on CT or EUS. If at any point abnormal lymph nodes are identified, I would proceed with a course of neoadjuvant CRT followed by the appropriate transabdominal resection. This approach has been shown to increase local control as well as the rate of sphincter preservation, while at the same time decreasing toxicity [42]. The potential downside of this treatment approach is the potential for overtreating patients who have been clinically "over-staged." Incorrect tumor staging occurs in 17% of cases in low-lying rectal tumors and the sensitivity and specificity of EUS for nodal staging is 67% and 78%, respectively [38].

For stage I adenocarcinoma of the rectum, neoadjuvant treatment is not normally indicated. Conversely, for patients with low-lying lesions or rectal lesions requiring an APR, neoadjuvant radiation or CRT can be used to sometimes help make the patient a candidate for a sphincter-sparing LAR [43,44]. For these patients, my preference is to proceed with a course of neoadjuvant CRT with concurrent infusional 5-FU or oral capecitabine-based chemotherapy to maximize their chances of sphincter preservation. I would treat the patient using IMRT to 4500 cGy to the pelvis followed by a boost to the mesorectum and pre-sacral space to an additional 540 cGy. Although IMRT is not considered the standard of care, it has been shown to decrease radiation dose to adjacent normal structures (small bowel, femoral heads) when compared to conformal radiation [45]. Because LE candidates have a better prognosis than patients with T3–T4 lesions, IMRT may be warranted. At my institution, surgery then takes place within 6 to 8 weeks after completion of neoadjuvant CRT. In a subset of stage I patients, sphincter preservation can also be achieved with upfront full thickness excision. Patients must meet certain criteria in order to qualify for this approach. These criteria include: mobile, nonfixed tumor less than 3 cm and involving less than one-third of the luminal circumference; well to moderate differentiation without LVSI; and tumor location within 8 cm of the anal verge. The only patients not requiring additional therapy are those who are found after surgery to have true T1 lesions, negative margins, and none of the high-risk features mentioned earlier. For patients upstaged to T2 on final pathologic analysis or those with high-risk features, additional treatment is needed. This is further discussed subsequently.

For a patient with a uT2 lesion and none of the high-risk features discussed earlier, it is reasonable to proceed with a full thickness excision if the patient is well informed on the potential outcomes and additional treatments that may be required. If the patient is found to have a pT1 tumor on the final pathologic analysis and no high-risk features, no further treatment is needed. If the patient is found to indeed have a pT2 lesion, NCCN guidelines only give the option of proceeding with completion transabdominal resection as local recurrence rates of 11% to 45% have been observed [46–48]. In this case, if the patient is found to have negative lymph nodes, no further treatment is needed. However, in patients with high risk pT1 or pT2 lesions who have undergone upfront full thickness excision, phase 2 data support the use of adjuvant CRT instead of completion transabdominal resection with local recurrence rates of 7% and 8%, respectively [49]. Further investigation is needed to evaluate whether a neoadjuvant CRT approach for high risk T1, T2, or even T3N0 patients followed by full thickness excision would provide similar benefits to the ones seen in T3 and node-positive patients who undergo transabdominal resection [30,34].

SECTION EDITOR'S NOTE

Joseph M. Herman

The results of the recently published ACOSOG Z6041 study demonstrated excellent rates of pathologic complete response and negative resection margins in patients with uT2 rectal cancer following neoadjuvant CRT. This trial established neoadjuvant capecitabine-based CRT as a potential standard of care for localized T1-T2 rectal cancer. However, it is important to stress that this regimen does result in higher rates of toxicity and postsurgical complications when compared

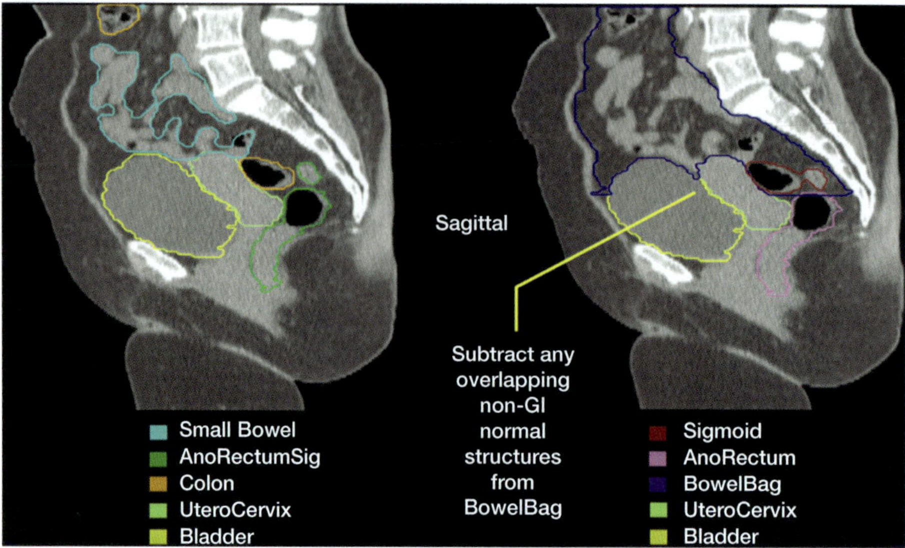

FIGURE 3.2.3 ■ RTOG normal tissue contouring atlas, female. Found at www.rtog.org/CoreLab/Contouring Atlases/FemaleRTOGNormalPelvisAtlas.aspx

to TEM alone. There are limited data to support upfront LE followed by adjuvant CRT and it is unlikely that a randomized study will compare pre- versus postoperative CRT; therefore, these patients should ideally be discussed in a multidisciplinary setting where the final treatment plan can be determined by clinicians, patients, and families. When possible, patients should be enrolled in clinical trials. As with locally advanced rectal cancer (T3-T4), use of neoadjuvant chemotherapy prior to CRT could be used to downstage T1-T2 rectal tumors and select patients who are more likely to benefit from neoadjuvant versus adjuvant CRT-based on the criteria mentioned in the review. This approach is being considered in the cooperative group setting. The role of IMRT is controversial, but should be considered in younger patients where long-term effects of radiation can be substantial. If one uses IMRT, existing atlases should be used to ensure correct contouring of organs at risk (Figure 3.2.3).

In the future, novel biomarkers and imaging correlates are likely to play a key role in determining which patients should receive more or less aggressive treatment. Strides made in surgical and radiation technology should also improve rectal tumor control while limiting treatment-related toxicity. For example, con-tact, high dose rate endorectal brachytherapy, or stereotactic body radiation therapy may have a role in downstaging or sterilizing intact tumors and residual disease following surgery. However, prospective data are needed to determine the efficacy of these technologies in early stage rectal cancer management.

REFERENCES

1. Blackstock W, Russo SM, Suh WW, et al. ACR appropriateness criteria: Local excision in early-stage rectal cancer. *Curr Probl Cancer.* 2010;34:193–200.
2. NCCN practice guidelines for rectal cancer. 2011. www.nccn.org. Accessed July 1, 2011.
3. Cho YB, Chun HK, Kim MJ, et al. Accuracy of MRI and 18F-FDG PET/CT for restaging after preoperative concurrent chemoradiotherapy for rectal cancer. *World J Surg.* 2009;33:2688–2694.
4. Pahlman L, Torkzad MR. Rectal cancer staging: Is there an optimal method? *Future Oncol.* 2011;7:93–100.
5. Lezoche G, Guerrieri M, Baldarelli M, et al. Transanal endoscopic microsurgery for 135 patients with small nonadvanced low rectal cancer (iT1-iT2, iN0): Short- and long-term results. *Surg Endosc.* 2011;25:1222–1229.

6. Ota DM, Nelson H, ACOSOG Group Co-Chairs. Local excision of rectal cancer revisited: ACOSOG protocol Z6041. *Ann Surg Oncol.* 2007;14:271.

7. Eglinton T, Luck A, Bartholomeusz D, et al. Positron-emission tomography/computed tomography (PET/CT) in the initial staging of primary rectal cancer. *Colorectal Dis.* 2010;12:667–673.

8. Marks J, Mizrahi B, Dalane S, et al. Laparoscopic transanal abdominal transanal resection with sphincter preservation for rectal cancer in the distal 3 cm of the rectum after neoadjuvant therapy. *Surg Endosc.* 2010;24:2700–2707.

9. Bach SP, Hill J, Monson JR, et al. A predictive model for local recurrence after transanal endoscopic microsurgery for rectal cancer. *Br J Surg.* 2009;96:280–290.

10. Kajiwara Y, Ueno H, Hashiguchi Y, et al. Risk factors of nodal involvement in T2 colorectal cancer. *Dis Colon Rectum.* 2010;53:1393–1399.

11. Peng J, Chen W, Sheng W, et al. Oncological outcome of T1 rectal cancer undergoing standard resection and local excision. *Colorectal Dis.* 2011;13:e14–e19.

12. Sato T, Ueno H, Mochizuki H, et al. Objective criteria for the grading of venous invasion in colorectal cancer. *Am J Surg Pathol.* 2010;34:454–462.

13. Ueno H, Hashiguchi Y, Kajiwara Y, et al. Proposed objective criteria for "grade 3" in early invasive colorectal cancer. *Am J Clin Pathol.* 2010;134:312–322.

14. Borschitz T, Heintz A, Junginger T. Transanal endoscopic microsurgical excision of pT2 rectal cancer: Results and possible indications. *Dis Colon Rectum.* 2007;50:292–301.

15. Ding PR, An X, Cao Y, et al. Depth of tumor invasion independently predicts lymph node metastasis in T2 rectal cancer. *J Gastrointest Surg.* 2011;15:130–136.

16. Nair RM, Siegel EM, Chen DT, et al. Long-term results of transanal excision after neoadjuvant chemoradiation for T2 and T3 adenocarcinomas of the rectum. *J Gastrointest Surg.* 2008;12:1797,805; discussion 1805–1806.

17. Christoforidis D, Cho HM, Dixon MR, et al. Transanal endoscopic microsurgery versus conventional transanal excision for patients with early rectal cancer. *Ann Surg.* 2009;249:776–782.

18. Caricato M, Borzomati D, Ausania F, et al. Prognostic factors after surgery for locally recurrent rectal cancer: an overview. *Eur J Surg Oncol.* 2006;32:126–132.

19. Duek SD, Issa N, Hershko DD, Krausz MM. Outcome of transanal endoscopic microsurgery and adjuvant radiotherapy in patients with T2 rectal cancer. *Dis Colon Rectum.* 2008;51:379,84; discussion 384.

20. Allaix ME, Arezzo A, Caldart M, et al. Transanal endoscopic microsurgery for rectal neoplasms: Experience of 300 consecutive cases. *Dis Colon Rectum.* 2009;52:1831–1836.

21. Stipa F, Lucandri G, Ferri M, et al. Local excision of rectal cancer with transanal endoscopic microsurgery (TEM). *Anticancer Res.* 2004;24:1167–1172.

22. Garcia-Aguilar J, Holt A. Optimal management of small rectal cancers: TAE, TEM, or TME? *Surg Oncol Clin N Am.* 2010;19:743–760.

23. Tsai BM, Finne CO, Nordenstam JF, et al. Transanal endoscopic microsurgery resection of rectal tumors: Outcomes and recommendations. *Dis Colon Rectum.* 2010;53:16–23.

24. Moore JS, Cataldo PA, Osler T, Hyman NH. Transanal endoscopic microsurgery is more effective than traditional transanal excision for resection of rectal masses. *Dis Colon Rectum.* 2008;51:1026,30; discussion 1030–1031.

25. Ramirez JM, Aguilella V, Valencia J, et al. Transanal endoscopic microsurgery for rectal cancer. Long-term oncologic results. *Int J Colorectal Dis.* 2011;26:437–443.

26. Whitehouse PA, Armitage JN, Tilney HS, Simson JN. Transanal endoscopic microsurgery: Local recurrence rate following resection of rectal cancer. *Colorectal Dis.* 2008;10:187–193.

27. Guerrieri M, Baldarelli M, Organetti L, et al. Transanal endoscopic microsurgery for the treatment of selected patients with distal rectal cancer: 15 years experience. *Surg Endosc.* 2008;22:2030–2035.

28. Callender GG, Das P, Rodriguez-Bigas MA, et al. Local excision after preoperative chemoradiation results in an equivalent outcome to total mesorectal excision in selected patients with T3 rectal cancer. *Ann Surg Oncol.* 2010;17:441–447.

29. Marks JH, Valsdottir EB, DeNittis A, et al. Transanal endoscopic microsurgery for the treatment of rectal cancer: Comparison of wound complication rates with and without neoadjuvant radiation therapy. *Surg Endosc.* 2009;23:1081–1087.

30. Park C, Lee W, Han S, et al. Transanal local excision for preoperative concurrent chemoradiation therapy for distal rectal cancer in selected patients. *Surg Today.* 2007;37:1068–1072.

31. Habr-Gama A, Perez RO, Wynn G, et al. Complete clinical response after neoadjuvant chemoradiation therapy for distal rectal cancer: Characterization of clinical and endoscopic

findings for standardization. *Dis Colon Rectum.* 2010;53:1692–1698.

32. Meadows K, Morris CG, Rout WR, et al. Preoperative radiotherapy alone or combined with chemotherapy followed by transanal excision for rectal adenocarcinoma. *Am J Clin Oncol.* 2006;29:430–434.

33. Smith FM, Waldron D, Winter DC. Rectum-conserving surgery in the era of chemoradiotherapy. *Br J Surg.* 2010;97:1752–1764.

34. Caricato M, Borzomati D, Ausania F, et al. Complementary use of local excision and transanal endoscopic microsurgery for rectal cancer after neoadjuvant chemoradiation. *Surg Endosc.* 2006;20:1203–1207.

35. Habr-Gama A, Perez R, Proscurshim I, Gama-Rodrigues J. Complete clinical response after neoadjuvant chemoradiation for distal rectal cancer. *Surg Oncol Clin N Am.* 2010;19:829–845.

36. Hazard LJ, Shrieve DC, Sklow B, et al. Local excision vs. radical resection in T1-2 rectal carcinoma: Results of a study from the Surveillance, Epidemiology, and End Results (SEER) registry data. *Gastrointest Cancer Res.* 2009;3(3):105–114.

37. Baxter NN, Steward AK, Nelson H. Oncological outcome of T1 rectal cancer undergoing standard resection and local excision. *J Clin Oncol.* 2004;22:14S.

38. Bipat S, Glas A, Slors F, et al. Rectal cancer: Local staging and assessment of lymph node involvement with endoluminal US, CT, and MR imaging—a meta-analysis. *Radiology.* 2004;232:773–783.

39. Gowdra Halappa V, Corona Villalobos CP, Bonekamp S, et al. Rectal imagining: High-resolution MRI of carcinoma of the rectum at 3 T. *AJR Am J Roentgenol.* 2012 Jul;199(1):W35–W42.

40. Garcia-Aguilar J, Shi Q, Thomas CR Jr, et al. A phase II trial of neoadjuvant chemoradiation and local excision for T2N0 rectal cancer: Preliminary results of the ACOSOG Z6041 trial. *Ann Surg Oncol.* 2012 Feb;19(2):384–391.

41. Greenberg JA, Shibata D, Herndon JE 2nd, et al. Local excision of distal rectal cancer: An update of cancer and leukemia group B 8984. *Dis Colon Rectum.* 2008;51(8):1185–1191.

42. Sauer R, Becker H, Hohenberger W, et al. Preoperative versus postoperative chemoradiotherapy for rectal cancer. *N Engl J Med.* 2004;351:1731–1740.

43. Gérard JP, Azria D, Gourgou-Bourgade S, et al. Comparison of two neoadjuvant chemoradiotherapy regimens for locally advanced rectal cancer: Results of the phase III trial ACCORD 12/0405-Prodige 2. J Clin Oncol. 2010 Apr 1;28(10):1638–1644. Epub 2010 Mar 1.

44. Gérard JP, Chapet O, Nemoz C, et al. Improved sphincter preservation in low rectal cancer with high-dose preoperative radiotherapy: The lyon R96-02 randomized trial. J Clin Oncol. 2004 Jun 15;22(12):2404–2409.

45. Jones WE, 3rd, Thomas CR Jr, Herman JM, et al. ACR appropriateness criteria® resectable cancer. *Radiat Oncol.* 2012 Sep 24;7:161. doi: 10.1186/1748-717X-7-161.

46. Baxter N, Aguilar J. Organ preservation for rectal cancer. *J Clin Oncol.* 2007;25:1014–1020.

47. Garcia-Aguilar J, Mellgren A, Sirivongs P, et al. Local excision of rectal cancer without adjuvant therapy: A word of caution. *Ann Surg.* 2000;231:345–351

48. Sengupta S, Tjandra JJ. Local excision of rectal cancer: What is the evidence? *Dis Colon Rectum.* 2001;44:1345–1361.

49. Russell AH, Harris J, Rosenberg PJ, et al. Anal sphincter conservation for patients with adenocarcinoma of the distal rectum: Long-term results of radiation therapy oncology group protocol 89-02. *Int J Radiat Oncol Biol Phys.* 2000;46:313–322.

■ CASE 3 ■

Anal Cancer

CLINICAL PROBLEM

It is well established that squamous cell carcinoma (SCC) of the anal canal can be treated with definitive chemoradiation (CRT), and that abdominoperineal resection (APR) is reserved for salvage only. The 5-year survival rate for patients who receive standard CRT approaches 70%; however, 20% to 40% experience grade 3 to grade 4 toxicity and administration with concurrent mitomycin-C (MMC) causes significant hematological toxicity. It has been suggested that treating anal SCC with intensity-modulated radiation therapy (IMRT) will decrease acute toxicities while maintaining similar treatment efficacy. Although IMRT may decrease toxicity, many question whether IMRT may result in higher local recurrence rates.

CASE EXAMPLE

A 45-year-old female presents with a 3-month history of rectal bleeding. She undergoes a colonoscopy and anoscopy and is found to have a circumferential anal canal tumor measuring 1.8 cm with a palpable 1.5 cm right-sided inguinal lymph node. She is staged as T1N2M0, is HIV negative, and has a Karnofsky performance status (KPS) score of 90.

Management Decisions

- Should a PET/CT or CT be ordered for staging? Is it necessary to biopsy the palpable or PET-avid inguinal lymph nodes?
- What type of pelvic radiotherapy should be accomplished—IMRT versus 3-D conformal? If the patient were an older male, would IMRT be necessary?
- Should radiation be given concurrently with 5-fluorouracil (5-FU) and MMC or 5-FU and cisplatin?
- Would the patient be managed differently if she were HIV positive?
- What final radiation dose should be delivered to the primary tumor and palpable inguinal node?

MAJOR OPINION

Salma K. Jabbour

Should a PET/CT or CT Be Ordered for Staging? Is It Necessary to Biopsy the Palpable or PET-Avid Inguinal Lymph Nodes?

The standard of care for radiographic staging of anal canal carcinoma is a CT scan or MRI of the abdomen and pelvis along with either a chest x-ray or chest CT scan. According to the 2011 National Comprehensive Cancer Network (NCCN) guidelines, a PET scan can be considered, but should not replace a CT scan, for staging or treatment planning as it has not been validated [1]. PET scans are promising because of their apparent ability to aid in staging and treatment planning and may also be of prognostic significance. They probably are best used in conjunction with routine contrast-enhanced CT imaging.

With regard to staging, multiple studies have demonstrated that PET scans can change the stage of the tumor in about 25% of cases [2] and identify positive pelvic or inguinal nodes in 10% to 20% of cases [3,4] and metastases in about 25% of cases in comparison to CT alone or physical examination [5]. Also, PET/CT detected 91% of nonexcised primary tumors, whereas CT visualized 59% of them [4].

Given the discrepancies seen between PET and CT scans in staging, accessible lymph nodes should be biopsied or should undergo fine needle aspiration (FNA), particularly for those in the inguinal regions. This need for biopsy is confirmed by Mistrangelo et al., who studied patients who underwent both sentinel lymph node biopsy and PET scans. PET-CT scans detected no inguinal metastases in 74% of cases and found metastases in the remaining 26% [6]. Histological analyses of the sentinel lymph nodes detected metastases in only 11% (4 of 27 false positive cases) of cases. PET-CT had a sensitivity of 100%, with a negative predictive value of 100%. Owing to the high number of false positives, PET-CT specificity was 83%, and positive predictive value was 43% [6]. Therefore, biopsy should still be performed if a PET scan is avid or lymph nodes are palpable in the groin.

PET scans may also alter treatment planning volumes, including the gross tumor volume (GTV) in 56% of cases and clinical target volume (CTV) in 37% of cases, especially with a fusion of both PET and CT, which increased the size of GTV and CTV [3], but these results have not been validated pathologically. PET scan may also help predict prognosis, as patients with a complete response (CR) following CRT were found to have a 2-year cause-specific survival rate of 94% versus 39% with a partial metabolic response, and 2-year progression-free survival rate of 95% with CR versus 22% of those with partial metabolic response in the anal tumor [7]. Moreover, higher standardized uptake value (SUV) (max) was significantly associated with an increased risk of nodal metastasis at diagnosis and worse disease-free survival (DFS) rates [8]. In sum, these pilot results evaluating PET scans demonstrate potential benefit in staging, radiation field design, and predicting prognosis, but should be used with caution as histopathologic confirmation is limited.

It is preferred to obtain a PET-CT scan along with a CT or MRI of the abdomen and pelvis with contrast. If PET alone is performed without CT fusion, an entire CT of the chest, abdomen, and pelvis with IV contrast would be necessary. As smoking is a risk factor for anal canal carcinoma, a chest CT rather than chest x-ray is favored as primary lung cancers have been discovered during the workup for these patients. PET-CT scans, all available imaging, and anoscopy/colonoscopy should be used in conjunction with clinical exam findings including pelvic examination in women and a prostate-specific antigen (PSA) in men to help plan target

volumes. PET scanning is also useful to trigger appropriate inguinal lymph node biopsies, which should be performed as there is a remarkable rate of false positive lymph nodes detected on PET scan alone. Whether a lymph node is truly malignant or simply reactive will alter planning volumes, doses, and prognosis.

What Type of Pelvic Radiotherapy Should Be Accomplished—IMRT Versus 3-D Conformal? If the Patient Were an Older Male, Would IMRT Be Necessary?

Organ-preserving CRT, the standard of care for definitive therapy of anal canal carcinoma, is successful in approximately 70% of cases, and avoids a permanent colostomy via APR. The downside of CRT with radiosensitizing 5-FU and mitomycin is the significant acute toxicity including moist desquamation of the perineum, cytopenias, and gastrointestinal (GI) side effects. These side effects can result in treatment breaks and compromise local control rates [9]. Dosimetric studies have confirmed a hypothetical benefit of IMRT by reduced radiation doses to small bowel, bladder, external genitalia, femoral heads, and iliac crests over 3D-conformal radiation therapy (3D-CRT) [10].

Examining the toxicity rates from the Radiation Therapy Oncology Group (RTOG) 98-11 trial demonstrated that 61% of patients treated on the MMC and 5-FU arm experienced grade 3 to grade 4 hematologic toxicities, 48% of patients had grade 3 to grade 4 skin toxicities, and 35% of patients had grade 3 to grade 4 GI toxicities [11,39]. Again, it is of concern that high rates of acute treatment-related toxicities may cause unintended treatment breaks, reducing efficacy of therapy [9].

Clinical experiences with IMRT have demonstrated a reduction in side effects. A series from the University of Chicago evaluating 17 patients treated with IMRT showed that all patients experienced acute grade 2 dermatitis, namely moist desquamation in the perianal and intergluteal areas. Nine patients who experienced acute grade 2 GI toxicity developed easily controllable diarrhea requiring antimotility agents. No patients developed any grade 3 or grade 4 toxicities [12]. Other series have verified the improvement in the side-effect profile with the use of IMRT as shown in Table 3.3.1.

TABLE 3.3.1 ◼ *Summary of Trials Incorporating IMRT in Anal Cancer*

AUTHOR	N	CONCURRENT CRT REGIMEN	DOSE TO REGIONAL UNINVOLVED LN (GY)	DOSE TO TUMOR/ POSITIVE LN (GY)	MEDIAN F/U (MONTHS)	TOXICITY	TREATMENT BREAKS	OUTCOMES
Salama et al. [13]	53	MMC/5-FU (90%) 5-FU or 5-FU/ CDDP (10%)	45/25 fx	51.5	14.5	Grade 3+ GI: 15% Derm: 38% Grade 4 Heme: 58%	42% Median 4 days	18 months CFS: 84% OS: 93% LRC: 84% FFDF: 93%
Pepek et al. [14]	31 with SCC, 47 with anal canal and perianal skin cancers	MMC/5-FU (62%) Other chemo (27%)	45/25 fx	54	19 (SCC)	Grade 3+ GI: 16% (N/V/D) Derm: 0% Grade 3+ Heme: 30%	18% Median 5 days	2 years (SCC) CFS: 91% OS: 100% LRC: 95% FFDF: 100%
Kachnic et al. [15]	43	MMC/5-FU (81%) 5-FU or 5-FU/ CDDP (19%)	T2N0: 42 (1.5 Gy/fx) T3-T4N0-N3: 45 (1.5 Gy/fx) Dose-painted	T2N0: 50.4 (1.8 Gy/fx) T3-T4N0-N3: 54 (1.8 Gy/fx) LN > 3 cm and 50.4 for LN ≤ 3 cm	24	Grade 3+ GI: 7% Derm: 10% Grade 3+ Heme: 51%	40% Median 2 days	2 years CFS: 90% OS: 94% LRC: 95% FFDF: 92%
Bazan et al. [16]	29	MMC/5-FU (85%) 5-FU/CDDP (13%)	Low risk PTV: 40 (1.6 Gy/fx) Intermediate risk PTV: 45 (1.8 Gy/fx) Dose-painted	54	32	Grade 3+ GI: 7% Derm: 21% Grade 3+ Heme: 21%	34% Median 1.5 days	3 years CFS: 91% OS: 88% LRC: 92% PFS: 84%
Kachnic et al. (RTOG 0529) [17,18,40] Red journal 2012	52	MMC/5-FU (100%)	T2N0: 42 (1.5 Gy/fx) T3-T4N0-N3: 45 (1.5 Gy/fx) Dose-painted	T2N0: 50.4 (1.8 Gy/fx) T3-T4N0-N3: 54 (1.8 Gy/fx) LN > 3 cm and 50.4 for LN ≤ 3 cm	23	Grade 3+ GI: 21% Derm: 23% Grade 2+ Heme: 73%	NR in available abstracts	2 years CFS: 86% OS: 88% DFS: 77% (abstract only)

5-FU, 5-fluorouracil; CDDP, cisplatin; CFS, colostomy-free survival; CRT, chemoradiation; Derm, dermatologic; DFS, disease-free survival; FFDF, freedom from distant failure; F/U, follow-up; fx, number of fractions; GI, gastrointestinal; Gy, gray; Heme, hematologic; LN, lymph nodes; LRC, local–regional control; MMC: mitomycin-C; NR, not reported; N/V/D: nausea, vomiting, diarrhea; OS, overall survival; PFS, progression-free survival; PTV, planning target volume; SCC, squamous cell carcinoma.

Based on these studies, IMRT appears to decrease acute toxicity in anal cancer patients and should be considered an emerging standard of care for this disease. Care, however, must be taken when contouring structures. In RTOG 0529, with real-time quality assurance, 81% of cases required recontouring prior to treatment [17,40].

Wright et al. quantified patterns of failure in 180 patients treated with conventional radiation therapy for anal canal SCC and showed that 45 patients had local–regional failure—78% of failures occurred at the primary site (56% local only and 22% with local and regional failure) and 22% had regional-only failure [19]. In another study by Das et al., the primary pattern of local–regional failure involved the anus or rectum. Another problematic site of failure was the pre-sacral and iliac regions for patients in whom the superior border of the pelvic field was placed at the bottom of the sacroiliac joints [20].

In the Wright study, among 20 patients who had a component of regional failure, 8 experienced failure in the inguinal nodes, 4 of whom were clinically node negative and 4 clinically positive, contributing to 40% of patients with regional failure. These inguinal recurrences could be quite superficial implying the need for generous margins on the femoral vessels to just below the level of the skin [19]. In the Das study, inguinal lymph node failures occurred in only 1 of 18 local–regional failures, but patients in the study received higher doses to grossly involved lymph nodes of 55 Gy compared to 45 to 50.4 Gy in the Wright study [20]. Common iliac failures occurred in 4 patients, all of whom had T3 disease and 3 of 4 had node-positive disease, so it was recommended that common iliac nodes should be included in the CTV for cT3, cT4, or node-positive disease. Internal and external iliac lymph nodes and the pre-sacral space must be included in the CTV in all cases. Failure in the perianal region was common and highlighted the need to respect a 2-cm margin on the tumor and anal margin in the CTV, even if this causes difficulty with the genital dose constraints [19]. Patients with a more advanced T-stage were more likely to have local–regional failure, calling for possible dose-escalation to the primary site and grossly involved lymph nodes [20].

In summary, carefully designed IMRT for anal canal cancer (ACC) is safe and has comparable efficacy to 3D-CRT with the benefit of reduction in acute toxicity. Knowledge of patterns of failure is vital to accurately delineate treatment volumes and avoid marginal misses. Recently published results from the RTOG 0529 phase 2 trial that evaluated IMRT show a significant reduction in acute grade 2+ hematologic adverse events (AEs), 73% (9811 85%, p = .032); grade 3+ GI AEs, 21% (9811 36%, p = .0082); and grade 3+ dermatologic AEs, 23% (9811 49%, P < .0001), with DP-IMRT [17,40].

Given the available data and effectiveness, IMRT is recommended for anal carcinoma cases as it should be of benefit to patients of all age groups and genders to help lessen acute side effects and potential long-term toxicities by reducing dose to bowel, bone marrow, femoral heads, genitalia, and skin.

Should Radiation Be Given Concurrently With 5-FU and MMC or 5-FU and Cisplatin?

Owing to the high level of hematologic toxicity with MMC, multiple phase 2 studies [21–24] have evaluated cisplatin as a possible radiosensitizer in combination with 5-FU and radiation and this question prompted RTOG 98-11. RTOG 98-11, a phase 3 randomized trial, compared standard CRT with MMC, 5-FU, and radiation therapy (n = 324) to 2 cycles of induction cisplatin and 5-FU followed by CRT with cisplatin and 5-FU (n = 320) [11,39]. The initial report showed no significant differences in 5-year overall survival (OS), 5-year local–regional recurrence, and distant metastases; however, the cumulative rate of colostomy was significantly less for mitomycin-based (10%) than cisplatin-based (19%) treatment. Severe hematological toxicity was indeed worse with mitomycin-based therapy [11,39]. This trial has been criticized for the induction cisplatin/5-FU portion, which prohibited direct comparison of radiation with cisplatin or mitomycin. It is not clear if the delay in initiating radiation therapy led to worse outcomes by prolonging duration of therapy by 56 days, especially if patients were unresponsive to this induction chemotherapy regimen [25].

Published only as an abstract at the American Society of Clinical Oncology (ASCO) conference in 2009, the U.K. Anal Cancer Trial (ACT II) is a phase 3 trial that evaluated whether replacing MMC (n = 471) with cisplatin (n = 469) improved CR rates and whether 2 cycles of maintenance chemotherapy or no additional therapy after CRT reduced recurrence. Grade 3 or greater hematological toxicity was higher with the use of mitomycin (25% with mitomycin compared to 13% with cisplatin). Neither the CR (95%), recurrence-free survival (RFS) (75% at 3 years), OS rates, nor colostomy requirements were different among groups. Maintenance chemotherapy did not improve outcomes. The authors concluded that 5-FU and MMC with radiation therapy (RT) remains the standard of care [26]. Therefore, cisplatin should be used only for selected patients in whom hematological toxicity may be truly significant, such as patients with HIV/AIDS-related complications or a history of complications (ie, malignancies, opportunistic infections). At this junction, because of the colostomy-free and overall survival benefit reported in the update of RTOG 98-11, it is recommended that MMC, and not cisplatin, be employed together with 5-FU as the preferred radiosensitizer for anal cancer.

Would the Patient Be Managed Differently if She Were HIV Positive?

Patients who are HIV positive can be treated safely and effectively with CRT for anal cancer. Hesitancy to administer CRT in patients who are HIV positive stems from toxicity, particularly lowered blood counts, or possible opportunistic infections during treatment, and a poorer ability to recover from treatment toxicity in the face of chronic immunosuppression.

With the use of highly active antiretroviral therapy (HAART), CRT (even if the CD4 count is less than 200/mL) may be given safely at conventional doses to patients who are HIV positive with comparable CR rates to patients who are HIV negative [27–29]. However, for patients with CD4 counts of 200/mL or less, increased morbidity may require prolonged treatment breaks [30]. In this population with low CD4 counts that is not on HAART, decreasing chemotherapy doses, not delivering mitomycin, or giving a lower dose treatment (30 Gy) may be considered [31].

In another study by Oehler-Janne et al. comparing patients who are HIV negative to those who are HIV positive, patients who are HIV positive were able to receive standard CRT with good CR rates and similar 5-year OS rates as patients who are HIV negative, but the major cause of death in patients who are HIV positive was anal cancer. Local control and long-term sphincter preservation remained problematic. Adherence to standard treatment was frequently jeopardized in patients who are HIV positive who were at risk of not obtaining the optimal treatment (longer RT duration, lower equivalent dose, and less mitomycin-based therapy). In addition, patients who are HIV positive required inguinal RT more often because of advanced disease, which can further contribute to toxicity [32].

In summary, the available data support the use of CRT in patients who are HIV positive. It appears that outcomes should be comparable in patients who are HIV positive to those who are HIV negative, but there is a chance of greater toxicity and relapse. IMRT may be well suited to this population of patients with the potential to reduce acute morbidities making CRT more tolerable.

It is favored that patients with HIV be managed with CRT incorporating IMRT, MMC, and 5-FU, if possible, on the basis of CD4 counts and performance status. HAART should also be initiated. If the patient has a borderline CD4 count of 200/mL or lesser, cisplatin may be considered to replace MMC, or reduced doses of chemotherapy can be used. Blood counts should be monitored weekly during CRT for all patients with a low threshold to suspect neutropenia, especially in a patient who is HIV positive.

What Final Radiation Dose Should Be Delivered to the Primary Tumor and Palpable Inguinal Node?

For this T1N2M0 anal cancer, if standard 3D-CRT is delivered, the final dose to the primary tumor should be 55 to 59 Gy and the positive lymph nodes should be boosted to 55 to 59 Gy as well, as per RTOG 98-11. If IMRT is used, as per RTOG 0529, with a dose-painted technique, the positive lymph node may receive a dose of 50.4 Gy in 30 fractions and the primary tumor should be treated to 54 Gy in 1.8 Gy per fraction. The RTOG 0529 paradigm is to be followed and treated with dose-painted IMRT (Figure 3.3.1). It is preferred for patients to be simulated supine as this is most reproducible with respect to pelvic tilt, presacral volumes, and inguinal volume alignment. Patients receive oral and IV contrast during simulation and a custom mold is created. A frog-legged position would be reasonable for this patient with involved inguinal lymph nodes. In vivo dose measurements (TLDs or diodes) are recommended to ensure accuracy of treatment to within 20% of the calculated dose. If the dose is below the prescription dose, bolus may need to be incorporated into the treatment plan, with a second in vivo dose measurement for verification.

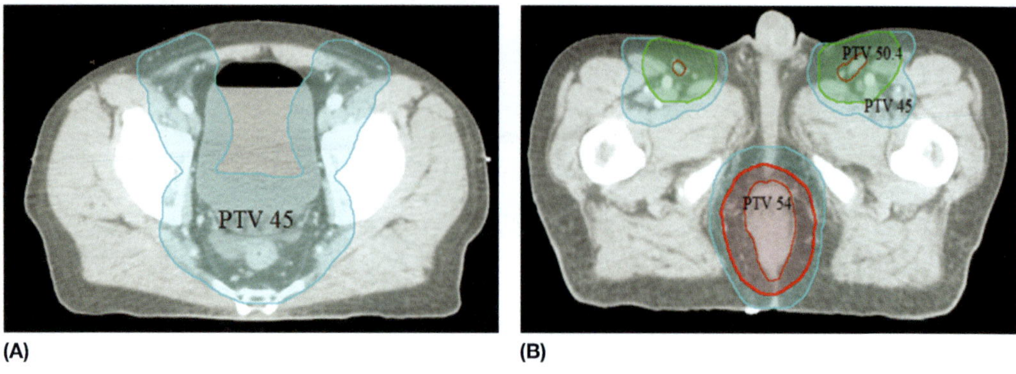

FIGURE 3.3.1 ■ Dose painted intensity modulated IMRT following RTOG 0529. Representative figures from target volumes and doses of a cT3N3M0 stage IIIB anal squamous cell carcinoma. The above figures demonstrate the Planning Target Volumes (PTVs). Figure 3.3.1A shows the PTV 45 (blue colorwash), treating all elective nodal volumes including inguinal, mesorectal, presacral, perirectal and internal/external iliac lymph nodes. Figure 3.3.1B shows the PTV 50.4 (green colorwash) which treats the involved bilateral inguinal nodal volumes. PTV 54 (red colorwash) treats the primary anal tumor volume. PTV 45 is also demonstrated (blue colorwash).

ACADEMIC COMMMENT

Karyn A. Goodman

Treatment for anal SCC is an example of the success of CRT in organ preservation. A woman with a cT1N2 stage anal cancer has an excellent chance of cure with concurrent chemotherapy and pelvic radiotherapy; however, the acute and late toxicities of therapy can be significant. In order to minimize the impact of therapy on long-term quality of life in our patients, I use many of the tools available in diagnostic imaging and treatment planning to better target pelvic radiotherapy, as well as post-treatment interventions to address potential late effects.

The work-up for this patient should include a baseline CT of the chest/abdomen/pelvis, routine laboratory tests, including a hemoglobin, given her history of bleeding. I also have all of our patients evaluated by a colorectal surgeon who performs a rigid proctoscopy or sigmoidoscopy and endorectal ultrasound to evaluate the size of the lesion and to identify any perirectal lymphadenopathy in order to refine our clinical staging of the patient. The surgeons are also involved in the close follow-up of these patients after therapy, so a baseline exam is essential for comparison with the posttreatment exams. I also routinely perform an FNA of any palpable inguinal lymphadenopathy to determine if the enlarged node(s) is reactive or has evidence of metastatic SCC because the sensitivity of clinical examination and CT imaging is poor and the involvement of inguinal nodes will impact on both treatment decisions and prognosis. While PET/CT is not standard for staging anal cancer, it can be very helpful for treatment planning purposes, improving the delineation of the primary tumor extent, and identifying potentially positive lymph nodes. However, the specificity of PET/CT is 83% and positive predictive value is only 43% for detecting metastatic inguinal nodes [6], so PET-positive inguinal nodes should be confirmed by FNA. I routinely perform a PET/CT simulation for patients who have not undergone a prior PET/CT scan.

Radiation treatment planning for anal cancer has evolved from standard 2-dimensional AP-PA or 3-dimensional 4-field plans that were described in the RTOG 98-11 trial [11,39], to conformal, anatomy-based plans delivered using IMRT. At Memorial Sloan-Kettering Cancer Center (MSKCC), I treat all patients, male and female, with anal cancer using IMRT to minimize the radiation dose to the normal tissues of the pelvis, particularly the small bowel, bladder, external genitalia, vagina for women, femoral heads, and pelvic bones. The RTOG 0529 study has nicely demonstrated a statistically significant reduction in grade 3 or higher acute GI and skin toxicity using IMRT as compared with the toxicity associated with conventional pelvic radiotherapy used in RTOG 98-11 [17,40]. To further reduce the dose to the bowel, our patients are treated with a full bladder and in the prone position. As we have initiated the use of IMRT planning for anal cancer, our GI and skin toxicities have been significantly less and we no longer have to give treatment breaks for these toxicities. However, we do still have treatment breaks related to hematologic toxicity from MMC. This typically occurs approximately 14 days after administration of MMC at 10 mg/m^2. Although the hematologic toxicity of MMC is considerable, the omission of MMC was associated with a significantly worse colostomy-free survival [33]. Moreover, the replacement of MMC by cisplatin has not been associated with any improvement in outcomes in 2 randomized trials [26,34] and may have been associated with an inferior colostomy rate in a third randomized trial [2]. Thus, although we had used an induction approach with cisplatin and 5-FU followed by concurrent MMC/5-FU/ pelvic radiation for patients with advanced anal cancers per the Cancer and Leukemia Group B (CALGB) phase 2 study for several years at MSKCC, when the results of the RTOG 98-11 study were reported, we returned to the standard chemotherapy regimen of 5-FU 1000 mg/m^2 continuous venous infusion with MMC 10 mg/m^2.

If this patient were HIV positive and had been on HAART such that her CD4 count was greater than 200/mL and her viral load was low or undetectable, I would treat her similarly to any patient with anal cancer, although we would be vigilant about following her counts to detect if she became neutropenic and would have a low threshold for using growth factors. However, if her HIV infection was not well controlled and/or her CD4 count was less than 200/mL, I would send her for a consultation with an infectious disease physician who specializes in the management of patients who are HIV positive to consider changing her medications. We would treat her with dose-reduced 5-FU, omitting MMC and possibly using cisplatin instead, per the AIDS Malignancy Consortium trial for patients with HIV-associated anal carcinoma, which is looking at the combination of cisplatin, 5-FU, and cetuximab with pelvic radiation [35].

The dose of radiation is stage dependent. At MSKCC, I treat the uninvolved elective pelvic and inguinal nodes to a dose of 45 Gy at 1.8 Gy per fraction, without a cone-down to the "true pelvis" after 30.6 Gy. With IMRT, the bowel can be spared more efficiently, as demonstrated by several dosimetric studies [12], and therefore the toxicity of taking the pelvic nodes to the full dose of 45 Gy has been relatively minimal. While the RTOG

0529 study used a lower dose per fraction (1.6 Gy) to the pelvic nodes for patients with early stage disease, I have kept a standard 1.8 Gy/fraction for all patients when treating the elective nodes. For this patient, with a T1 primary tumor, I would use an integrated boost to treat her primary tumor to a dose of 50 Gy in 2 Gy fractions. If her tumor had been 2 cm or larger, I would have boosted with an additional 6 Gy in 3 fractions. In patients with T1 primary tumors and involved inguinal nodes, I will often boost the inguinal nodes using an integrated boost at 2.12 Gy over 25 fractions to 53 Gy while treating the primary site to 50 Gy in 2 Gy fractions. If the primary is going to 56 Gy in 2 Gy fractions, I will take the involved node(s) to 56 Gy in 2 Gy fractions as well using the sequential boost of 6 Gy.

The patient would be followed closely with digital rectal exams, anoscopy, and proctoscopy/ EUS by me and a colorectal surgeon. A follow-up PET/CT is performed at 3 months posttreatment and then if the uptake has resolved, the patient is followed with an annual CT of the chest, abdomen, and pelvis. We also have all of our female patients counseled on the use of vaginal dilators and we are currently studying the compliance of women with the use of these dilators. We also recommend bone density scans and evaluation of vitamin D levels for women, particularly those who have preexisting osteoporosis. We recommend vitamin D and calcium supplementation for all patients to reduce the risk of radiation-induced sacral insufficiency fractures.

COMMUNITY PRACTITIONER COMMENT

Sameer Keole

Should a PET/CT or CT Be Ordered for Staging?

Our practice standard is to order a PET/CT scan for ACC staging and workup. While the role of CT in ACC is well established and is considered the standard of care, the role of PET scans is still unclear and has not been validated in a prospective trial [1]. It docs appear that PET scans, in conjunction with CT scans, will improve sensitivity for nodal disease, particularly in the groin [4]. This benefit may be more pronounced in patients who are HIV positive. Furthermore, PET scans may change management and radiation fields in a significant number of patients as well [2].

What Type of Pelvic Radiotherapy Should Be Accomplished—IMRT Versus 3-D Conformal Therapy?

3D-CRT is the current standard of care in ACC and has been shown to decrease toxicity while not compromising local control versus 2-D RT [36]. Despite this improvement, toxicities are still common and sometimes patients require a treatment break, which can compromise local control. IMRT has the promise of being able to deliver the same dose while minimizing toxicity. Several early series of IMRT for ACC have been reported with excellent results [13–16]. The RTOG 0529 trial was a phase 2 study that evaluated dose-painting IMRT in combination with 5-FU and MMC in hopes of decreasing acute toxicities while delivering RT for ACC. Perhaps the most important early report from this trial was that nearly 81% of the patient plans in this trial required revision during central review prior to delivery [17,40]. Our group's current standard is evolving, but in recent years, we have been using IMRT more often in the setting of ACC. We use the RTOG contouring atlas (available on-line at www.rtog.org) to help define nodal volumes. We recently used proton therapy for the treatment of a man with T2N0 ACC in an attempt to decrease acute toxicities. The use of proton therapy versus IMRT decreased small bowel dose by 60% and bladder dose by 40% while using the same target volumes. A phase 2 trial to further study the role of proton therapy in ACC is in the design process.

If the Patient Were an Older Male, Would IMRT Be Necessary?

Age, performance status, or comorbid conditions would not influence our choice of radiation therapy delivery. Given the emerging data and decreased toxicity, I would treat all patients with IMRT if allowable by insurance.

Should Radiation Be Given Concurrently With 5-FU and MMC or 5-FU and Cisplatin?

The question of MMC versus cisplatin is a dilemma facing many practitioners in the community setting. While RTOG 98-11 was designed to answer this question, its design of allowing induction chemotherapy for cisplatin, but not for MMC, makes the conclusions difficult to interpret [11,39]. In RTOG 98-11, higher locoregional recurrence rates (33% vs. 25%) and colostomy rates (19% vs. 10%) were seen in the cisplatin arm. But the question for many was whether or not the poor outcomes seen in the cisplatin arm were due to the drug itself or due to induction therapy. The recently published long-term results of RTOG 98-11 demonstrated that DFS and OS were statistically better for RT + 5-FU/MMC versus RT + 5-FU/cisplatin. This firmly establishes the standard of care chemotherapy as 5-FU/MMC. The ACT II trial, reported in an abstract only at the 2009 ASCO meeting, was a 2 x 2 randomization [26]. The first randomization was MMC versus cisplatin. The second randomization was a no-maintenance chemotherapy versus 2 cycles of 5-FU and cisplatin given post-CRT. In this trial, MMC and cisplatin were equivalent in terms of CR (94% MMC, 95% cisplatin at 3 years). The patients receiving cisplatin had a lower rate of grade 3 or higher hematologic toxicity (12% vs. 25%, $p < .001$). There was also no benefit from maintenance chemotherapy. In reviewing these 2 studies, it can be safely said that there is no role for either induction or maintenance chemotherapy in ACC and that any chemotherapy that is given should be done so in conjunction with RT. Substituting cisplatin for MMC is reasonable and probably well within the standard of care. At our institution, our multidisciplinary team still chooses to prescribe MMC in conjunction with 5-FU. Perhaps the next question will be the substitution of 5-FU for oral capecitabine. There is at least 1 reported study that demonstrates the feasibility of this approach [37]. At this time, however, it would be difficult to say that the substitution of capecitabine for 5-FU, in the setting of CRT for ACC, should be done routinely.

Would the Patient Be Managed Differently if She Were HIV Positive?

HIV status alone does not impact our management status. In the patient who is HIV positive, we carefully examine the patient's performance status and CD4 count, as early data found that these parameters may be correlated with the outcomes [13]. More modern series have shown that the CD4 count of a patient does not always correlate with either tolerance to treatment or end outcome [29,38]. Our current practice is to make sure that patients who are HIV positive are currently taking HAART and to include the patient's infectious disease and/or primary care team in his or her multidisciplinary management. Depending on the case, our group may have a lower threshold to use IMRT over 3D-CRT and cisplatin over MMC in a patient who is HIV positive.

Is It Necessary to Biopsy the Palpable Inguinal Lymph Node?

Owing to the discordance of imaging studies and the implications of a positive inguinal lymph node, we would biopsy in this setting. We have the luxury of having dedicated colorectal surgeons, interventional radiology, and a multidisciplinary GI tumor board to discuss such cases and the expertise to perform procedures, from simple to complex, in our hospital. In simple terms, an inguinal lymph node biopsy could be easily obtained and we would expect the morbidity to be low in experienced hands. Alternatively, if a lymph node is highly fluorodeoxyglucose (FDG)-avid and a biopsy cannot be obtained in a timely manner, I would typically treat the node definitively as long as normal tissue constraints could be obtained.

What Final Radiation Dose Should Be Delivered to the Primary Tumor and Palpable Inguinal Node?

Based on RTOG 0529 and RTOG 98-11, primary target volume (PTV) doses should be between 54 Gy and 59.4 Gy, positive lymph node volume doses should be between 50.4 Gy and 59.4 Gy (depending largely on size), and elective nodal irradiation to the remainder of the clinically negative pelvic lymph nodes should be between 45 Gy and 50.4 Gy. When using IMRT, we follow RTOG 0529 volume definitions but we do not use dose-painting. Rather, we give all fractions at 1.8 Gy and boost isolated areas as needed. For this patient, we would prescribe a minimum of 54 Gy to the primary target, 50.4 Gy to the positive lymph node plus margin, and 45 Gy to the remainder of the pelvic lymph nodes and left inguinal lymph nodes. Discretion is left to the attending physician to increase the dose and he or she may make the target doses slightly higher on the basis of the patient's tolerance to combined modality therapy. It is reasonable to make this decision a few weeks into therapy rather than committing to it up front.

SECTION EDITOR'S NOTE

Joseph M. Herman

All 3 opinions agree on the use of IMRT for the treatment of ACC, especially when inguinal lymph nodal coverage is necessary. While the total dose and dose per fraction may differ, the opinions are within the range of the standard of care. If IMRT is to be used (per RTOG 0529), I would favor PET/CT to ensure that all pelvic lymph nodes that appear suspicious are included in the final PTV. If there are any inguinal lymph nodes that are equivocal based on PET/CT, I would perform an FNA as it would result in a higher radiation dose to that region and greater risk of short- and long-term toxicity. Given the updated results of RTOG 98-11, the standard chemotherapy with radiation should be 5-FU and MMC, although 5-FU and cisplatin is reasonable in specific cases. A patient who is HIV positive should receive HAART medications and be treated per the standard of care unless the patient has a very low CD4 count, insufficient counts to receive MMC, and/or insufficient performance status to tolerate aggressive management. Patients should be monitored closely by a multidisciplinary team and receive necessary restaging per the NCCN guidelines. Women should be provided with a dilator and/or counseling regarding sexual activity following CRT. Older women should be counseled regarding risks of subsequent fractures and preventive measures.

REFERENCES

1. NCCN practice guidelines for anal cancer. 2011. www.nccn.org. Accessed July 1, 2011.
2. Winton E, Heriot AG, Ng M, et al. The impact of 18-fluorodeoxyglucose positron emission tomography on the staging, management and outcome of anal cancer. *Br J Cancer.* 2009;100:693–700.
3. Krengli M, Milia ME, Turri L, et al. FDG-PET/CT imaging for staging and target volume delineation in conformal radiotherapy of anal carcinoma. *Radiat Oncol.* 2010;5:10.
4. Cotter SE, Grigsby PW, Siegel BA, et al. FDG-PET/CT in the evaluation of anal carcinoma. *Int J Radiat Oncol Biol Phys.* 2006;65:720–725.
5. Trautmann TG, Zuger JH. Positron emission tomography for pretreatment staging and post-treatment evaluation in cancer of the anal canal. *Mol Imaging Biol.* 2005;7:309–313.
6. Mistrangelo M, Pelosi E, Bello M, et al. Comparison of positron emission tomography

scanning and sentinel node biopsy in the detection of inguinal node metastases in patients with anal cancer. *Int J Radiat Oncol Biol Phys.* 2010;77: 73–78.

7. Schwarz JK, Siegel BA, Dehdashti F, et al. Tumor response and survival predicted by post-therapy FDG-PET/CT in anal cancer. *Int J Radiat Oncol Biol Phys.* 2008;71:180–186.

8. Kidd EA, Dehdashti F, Siegel BA, Grigsby PW. Anal cancer maximum F-18 fluorodeoxyglucose uptake on positron emission tomography is correlated with prognosis. *Radiother Oncol.* 2010;95:288–291.

9. Ben-Josef E, Moughan J, Ajani JA, et al. Impact of overall treatment time on survival and local control in patients with anal cancer: A pooled data analysis of Radiation Therapy Oncology Group trials 87-04 and 98-11. *J Clin Oncol.* 2010 Dec 1;28:5061–5066.

10. Menkarios C, Azria D, Laliberte B, et al. Optimal organ-sparing intensity-modulated radiation therapy (IMRT) regimen for the treatment of locally advanced anal canal carcinoma: A comparison of conventional and IMRT plans. *Radiat Oncol.* 2007;2:41.

11. Ajani JA, Winter KA, Gunderson LL, et al. Fluorouracil, mitomycin, and radiotherapy vs fluorouracil, cisplatin, and radiotherapy for carcinoma of the anal canal: A randomized controlled trial. *JAMA.* 2008;299:1914–1921.

12. Milano MT, Jani AB, Farrey KJ, et al. Intensity-modulated radiation therapy (IMRT) in the treatment of anal cancer: Toxicity and clinical outcome. *Int J Radiat Oncol Biol Phys.* 2005;63:354–361.

13. Salama JK, Mell LK, Schomas DA, et al. Concurrent chemotherapy and intensity-modulated radiation therapy for anal canal cancer patients: A multicenter experience. *J Clin Oncol.* 2007;25:4581–4586.

14. Pepek JM, Willett CG, Wu QJ, et al. Intensity-modulated radiation therapy for anal malignancies: A preliminary toxicity and disease outcomes analysis. *Int J Radiat Oncol Biol Phys.* 2010 Dec 1;78:1413–1419.

15. Kachnic LA, Tsai HK, Coen JJ, et al. Dose-painted intensity-modulated radiation therapy for anal cancer: A multi-institutional report of acute toxicity and response to therapy. *Int J Radiat Oncol Biol Phys.* 2012 Jan 1;82(1): 153–158.

16. Bazan JG, Hara W, Hsu A, et al. Intensity-modulated radiation therapy versus conventional radiation therapy for squamous cell carcinoma of the anal canal. *Cancer.* 2011 Aug 1;117(15) 3342–3351.

17. Kachnic LA, Winter KA, Myerson R, et al. RTOG 0529: A phase II evaluation of dose-painted IMRT in combination with 5-fluorouracil and mitomycin-C for reduction of acute morbidity in carcinoma of the anal canal. In: *ASTRO.* Chicago, IL: International Journal of Radiation Oncology Biology Physics; 2009. p. S5.

18. Kachnic LA, Winter KA, Myerson R, et al. Early efficacy results of RTOG 0529: A phase II evaluation of dose-painted IMRT in combination with 5-Fluorouracil and mitomycin-C for the reduction of acute morbidity in carcinoma of the anal canal. In: *ASTRO.* San Diego, CA: International Journal of Radiation Oncology Biology Physics; 2010. p. S55.

19. Wright JL, Patil SM, Temple LK, et al. Squamous cell carcinoma of the anal canal: Patterns and predictors of failure and implications for intensity-modulated radiation treatment planning. *Int J Radiat Oncol Biol Phys.* 2010 Nov 15;78:1064–1072.

20. Das P, Bhatia S, Eng C, et al. Predictors and patterns of recurrence after definitive chemoradiation for anal cancer. *Int J Radiat Oncol Biol Phys.* 2007;68:794–800.

21. Martenson JA, Lipsitz SR, Wagner H Jr, et al. Initial results of a phase II trial of high dose radiation therapy, 5-fluorouracil, and cisplatin for patients with anal cancer (E4292): An Eastern Cooperative Oncology Group study. *Int J Radiat Oncol Biol Phys.* 1996;35:745–749.

22. Gerard JP, Ayzac L, Hun D, et al. Treatment of anal canal carcinoma with high dose radiation therapy and concomitant fluorouracil-cisplatinum. Long-term results in 95 patients. *Radiother Oncol.* 1998;46:249–256.

23. Peiffert D, Giovannini M, Ducreux M, et al. High-dose radiation therapy and neoadjuvant plus concomitant chemotherapy with 5-fluorouracil and cisplatin in patients with locally advanced squamous-cell anal canal cancer: Final results of a phase II study. *Ann Oncol.* 2001;12:397–404.

24. Hung A, Crane C, Delclos M, et al. Cisplatin-based combined modality therapy for anal carcinoma: A wider therapeutic index. *Cancer.* 2003;97:1195–202.

25. Abbas A, Yang G, Fakih M. Management of anal cancer in 2010. Part 2: Current treatment standards and future directions. *Oncology.* 2010 Apr 30;24:417–424.

26. James R, Wan S, Glynne-Jones R, et al. A randomized trial of chemoradiation using mitomycin or cisplatin, with or without maintenance cisplatin/5FU in squamous cell carcinoma of the anus (ACT II). In: *ASCO.* Chicago, IL: ASCO; 2009.

27. Blazy A, Hennequin C, Gornet JM, et al. Anal carcinomas in HIV-positive patients: High-dose chemoradiotherapy is feasible in the era of highly active antiretroviral therapy. *Dis Colon Rectum.* 2005;48:1176–1181.

28. Fraunholz I, Weiss C, Eberlein K, et al. Concurrent chemoradiotherapy with 5-fluorouracil and mitomycin C for invasive anal carcinoma in human immunodeficiency virus-positive patients receiving highly active antiretroviral therapy. *Int J Radiat Oncol Biol Phys.* 2010 Apr;76:1425–1432.

29. Seo Y, Kinsella MT, Reynolds HL, et al. Outcomes of chemoradiotherapy with 5-Fluorouracil and mitomycin C for anal cancer in immunocompetent versus immunodeficient patients. *Int J Radiat Oncol Biol Phys.* 2009;75:143–149.

30. Hoffman R, Welton ML, Klencke B, et al. The significance of pretreatment CD4 count on the outcome and treatment tolerance of HIV-positive patients with anal cancer. *Int J Radiat Oncol Biol Phys.* 1999;44:127–131.

31. Peddada AV, Smith DE, Rao AR, et al. Chemotherapy and low-dose radiotherapy in the treatment of HIV-infected patients with carcinoma of the anal canal. *Int J Radiat Oncol Biol Phys.* 1997;37:1101–1105.

32. Oehler-Janne C, Huguet F, Provencher S, et al. HIV-specific differences in outcome of squamous cell carcinoma of the anal canal: A multicentric cohort study of HIV-positive patients receiving highly active antiretroviral therapy. *J Clin Oncol.* 2008;26:2550–2257.

33. Flam M, John M, Pajak TF, et al. Role of mitomycin in combination with fluorouracil and radiotherapy, and of salvage chemoradiation in the definitive nonsurgical treatment of epidermoid carcinoma of the anal canal: Results of a phase III randomized intergroup study. *J Clin Oncol.* 1996;14:2527–2539.

34. Conroy T, Ducreux M, Lemanski C, et al. Treatment intensification by induction chemotherapy (ICT) and radiation dose escalation in locally advanced squamous cell anal canal carcinoma (LAAC): Definitive analysis of the intergroup ACCORD 03 trial (abstr 4035). *J Clin Oncol.* 2009;27(Suppl):15.

35. AIDS Consortium Trial. Retrieved from http://www.clinicaltrials.gov/ct2/show/NCT00324415?term=aids+consortium+anal+cancer&rank=4

36. Vuong T, Kopek N, Ducreut M, et al. Conformal therapy improves the therapeutic index of patients with anal canal cancer treated with combined chemotherapy and external beam radiotherapy. *Int J Radiat Oncol Biol Phys.* 2007;67(5):1394–1400.

37. Glynne-Jones R, Meadows H, Wan S, et al. EXTRA–a multicenter phase II study of chemoradiation using a 5 day per week oral regimen of capecitabine and intravenous mitomycin C in anal cancer. *Int J Radiat Oncol Biol Phys.* 2008;72(1):119–126.

38. Edelman S, Johnstone PA. Combined modality therapy for HIV-infected patients with squamous cell carcinoma of the anus: outcomes and toxicities. *Int J Radiat Oncol Biol Phys.* 2006;66(1):206–211.

39. Gunderson LL, Winter KA, Ajani JA, et al. Long-term update of US GI intergroup RTOG 98-11 phase III trial for anal carcinoma: Survival, relapse, and colostomy failure with concurrent chemoradiation involving fluorouracil/mitomycin versus fluorouracil/cisplatin. *J Clin Oncol.* 2012 Nov 13. [Epub ahead of print]

40. Kachnic LA, Winter K, Myerson RJ, et al. RTOG 0529: A phase 2 evaluation of dose-painted intensity modulated radiation therapy in combination with 5-fluorouracil and mitomycin-C for the reduction of acute morbidity in carcinoma of the anal canal. *Int J Radiat Oncol Biol Phys.* 2012 Nov 12. pii: S0360-3016(12)03601-2. doi: 10.1016/j.ijrobp.2012.09.023. [Epub ahead of print].

Section 4

▪ **GYNECOLOGIC** ▪

Section Editor: William Small, Jr.

Medically Inoperable Endometrial Cancer

CLINICAL PROBLEM

Obesity is becoming increasingly common in the United States. In addition, obesity is often associated with other medical conditions placing these obese patients at a higher risk of surgical complications. Endometrial cancer is often associated with obesity; so as the number of obese patients steadily increases, so too does the number of patients with endometrial cancer. Secondary to their medical comorbidities, obese patients with endometrial cancer are increasingly deemed medically inoperable. In addition, nonobese patients can also present with significant medical comorbidities. These so-called "medically inoperable" patients are an increasing patient population and often are referred to radiation oncology for definitive management.

CASE EXAMPLE

A 350 lb, 4'10", 52-year-old female presents with vaginal bleeding with a biopsy positive for grade 1 endometrioid adenocarcinoma. The patient's medical history is significant for hypertension (HTN) and diabetes mellitus (DM). The patient's general gynecologist considers her medically inoperable and refers her to radiation oncology for definitive therapy.

Management Decisions

- Should the patient be referred to a gynecologic oncologist?
- Should there be a consideration for hormonal therapy?
- If radiotherapy is delivered, should external beam radiation therapy (EBRT) be utilized?
- What type of boost—intensity-modulated radiation therapy (IMRT) versus brachytherapy—should be given?
- If brachytherapy is chosen, how would you deliver it?

MAJOR OPINION

Jessica Hunn and David K. Gaffney

Management

A number of different physician specialties encounter women with benign and malignant tumors of the endometrium. Physicians with specific training and the greatest expertise in the management of these conditions are the gynecologic oncologists. Current practice guidelines recommend that patients diagnosed with endometrial cancer be referred to a gynecologic oncologist for preoperative consultation and treatment. The American Congress of Obstetrics and Gynecology especially recommends that a consultation is particularly beneficial in cases where nonoperative therapy is contemplated [1]. A number of retrospective reviews document superior outcomes for endometrial cancer and reduced use of adjuvant therapy if the surgeon is a gynecologic oncologist [2].

In the normal menstrual cycle, steroid hormones control the cyclic changes in the endometrium. Estrogen drives proliferation of the endometrial glandular epithelium and progesterone counteracts the effects of estrogen [3]. A gain of estrogen, or a loss of progesterone, can cause a loss of equilibrium and stimulate oncogenesis [3]. Endometrial carcinoma has long been associated with the presence of excessive or unopposed estrogen [4]. It has been known for many decades that large doses of estrogen induce endometrial hyperplasia and carcinomatous alterations in animals [4]. More recent studies corroborated the unopposed estrogen hypothesis, showing that exposure to exogenous estrogens, not opposed by progesterone, leads to endometrial hyperplasia and a malignant phenotype [5–7]. Tumors arising in conditions of elevated estrogen are classified as type 1 and typically characterized by low-grade endometrioid histology. In addition, these malignancies are usually found to have positive hormone receptor status [8]. Type 1 tumors represent 70% to 80% of endometrial cancers and patients in an early stage have a good prognosis [3,9]. On the other hand, type 2 endometrial cancers are typically not estrogen driven, are high grade, and are hormone receptor negative [8]. Type 2 tumors are generally more aggressive and have papillary serous or clear cell morphology. They are typically not hormone responsive and outcomes are generally poor with frequent recurrences [3,9].

Immunohistochemical analyses of these tumors have shown expression of estrogen receptors (ER) and progesterone receptors (PR) in low-grade, early stage endometrial cancers [10–12]. Receptor concentrations may be an indication of hormone responsiveness [10,13]. During the progression of endometrial cancer, the expression of PR often decreases [14]. Studies have also shown that progestins have an effect on tumor integrity in endometrial cancer by inhibiting estrogen-induced suppression of cell-to-cell aggregation of well-differentiated endometrial cancer cells [14].

Overall Treatment

The primary treatment for patients diagnosed with endometrial adenocarcinoma is a staging laparotomy/laparoscopy, total abdominal hysterectomy, bilateral salpingo-oophorectomy (BSO), and lymphadenectomy, depending on the pathological risk profile [15,16]. In some cases, however, surgery is not recommended because of poor medical conditions and potentially unacceptable morbidity and mortality, so alternate treatment strategies must be considered [17]. Perioperative risk assessment serves as a basis for appropriate patient counseling of the risks and benefits of the available treatment options [1]. Severe or fatal perioperative complications have been observed in patients with comorbid conditions such as marked obesity, DM, HTN, and cardiopulmonary dysfunction [18]. Patients

diagnosed with type 1 endometrial cancer often have such risk factors.

Progesterone has long been used in hormone-based therapies for endometrial carcinomas [3]. Oral, parenteral, or intrauterine device (IUD) deliveries of progestins have been successful [19–22]. Most of the literature and outcomes are based on women who wish to preserve fertility and while this approach is not standard, hormonal treatment is supported by isolated reports describing successful treatment with progestin alone [23]. From these data, possible success in women who have early cancers, but are not appropriate surgical candidates, can be extrapolated.

In 1962, one of the first successful uses of progestin as a treatment modality was in advanced or recurrent endometrial cancer [24]. Later, Podratz et al. found that progestational agents induced an objective response in 11% of 155 patients with advanced primary or recurrent endometrial cancer. The response rates decreased with decreasing tumor differentiation and survival was highly dependent on the degree of tumor differentiation [25]. Approximately 70% of endometrial carcinomas change their morphologic appearance in response to progesterone therapy because of the PR on the surfaces of the endometrial cancer cells [26]. In a review of the literature, the cumulative clinical response rate to progestin therapy was 72% in PR-positive tumors and 12% for PR-negative tumors [12].

One of the most important considerations for primary hormonal treatment of endometrial cancer is patient selection. The first criterion for hormonal treatment is an accurate diagnosis of a well-differentiated endometrial carcinoma by an expert pathologist [27]. Other criteria proposed include: well-differentiated carcinoma; no deep invasion of the myometrium visible on an MRI; absence of suspicious pelvic and para-aortic lymph nodes; absence of synchronous ovarian tumor; no contraindications for medical treatment; understanding, acceptance, and informed consent from the patient that this is not standard treatment; and that the patient will be compliant with follow-up [28].

Outcome data have been pooled from small studies over the past 4 decades. A review of the literature through 2007 showed a cumulative 76% complete response (CR) or partial response (PR) for patients treated with hormones, and the other 24% did not respond to treatment or had no response (NR). Of those who initially responded, 66% did not have a recurrence of the disease and

34% had a relapse. There have been 4 published deaths with conservative management [28]. The average response time is 12 weeks with an average duration of hormonal therapy of 6 months. The mean relapse time for recurrence was 20 months and the majority of patients underwent standard surgical therapy at the time of recurrence [28].

In addition to the lack of randomized control trials assessing the efficacy and feasibility of hormonal treatment for endometrial cancer, there is also a lack of consistent treatment. Most of the conservative treatment was either medroxyprogesterone acetate (MPA) or megestrol acetate [16]. A variety of other progestins were used in small patient groups, mostly before the 1980s. A multicenter phase 2 study with MPA as treatment for endometrial carcinoma and atypical hyperplasia found a 67% overall CR (55% of patients had endometrial cancer and 82% had atypical hyperplasia) [29]. The patients were given a daily oral dose of 600 mg of MPA with a low dose of aspirin. The treatment continued for 26 weeks with the primary end point being a pathologic CR.

More recently, the use of the progesterone IUD has been evaluated as a potential treatment modality. One of the advantages is the lower systemic progesterone for women who cannot tolerate the adverse affects of oral progestins. Progestasert, a progesterone-containing IUD, was evaluated in the primary treatment of early endometrial cancer in the United Kingdom [19]. The results showed a CR in 6 out of 8 women (75%) at the end of 12 months. However, a report of 4 cases of the Mirena, a levonorgestrel IUD, showed only a 25% response rate [30]. These are small studies and further investigation is needed to truly evaluate the safety of the progesterone/progestin IUD in the treatment of early endometrial cancer.

In addition to hormone treatment alone, some groups are evaluating the hysteroscopic resection of tumor in conjunction with hormone treatment. A hysteroscopy is generally a much less morbid surgical procedure and poor operative candidates may tolerate this better than the more extensive standard surgery. In a 2011 pilot study, combined operative hysteroscopy and progestin therapy showed only 1 recurrence in the 14 patients with early endometrial cancer [15].

Because of the concerns of failure of treatment and the substantial rates of recurrence with hormonal therapy, close surveillance and follow-up is required [23,31]. If this is not feasible or the patient is unreliable, then the patient is not a good candidate for hormone treatment. Recurrence may approach 50% and therefore histologic monitoring is a vital aspect of surveillance [20]. Following therapy, patients should undergo serial complete uterine evaluation approximately every 3 months to document response [1]. Furthermore, many women who begin with hormonal treatment ultimately need definitive treatment with surgery or radiation. If comorbidities preclude surgery, the radiotherapeutic options for definitive treatment need to be addressed.

Radiation Therapy

As discussed earlier, hormonal management works most effectively in low-grade tumors, and in select cases, hormonal management alone could be the preferred option. Radiotherapy is an appropriate option for medically inoperable patients with cancer of the uterus. Inoperability of uterine cancer is most appropriately determined by a gynecologic oncologist. Uterine cancer is a disease largely among the elderly and the survival rates of the general population are increasing in the United States. Correspondingly, medical comorbidities are an increasing problem in the endometrial cancer population. Obesity is becoming more common in this patient population, and consequently, there can be substantial morbidity associated with hysterectomy. Also, many, if not most, patients with comorbid conditions will die of intercurrent disease and not secondary to endometrial carcinoma. Conditions most frequently resulting in medical inoperability include HTN, DM, coronary artery disease, stroke, pulmonary disease, and hyperlipidemia.

There are a number of prognostic features that can be utilized to appropriately select patients for brachytherapy or external beam radiotherapy plus brachytherapy. Brachytherapy alone is most successful in clinical stage I and low-to-intermediate grade tumors. Nevertheless, brachytherapy alone has been utilized in grade 3 endometrioid histologies, as well as clear cell and uterine papillary serous cancers. For grade 3 tumors, adverse histologies, or stage II disease, in most cases a combination of external beam radiotherapy and brachytherapy is recommended.

Radiotherapy has been used extensively in the treatment of medically inoperable patients with endometrial cancer. A review of the modern literature is performed and presented in Table 4.1.1 and shows 5-year disease-free survival ranging from 80% to 88% and 5-year overall survival

TABLE 4.1.1 ■ *Radiotherapy in Medically Inoperable Endometrial Cancer*

| AUTHOR | INSTITUTION | N | % EBRT AND B | OS (%) | | | DSS (%) | | | LATE TOXICITY (%) | LF (%) | RF (%) | DF (%) | ICBT DOSE |
				2–3 YEAR	5 YEAR	10 YEAR	2–3 YEAR	5 YEAR	10 YEAR					
Wegner et al. [39]	University of Pittsburgh	26	73	28			73			8	8	0		7 × 5 Gy HDR
Shenfield et al. [38]	University of Alberta	44	0		60	24		88	80	11	9	0	2	30 × 2 Gy LDR
Coon et al. [37]	University of Pittsburgh	49	71	83	42		93	87		8	6	0	4	7 × 5 Gy HDR
Niazi et al. [36]	McGill University	38	21						78[†]	12	16		14	8 × 3 Gy HDR
Kucera et al. [35]	University of Vienna	228	0		60	30		85	75	4.6	17.5	1.3	2.2	8.5 × 4 Gy HDR
Nguyen and Petereit [34]	University of Wisconsin	36	100	65			85			21	12	3	6	7 × 5 Gy HDR
Fishman et al. [33]	Yale University	54	28		30/24*			80/85*		26[¶]				7058 mghr Ra eq
Chao et al. [32]	Washington University	101	75		66	38		84	82	5		10[‡]	13	

* indicates stage I/II.

[†] indicates 15 year rate.

[¶] includes diarrhea that responded to conservative outpatient management.

[‡] indicates total pelvic failures.

B, brachytherapy; DF, distant failure; DSS, disease-specific survival; EBRT, external beam radiation therapy; HDR, high-dose rate; ICBT, intracavitary brachytherapy; LDR, low-dose rate; LF, local failure; mghr Ra eq, milligram hour Radium equivalents; RF, regional failure; OS, overall survival.

Site specific failure rates are total, crude failure rates for LF, RF, and DF.

ranging from 24% to 66% [32–39]. Adverse features for relapse include increasing stage and grade, size of the uterus, and increasing age. As seen in Table 4.1.1, in patients with inoperable endometrial cancer, intercurrent disease far outpaces endometrial cancer as the most significant cause of death.

A variety of brachytherapy techniques have been employed, from low-dose rate intracavitary procedures such as Heyman capsules alone, tandem and ovoids, tandem and ring, tandem and cylinder, or various combinations. Also, low-dose-rate (LDR), pulse-dose-rate (PDR), and high-dose-rate (HDR) brachytherapy have been used either alone or in combination with external beam. A number of intrauterine-specific applicators have been developed, and the American Brachytherapy Society (ABS) specifically recommends dedicated IUDs for the treatment of these patients [40]. The ABS also recommends 3-D imaging to determine endometrial thickness and has made specific recommendations regarding dose fractionation. MRI can be particularly helpful in identifying the specific tumor site. In one series where MRI was used for tumor identification in stage I cases, the survival rate was 100% [36]. A particular advantage of brachytherapy alone in select patients is the reduced number of fractions or treatment visits required. The uterine cavity is well suited for brachytherapy applications and brachytherapy eliminates concerns regarding organ motion. In addition, given the inverse square law, very high doses can be delivered to the endometrial lining with brachytherapy, which would be difficult-to-impossible to reproduce with external beam approaches while maintaining safe doses to organs at risk.

As seen in Table 4.1.1, local control can be achieved in 81% to 91% of cases. Disease-specific survival has ranged from 80% to 88% and 75% to 82% at 5 and 10 years, respectively. Regional failure rates have been reported to be low (0–3%) and distant rates of failure have ranged from 2% to 14%. Patients with inoperable endometrial cancer are at high risk for perioperative complications and several series have recommended HDR over LDR to decrease the time required to lie supine in a hospital bed. For example, Shenfield et al. documented a high rate of pulmonary emboli in patients undergoing LDR brachytherapy [38]. Secondary to this, Nguyen et al. and Nag et al. have recommended that brachytherapy for this indication be performed in hospital-based settings where anesthesia, radiology, and other services are widely available [34,40].

In summary, patients with inoperable uterine cancer should have a consultation with a gynecologic oncologist. In select patients with grade 1 disease, hormonal therapy may be an option. Radiotherapy has a long history in the treatment of medically inoperable patients, and outcomes generally range from good to excellent. The major cause of death in this population is intercurrent disease. For this patient, imaging with MRI is advocated. T2-weighted images nicely show uterine tumors. If there is clearly a greater than 50% penetration of the myometrium, she would be treated with external beam and HDR brachytherapy. If the lesion penetration is less than 50% of the myometrium, HDR brachytherapy alone would be advocated.

ACADEMIC COMMENT

Kristin A. Bradley

Clinical Problem 1—Obesity and "Medically Inoperable" Endometrial Cancer

Endometrial cancer is the most common gynecologic malignancy, with an estimated incidence of 46,470 new cases in the United States in 2011 [41]. The incidence is rising as obesity, a risk factor for developing endometrial cancer, continues to increase. Fortunately, the majority of patients are diagnosed with early-stage disease after presenting with postmenopausal bleeding. The standard of care for early-stage uterine cancer is a surgical approach with hysterectomy and BSO. The role of surgical nodal staging is a topic of current debate and investigation, but in the United States it is most commonly performed at the time of hysterectomy. Owing to the rise of obesity, radiation oncologists are increasingly seeing patients considered poor surgical candidates, or deemed "medically inoperable." Patients who are obese often have other medical comorbidities, including DM, HTN, heart disease, and lung disease, which increase the operative risk and put them at an increased risk for perioperative mortality and morbidity.

In this difficult gynecologic case, the scenario of a 52-year-old female who is 4'10" and 350 lb (BMI 73—morbidly obese) with a diagnosis of "medically inoperable" endometrial cancer, grade 1 is considered. She has HTN and diabetes, and her general gynecologist refers her for definitive radiation therapy. In discussing this case, there are several questions to consider.

Should the Patient Be Referred to a Gynecologic Oncologist?

In the United States, surgery for endometrial cancer is performed by either gynecologic oncologists or by general gynecologists, sometimes with the assistance of general surgeons for the surgical nodal assessment. The decision about referral to a gynecologic oncologist may be made on accessibility and availability of a subspecialty surgeon, patient preference, the general gynecologist's experience and skill, the patient's risk level, and other factors. In this case and others that are similar, it is important that a gynecologic oncologist evaluate the patient prior to labeling the patient as "medically inoperable." The gynecologic oncologist may have more experience operating on patients who are obese/morbidly obese, and may have the added support of anesthesia and other medical teams experienced in managing the increased complications that can be encountered while taking care of these patients in the perioperative period. In a study evaluating whether oncologic specialization influences outcomes following surgery for early-stage endometrial cancer, it was found that primary surgical treatment by a gynecologic oncologist compared to that by a general gynecologist improved disease-free survival (DFS) [42]. This was despite significantly worse pathologic tumor characteristics and lesser use of adjuvant radiation therapy in the patients seen by gynecologic oncologists. In addition, higher rates of complete surgical staging are achieved when a gynecologic oncologist is involved in the management of patients with endometrial cancer [42,43].

Should There Be Consideration for Hormonal Therapy?

Conservative management with progestin therapy in young, premenopausal women diagnosed with early-stage endometrial cancer is being investigated with the goal of delaying definitive surgery for fertility sparing [44,45]. Outside of this unique patient population, the use of adjuvant progestin therapy also has been advocated to reduce the risk of recurrence following surgery for endometrial cancer. A Cochrane meta-analysis that included over 4,500 women found no significant difference in the risk of death from endometrial cancer at 5 years with the use of progestin therapy [46]. In our institution's management of patients with "medically inoperable" endometrial cancer, we may use progestin-based hormone therapy to help control heavy vaginal bleeding prior to definitive therapy, but do not consider it as a substitute for surgery or radiation therapy.

If Radiotherapy Is Delivered, Should External Beam Radiotherapy Be Utilized? What Type of Boost—IMRT Versus Brachytherapy? How to Deliver the Brachytherapy?

Despite standard consultation with a gynecologic oncologist at our institution, I increasingly am being asked to consider patients for definitive radiation therapy for "medically inoperable" endometrial cancer. Most commonly, the concerns of the gynecologic oncologist are related to comorbid conditions rather than relating solely to the patient's obesity. In the scenario of inoperable endometrial cancer, different approaches to radiation management have been employed and reported, including LDR brachytherapy with or without pelvic radiation [47], pelvic EBRT with HDR brachytherapy [36,37,39], and HDR brachytherapy alone [34–36,38,48].

At our institution, if a patient is being considered for definitive radiation therapy, we consider individual patient and disease characteristics to decide whether to treat with brachytherapy alone or EBRT plus brachytherapy. For patients with tumor factors that increase the risk for extrauterine spread, such as outer ½ myometrial invasion identified on imaging, grade 3 tumors, or clinical stage II disease, we use a combination of EBRT (typically a 45 Gy dose) followed by consolidative HDR brachytherapy (20–25 Gy in 5 fractions). We have used brachytherapy alone (45 Gy in 5 fractions) for patients without these risk factors, or for patients considered poor candidates to receive EBRT owing to concerns about tolerability. Although EBRT may improve the outcome by addressing microscopic extrauterine disease, pelvic radiation therapy increases the toxicity profile of the radiation therapy [49]. Therefore, we have treated the majority of our clinical stage I patients with brachytherapy alone.

It is difficult to compare control rates and outcomes achieved by using brachytherapy alone to outcomes with EBRT plus brachytherapy because of the heterogeneity of radiation techniques used, the mix of both techniques in several of the reports, the inclusion of only stage I patients in some reports and stage I–II in others, the variability in reported follow-up and disease control rates, and the different techniques used to follow patients for recurrence after therapy. In general, however, single-institution series report cancer-specific outcomes [cause-specific survival (CSS), disease-specific survival (DSS), and disease-free survival (DFS)] of 70% to 85% at 5 years [34–38,47–49]. Owing to comorbidities with competing causes for death, overall survival rates are considerably lower in this patient population.

Different techniques for delivering the primary or consolidative brachytherapy have been used and reported. In 2000, the ABS published their recommendations for HDR brachytherapy for carcinoma of the endometrium, and provided suggested HDR fractionation and dose schedules with and without the use of pelvic EBRT [50]. The ABS guidelines recommend performing the procedure under spinal or conscious sedation anesthesia, or with some type of adequate analgesia. Use of tandem and ovoids, tandem and cylinders, tandem and ring, Rotte "Y" applicator, or Bauer endometrial applicator is endorsed by the ABS guidelines. Dual tandem applicators, such as the Rotte "Y" applicator, have the advantage of being able to provide better dosimetric coverage to the fundus in patients with larger uterine width. In addition to a variety of applicators, different approaches to dose prescription and fractionation have been used. The treatment should be "target-based" with the use of image guidance that may include ultrasound, orthogonal radiographs, CT, or MRI, depending on the availability of these resources and the patient's tolerance. In general, the target volume is the entire uterus, cervix, and upper vagina, with dose prescription most commonly reported at 2 cm from the central axis at the midpoint along the uterine applicator. Varying frequencies of brachytherapy application have been employed, ranging from twice-daily fractionation to 1-week intervals between treatments.

In "medically inoperable" patients who are unable to undergo brachytherapy procedures, EBRT alone may be considered, either in a palliative role or for definitive treatment. In my experience, patients who are considered to be too poor candidates for either surgery or brachytherapy may be best treated with a palliative intent if they have uterine bleeding that is bothersome or results in symptomatic anemia. Typically in this scenario, 30 to 37.5 Gy in 10 to 15 fractions is delivered. Although IMRT may be considered to escalate dose while respecting normal tissue tolerances, brachytherapy should be used instead of IMRT whenever possible. IMRT in these patients can be particularly challenging for a variety of reasons, including inability to fit through the CT bore, inability to see external contours in the planning system because of patient's size and the CT's limited field of view, difficulty in verifying positioning accuracy on a daily basis, and internal motion management challenges.

COMMUNITY PRACTITIONER COMMENT

Christian Hyde

Obesity is a major risk factor for endometrial cancer and is also a practical impediment to its treatment. The adipocytes produce estrogens that act as active promoters of cancer cell growth and development, but obesity also causes many other problems that preclude safe anesthesia, surgical intervention, and radiation therapy. For example, with intubation for general anesthesia, morbid obesity can alter the throat anatomy, making the angles of the intubation more difficult, requiring higher ventilation pressures to expand the chest, and the thickened neck makes emergency tracheostomy even riskier. Greater adipose tissue deposits can lead to third spacing of IV fluids and act as a storage reservoir for anesthetic gases, altering usual pharmacokinetics. For pelvic surgery, obesity increases the effective depth and narrowness of the pelvis and thus makes it more difficult to safely reach the uterus and associated vessels. Laparoscopic surgery may require longer instruments to traverse the abdominal fat, and higher CO_2 inflation pressures may be needed to inflate the abdomen of a patient who is morbidly obese.

EBRT typically relies on surface skin tattoos that are surrogates of internal anatomy (within a centimeter or so) in lean patients. However in obese patients, the larger distance between the skin and internal bony anatomy can lead to major anatomic shifts and geographic misses in delivery of EBRT. Obesity can also make it more difficult to visualize the cervix on a physical exam, requiring a longer speculum and more difficult angles for cannulation of the cervix to make the initial cancer biopsy, or to deliver brachytherapy.

In this clinical case, a 52-year-old female weighs 350 lb and is 4'10" tall. She presents with vaginal bleeding and a biopsy reveals grade 1 endometrioid adenocarcinoma. She has HTN and

DM. The community-based general gynecologist considers her medically inoperable and refers her to radiation oncology for definitive therapy.

This patient's grade 1 endometrioid adenocarcinoma would typically carry an excellent cure rate and not represent a major clinical problem, but because of her morbid obesity she is considered medically inoperable. Obesity is not the only reason a patient may be medically inoperable; other complicating factors may include the need for chronic anticoagulation due to recent deep venous thrombosis or pulmonary embolism, high risk coronary artery disease, oxygen dependence, multiple strokes, or chronic obstructive pulmonary disease (COPD). This particular patient raises multiple challenges regarding safe and practical radiation oncology in the obese patient.

Workup and Staging

Prior to starting radiation therapy, the patient should consult with a gynecologic oncologist to see whether the patient can be rendered operable. It would also be wise to obtain a full clinical staging to understand the extent of the patient's malignancy, so that all areas involved with the tumor will receive adequate surgery or radiation dose. Modification of scans may be required; for example, transpelvic ultrasound may not scan deeply enough, but transvaginal ultrasound would approach the tumor more directly. Similarly, an MRI may not be a practical option if the girth is too wide for the bore of the magnet, or she is too heavy for the MRI table's weight limit (typically 300–350 lb). However, if she were within the table weight limit, then an endorectal or endovaginal MRI coil may provide a closer view than the conventional pelvic MRI coil, similar to how endorectal MRI is commonly used for rectal and prostate cancer staging. CT staging may be less useful because of the typical table limits of 300 to 350 lb. The presence of DM may limit the use of intravenous iodine contrast; if on metformin she may need her metformin held, and IV hydration may need to be administered to protect against nephrotoxicity.

Hormonal Therapy

Hormonal therapy could be considered as definitive monotherapy although many patients eventually progress despite progestins, and therefore it could be considered for a second-line approach or palliation in case definitive radiation therapy fails. Unfortunately, the question of antihormonal therapy concurrently with definitive radiation has not been extensively investigated in endometrial cancer. If one were to extrapolate from prostate cancer, there may be a theoretical synergy between concurrent antihormonal therapies, but these inoperable cases occur too rarely for a large clinical trial.

EBRT Planning

If radiotherapy were to be utilized for definitive treatment, the patient would first need a simulation. These are usually performed on CT scanners and, therefore, may be limited by CT scanner table limits. Current linear accelerators have table limits in similar ranges, about 300 to 400 lb. Another limitation in simulating obese patients is that their surface anatomy is often not visible within the standard 50 cm displayed field of view obtainable by the CT machine. These patients often undergo 2 CT scans: one to show the thickness from the left hip skin to the bony pelvis, and the other from the right hip skin to the bony pelvis. The 2 images are then fused to produce a composite for which the skin-surface-distance (SSD) can be calculated, as this determines how much radiation must be given to overcome the attenuation through the tissue. IMRT, in particular, depends on exacting calculations and may be impractical for this patient in whom a considerable variation in set-up would be expected. Three-dimensional conformal radiation therapy to the pelvis can be given with some sparing of the bladder and rectum, albeit not as complete as would be available with IMRT.

One could overcome the daily shifting surface anatomy by using image-guided radiation therapy (IGRT), typically with daily kilovoltage x-rays used to localize the bony pelvis rather than relying solely on skin surface marks such as tattoos. An initial dose of 4500 cGy in 25 fractions of 180 cGy each could be administered using 3-D-conformal radiation therapy targeted to the vagina, uterus, and pelvic lymph nodes. If the patient were found to be a grade 1 or 2 and stage I with no visible extension beyond the endometrium, then treatment could consist of definitive brachytherapy without EBRT.

Brachytherapy

Many patients who are treated after total abdominal hysterectomy (TAH) and BSO will undergo adjuvant vaginal cuff brachytherapy, typically treating the top few centimeters of the vagina with a vaginal cylinder containing a temporary HDR iridium 192 radioactive seed. A similar approach in a tandem-plus-cylinder arrangement can be used for definitive brachytherapy in a patient who is morbidly obese. It consists of 1 or 2 central uterine tandems that carry the radioactive seed into the cornu of the endometrium and treat its entire length, integrated with a cylinder-shaped device to treat the upper 2 to 3 cm of the vagina. Definitive brachytherapy doses could consist of 5 Gy in 5 insertions to 5 mm depth from the vaginal surface, while simultaneously giving 7.3 Gy in 5 insertions via the uterine tandems. Using definitive HDR brachytherapy alone, Kucera et al. treated 228 patients with stage I primary inoperable endometrial cancer, achieving a 60% 5-year overall survival with only a 5% complication rate and 17.5% recurrence rate [34].

Most radiation departments have round-ended vaginal cuff cylinders for postoperative therapy, but not necessarily a tandem-and-cylinder arrangement. A more commonly employed set-up is a tandem and ring, which is frequently used for definitive HDR brachytherapy of cervical cancer. The tandem irradiates the endometrium centrally while the ring treats the cervix and proximal vagina. The ring treats only the uppermost 1 to 2 cm or so of the vagina, and so would not be appropriate in the presence of visible or likely vaginal spread, such as with papillary serous cancers of the endometrium, which have a higher propensity for drop metastases into the lower vagina.

For patients at higher risk of lymph node spread, bulky endometrial tumor, or cervical extension, external beam irradiation should precede brachytherapy in a fashion similar to that employed for definitive irradiation of cervical cancer. After 4500 cGy external beam, four insertions of 500 cGy HDR brachytherapy could be given for approximately 7500 cGy effective total dose, or higher, depending on tumor size. The vaginal epithelium can typically tolerate 100 Gy and the endometrium in excess of 100 Gy, as is commonly delivered during cervical cancer irradiation. The thickness of the myometrium acts as an internal buffer to displace the adjacent bowel and bladder. The main side effects for the patient may include vaginal stenosis, bladder and bowel frequency, and a 5% risk of chronic hematuria and/or hematochezia.

Practical Considerations for Planning and Treatment

Three-dimensional calculations of the doses for the rectum and bladder can be obtained by performing a CT simulation on the patient prior to each delivery of brachytherapy and then using 3-D planning computer software. However, if the patient were too obese for CT scan table limits, physics planning can be performed using traditional diagnostic x-ray equipment. Doses to the bladder and rectum can be calculated using a Foley catheter filled with iodine contrast and a rectal tube filled with metal marker BBs. Definitive radiation therapy can be delivered without general anesthesia, but typically 1 to 2 mg of Ativan and 2 hydrocodone/acetaminophen tablets are helpful to improve patient comfort during cannulation of the tandem(s) into the cervix. At the time of initial cannulation, placement of an endocervical plastic sleeve may facilitate the subsequent insertions and help protect against uterine perforation by the relatively narrow HDR tandem, if a single tandem is to be used. However, the advantage of dual tandems is the creation of a Y-shaped dose distribution that more closely follows the endometrial surface, ending in each cornu, and delivering more conformal dose to the tumor.

Patient Follow-Up

After delivery of definitive treatment, the patient should be followed up on a regular basis, with particular attention to return of any vaginal bleeding or discharge, which may indicate a recurrence. Periodic imaging to document initial tumor control, and perhaps annually thereafter, may be considered but in the absence of symptoms can be relatively low yield and of low practical value in the surgically unsalvageable patient. Progestin therapy should be considered if the cancer recurs, but data are lacking to support its use in the adjuvant setting.

SECTION EDITOR'S NOTE

William Small, Jr.

In general, I agree with the authors' approaches. I would obtain a gynecologic oncologist's opinion to confirm true medical unresectability. If this is conformed, if possible, I would obtain a pelvic MRI. Based on these findings, I would deliver definitive radiotherapy with brachytherapy, usually preceeded by EBRT.

REFERENCES

1. American College of Obstetricians and Gynecologists. ACOG practice bulletin, clinical management guidelines for obstetrician-gynecologists, number 65, August 2005: Management of endometrial cancer. *Obstet Gynecol.* 2005 Aug;106(2): 413–425.

2. Macdonald OK, Sause WT, Lee RJ, et al. Adjuvant radiotherapy and survival outcomes in early-stage endometrial cancer: A multi-institutional analysis of 608 women. *Gynecol Oncol.* 2006 Nov;103(2):661–666.

3. Yang S, Thiel KW, Leslie KK. Progesterone: The ultimate endometrial tumor suppressor. *Trends Endocrinol Metab.* 2011 Apr;22(4):145–152.

4. Kelley RM, Baker WH. The role of progesterone in human endometrial cancer. *Cancer Res.* 1965 Aug;25(7):1190–1192.

5. Akhmedkhanov A, Zeleniuch-Jacquotte A, Toniolo P. Role of exogenous and endogenous hormones in endometrial cancer: Review of the evidence and research perspectives. *Ann NY Acad Sci.* 2001 Sep;943:296–315.

6. Key TJ, Pike MC. The dose-effect relationship between 'unopposed' oestrogens and endometrial mitotic rate: Its central role in explaining and predicting endometrial cancer risk. *Br J Cancer.* 1988 Feb;57(2):205–212.

7. Henderson BE, Feigelson HS. Hormonal carcinogenesis. *Carcinogenesis.* 2000 Mar;21(3):427–433.

8. Mauland KK, Trovik J, Wik E, et al. High BMI is significantly associated with positive progesterone receptor status and clinico-pathological markers for non-aggressive disease in endometrial cancer. *Br J Cancer.* 2011 Mar 15;104(6):921–926.

9. Samarnthai N, Hall K, Yeh IT. Molecular profiling of endometrial malignancies. *Obstet Gynecol Int.* 2010;2010:162363.

10. Gates EJ, Hirschfield L, Matthews RP, Yap OW. Body mass index as a prognostic factor in endometrioid adenocarcinoma of the endometrium. *J Natl Med Assoc.* 2006 Nov;98(11):1814–1822.

11. Kauppila A, Kujansuu E, Vihko R. Cytosol estrogen and progestin receptors in endometrial carcinoma of patients treated with surgery, radiotherapy, and progestin. Clinical correlates. *Cancer.* 1982 Nov 15;50(10):2157–2162.

12. Ehrlich CE, Young PC, Stehman FB, et al. Steroid receptors and clinical outcome in patients with adenocarcinoma of the endometrium. *Am J Obstet Gynecol.* 1988 Apr;158(4):796–807.

13. Mortel R, Levy C, Wolff JP, et al. Female sex steroid receptors in postmenopausal endometrial carcinoma and biochemical response to an anti-estrogen. *Cancer Res.* 1981 Mar;41(3):1140–1147.

14. Hanekamp EE, Kuhne LM, Grootegoed JA, et al. Progesterone receptor A and B expression and progestagen treatment in growth and spread of endometrial cancer cells in nude mice. *Endocr Relat Cancer.* 2004 Dec;11(4):831–841.

15. Laurelli G, Di Vagno G, Scaffa C, et al. Conservative treatment of early endometrial cancer: Preliminary results of a pilot study. *Gynecol Oncol.* 2011 Jan;120(1):43–46.

16. Ramirez PT, Frumovitz M, Bodurka DC, et al. Hormonal therapy for the management of grade 1 endometrial adenocarcinoma: A literature review. *Gynecol Oncol.* 2004 Oct;95(1):133–138.

17. Bokhman JV, Chepick OF, Volkova AT, Vishnevsky AS. Can primary endometrial carcinoma stage I be cured without surgery and radiation therapy? *Gynecol Oncol.* 1985 Feb;20(2): 139–155.

18. Harris WJ. Complications of hysterectomy. *Clin Obstet Gynecol.* 1997 Dec;40(4):928–938.

19. Montz FJ, Bristow RE, Bovicelli A, et al. Intrauterine progesterone treatment of early endometrial cancer. *Am J Obstet Gynecol.* 2002 Apr;186(4):651–657.

20. Gotlieb WH, Beiner ME, Shalmon B, et al. Outcome of fertility-sparing treatment with progestins in young patients with endometrial cancer. *Obstet Gynecol.* 2003 Oct;102(4):718–725.

21. Imai M, Jobo T, Sato R, et al. Medroxyprogesterone acetate therapy for patients with adenocarcinoma of the endometrium who wish to preserve the uterus-usefulness and limitations. *Eur J Gynaecol Oncol.* 2001;22(3):217–220.

22. Kaku T, Yoshikawa H, Tsuda H, et al. Conservative therapy for adenocarcinoma and atypical endometrial hyperplasia of the endometrium in young women: Central pathologic review and treatment outcome. *Cancer Lett.* 2001 Jun 10;167(1):39–48.

23. Kim JJ, Chapman-Davis E. Role of progesterone in endometrial cancer. *Semin Reprod Med.* 2010 Jan;28(1):81–90.

24. Kelley RM, Baker WH. Progestational agents in the treatment of carcinoma of the endometrium. *N Engl J Med.* 1961 Feb 2;264:216–222.

25. Podratz KC, O'Brien PC, Malkasian GD Jr, et al. Effects of progestational agents in treatment of endometrial carcinoma. *Obstet Gynecol.* 1985 Jul;66(1):106–110.

26. Saegusa M, Okayasu I. Progesterone therapy for endometrial carcinoma reduces cell proliferation but does not alter apoptosis. *Cancer.* 1998 Jul 1;83(1):111–121.

27. Lee NK, Cheung MK, Shin JY, et al. Prognostic factors for uterine cancer in reproductive-aged women. *Obstet Gynecol.* 2007 Mar;109(3):655–662.

28. Chiva L, Lapuente F, Gonzalez-Cortijo L, et al. Sparing fertility in young patients with endometrial cancer. *Gynecol Oncol.* 2008 Nov;111(2 Suppl):S101–S104.

29. Ushijima K, Yahata H, Yoshikawa H, et al. Multicenter phase II study of fertility-sparing treatment with medroxyprogesterone acetate for endometrial carcinoma and atypical hyperplasia in young women. *J Clin Oncol.* 2007 Jul 1;25(19):2798–2803.

30. Dhar KK, NeedhiRajan T, Koslowski M, Woolas RP. Is levonorgestrel intrauterine system effective for treatment of early endometrial cancer? Report of four cases and review of the literature. *Gynecol Oncol.* 2005 Jun;97(3):924–927.

31. Kim YB, Holschneider CH, Ghosh K, et al. Progestin alone as primary treatment of endometrial carcinoma in premenopausal women. Report of seven cases and review of the literature. *Cancer.* 1997 Jan 15;79(2):320–327.

32. Chao CK, Grigsby PW, Perez CA, et al. Medically inoperable stage I endometrial carcinoma: A few dilemmas in radiotherapeutic management. *Int J Radiat Oncol Biol Phys.* 1996 Jan 1;34(1):27–31.

33. Fishman DA, Roberts KB, Chambers JT, et al. Radiation therapy as exclusive treatment for medically inoperable patients with stage I and II endometrioid carcinoma with endometrium. *Gynecol Oncol.* 1996 May;61(2):189–196.

34. Nguyen TV, Petereit DG. High-dose-rate brachytherapy for medically inoperable stage I endometrial cancer. *Gynecol Oncol.* 1998 Nov;71(2):196–203.

35. Kucera H, Knocke TH, Kucera E, Potter R. Treatment of endometrial carcinoma with high-dose-rate brachytherapy alone in medically inoperable stage I patients. *Acta Obstet Gynecol Scand.* 1998 Nov;77(10):1008–1012.

36. Niazi TM, Souhami L, Portelance L, et al. Long-term results of high-dose-rate brachytherapy in the primary treatment of medically inoperable stage I-II endometrial carcinoma. *Int J Radiat Oncol Biol Phys.* 2005 Nov 15;63(4):1108–1113.

37. Coon D, Beriwal S, Heron DE, et al. High-dose-rate Rotte "Y" applicator brachytherapy for definitive treatment of medically inoperable endometrial cancer: 10-year results. *Int J Radiat Oncol Biol Phys.* 2008 Jul 1;71(3):779–783.

38. Shenfield CB, Pearcey RG, Ghosh S, Dundas GS. The management of inoperable Stage I endometrial cancer using intracavitary brachytherapy alone: A 20-year institutional review. *Brachytherapy.* 2009 Jul–Sep;8(3):278–283.

39. Wegner RE, Beriwal S, Heron DE, et al. Definitive radiation therapy for endometrial cancer in medically inoperable elderly patients. *Brachytherapy.* Jul–Sep;9(3):260–265.

40. Nag S, Erickson B, Thomadsen B, et al. The American Brachytherapy Society recommendations for high-dose-rate brachytherapy for carcinoma of the cervix. *Int J Radiat Oncol Biol Phys.* 2000 Aug 1;48(1):201–211.

41. American Cancer Society. Cancer facts & figures 2011. Atlanta, GA: American Cancer Society; 2011, p. 4.

42. Macdonald OK, Sause WT, Lee RJ, et al. Does oncologic specialization influence outcomes following surgery in early stage adenocarcinoma of the endometrium? *Gynecol Oncol.* 2005 Dec; 99(3):730–735.

43. Roland PY, Kelly FJ, Kulwicki CY, et al. The benefits of a gynecologic oncologist: A pattern of care study for endometrial cancer treatment. *Gynecol Oncol.* 2004 Apr;93(1):125–130.

44. Park H, Seok JM, Yoon BS, et al. Effectiveness of high-dose progestin and long-term outcomes in young women with early-stage, well-differentiated endometrial adenocarcinoma of the uterine endometrium. *Arch Gynecol Obstet.* 2012;285(2):473–478.

45. Kalogiannidis I, Agorastos T. Conservative management of young patients with endometrial highly-differentiated adenocarcinoma. *J Obstet Gynaecol.* 2011;31(1):13–17.

46. Martin-Hirsch PL, Jarvis G, Kitchener H, Lilford R. Progestagens for endometrial cancer. *Cochrane Database Syst Rev.* 2011;6:CD001040.

47. Landgren RC, Fletcher GH, Delclos L, Wharton JT. Irradiation of endometrial cancer in patients with medical contraindication to surgery or with unresectable lesions. *AJR Am J Roentgenol.* 1976;126(1):148–154.

48. Sorbe B, Frankendai B, Risberg B. Intracavitary irradiation of endometrial carcinoma stage I by a high dose-rate afterloading technique. *Gynecol Oncol.* 1989;33(2):135–145.

49. Nout RA, Smit VT, Putter H, et al. Vaginal brachytherapy versus pelvic external beam radiotherapy for patients with endometrial cancer of high-intermediate risk (PORTEC-2): An open-label, non-inferiority, randomized trial; PORTEC Study Group. *Lancet.* 2010;375(9717):816–823.

50. Nag S, Erickson B, Parikh S, et al. The American Brachytherapy Society recommendations for high-dose-rate brachytherapy for carcinoma of the endometrium. *Int J Radiat Oncol Biol Phys.* 2000;48(3):779–790.

■ CASE 2 ■

Management of Stage IIIC Endometrial Cancer

CLINICAL PROBLEM

The "correct" treatment for a patient with endometrial cancer and positive lymph nodes at the time of surgery is a matter of intense debate and is currently the focus of an international randomized trial [1]. This dilemma is commonly seen in endometrial cancer and usually not referred to a "center of excellence."

CASE EXAMPLE

A 60-year-old White female, with a body mass index (BMI) of 31, presents with vaginal spotting, and an endometrial biopsy reveals a grade 2 endometrioid adenocarcinoma. The patient undergoes a total abdominal hysterectomy and bilateral salpingo-oophorectomy (TAH/BSO) and pelvic-only lymph node dissection and is found to have 1 of 3 left pelvic lymph node metastasis and 0 of 2 right pelvic lymph node metastasis. In addition, she has lymphovascular space invasion (LVSI) on final pathology; however, no invasion of the cervical stroma is seen.

Management Decisions

- Does the number of lymph nodes dissected influence the treatment decisions?
- Does the lack of para-aortic lymph node dissection influence the treatment decision?
- Should imaging be considered?
- Should surgical re-exploration be considered?
- How would a patient with a single lymph node metastasis be treated?

MAJOR OPINION

Jennifer F. De Los Santos

The case presented is of a patient with high-risk, node-positive endometrial cancer. There are several questions, some controversial, that surround this case that will be outlined and addressed here.

What Is the Incidence of Positive Para-Aortic Lymph Nodes (PALN) in Women With Endometrial Cancer Who Have Positive Pelvic Lymph Nodes (PLN)?

The incidence and distribution of nodal metastases in women with clinical stage I and occult stage II endometrial cancer was explored in Gynecologic Oncology Group (GOG) 33 [2]. In this study, 70 of 621 (11%) patients had evidence of pelvic and/or para-aortic nodal metastases. While 12 of 70 (17%) patients of these metastases occurred in PALN alone, the majority of PALN metastases [22 of 34 (65%)] occurred in patients who, in addition, had positive PLN. Thus, in patients who have nodal metastases, nearly half [34 of 70 (48.5%)] of them had a component of metastasis in the PALN, and having positive PLN appeared to be an additional risk factor for further nodal disease. In a more recent single institution series, lymphadenectomy (LND) was performed on 303 of 422 (72%) patients prospectively assessed for lymphatic dissemination by predefined guidelines that segregated patients into low and high risk. In the total of 63 of 303 (21%) patients presented with nodal metastases, 53 of 63 (84%) patients had positive PLN, 39 of 63 (62%) patients had positive PALN, and of those with involvement of PLN, 29 of 53 (55%), in addition, had concurrent PALN metastases [3]. A second retrospective study reviewing 42 patients with stage IIIC endometrial cancer and both PLN and PALN sampling noted positive PLN alone in 43% of the patients, positive PLN and PALN in 40% of the patients, and positive PALN alone in 17% of the patients [4].

88

Increasing numbers of positive PLN (p = .0001) as well as bilateral PLN involvement were associated with PALN metastases. These data closely mirror the data from the GOG study and suggest a significant risk of PALN involvement in patients who have positive PLN. Based on these data, the risk of this patient having positive PALN is approximately 50%.

Does LND Influence Outcome in Women With Endometrial Cancer?

Proponents of routine surgical staging, including both pelvic and para-aortic LND, assert that this is the most accurate way to assess risk and often leads to changes in postoperative therapeutic recommendations. Whether LND is of therapeutic value independent of nodal status is an issue of significant controversy. However, 2 recent phase 3 trials that investigated the survival benefit of LND in women with histologically proven endometrial cancer felt to be confined preoperatively to the uterus demonstrated no relapse-free, disease-free, or overall survival advantage [5,6]. The larger of these, the A Study in the Treatment of Endometrial Cancer (ASTEC) trial, randomized 1,408 women with histologically confirmed endometrial cancer felt to be confined to the uterus to standard surgery (hysterectomy, BSO, peritoneal washings and palpation of the PALN; n = 704) versus standard surgery plus LND (PLN and PALN; n = 704) [6]. In the LND arm, only 65% of women had at least 10 nodes removed (median, 12 nodes). The results demonstrated no significant difference in recurrence-free and overall survival. A second smaller trial randomized 514 women with clinical stage I endometrial cancer to pelvic LND (n = 264) or no LND (n = 250). Median number of nodes removed in the LND arm was 30. PALN sampling was at the discretion of the surgeon and occurred in 69 of 264 (26%) patients in the LND arm. In the no LND arm 194 of 250 (78%) had no lymph nodes removed and 56 of 250 (22%) had enlarged nodes necessitating sampling or LND. Adjuvant therapy did not differ between arms and no significant difference was seen in disease-free survival (DFS), overall survival (OS), or median time to relapse between arms. These findings were corroborated in a Cochrane meta-analysis, demonstrating no survival advantage for LND [7]. Although LND does not appear to improve survival in women with endometrial cancer limited to the uterus preoperatively, it does provide information that may alter treatment volumes for radiation, and may thus be helpful in women with at least high–intermediate risk disease (2 out of 3 factors including invasion in the outer half of the myometrium, grade 3 histology, and age greater than 60 years).

Does the Number of PLN and the Choice of Selective Nodal Dissection in the Pelvis Only Influence Treatment Decisions?

Involvement of PLN and/or PALN in patients with endometrial cancer is associated with poorer outcomes and is a marker for more aggressive disease [8]. Confirming the pathologic distribution of nodal involvement (pelvic alone versus para-aortic ± pelvic) helps the radiation oncologist determine the volumes that are necessary to encompass in their radiation portals to optimally reduce local regional recurrence risk. This is of particular importance as combined pelvic and para-aortic or extended-field treatment compared with pelvic radiation therapy (RT) alone in a prospective study in patients with cervical cancer resulted in a trend toward increased toxicity over treatment of pelvic fields alone [9]. It is notable that both acute and late toxicity appear increased as well, in comparison to historic data from a prospective phase 2 trial in patients with cervical cancer receiving daily extended-field RT with conventional techniques in combination with concurrent chemotherapy (CT) [10].

Additional features outside of positive PLN may be considered when selecting patients for para-aortic irradiation who are unable to receive surgical staging of the para-aortics, and who, in addition, have negative imaging. The presence of additional extra-uterine sites of disease, in addition to lymph node positivity (including positive peritoneal washings), portends a poorer prognosis than patients with disease limited to the nodes [8,11]. Patterns of failure for patients in this subset are predominated by distant failures, and this could be factored into a risk–benefit ratio when considering extended-field irradiation in a patient within this subset, with negative nodal imaging and no pathologic confirmation of PALN micrometastases. However, a single institution retrospective study in 17 women with positive PLN and *pathologically confirmed* negative PALN who received a median dose of 50.4 Gy to the pelvis demonstrated a 12% (2 of 17) rate of isolated failure in the PALN, suggesting risk is not completely mitigated by surgical staging alone, although the incidence is low [11].

How Accurate Are Imaging Studies in Assessing the Undissected Nodes? Which Imaging Studies Should be Used?

Small, single institutional studies investigating the sensitivity, specificity, and accuracy of F-FDG PET-CT for predicting nodal metastases in women with endometrial cancer have shown results ranging from 57% to 85%, 87.5% to 99%, and 80% to 7%, respectively [13–16]. One study showed a significant improvement in the sensitivity of detecting nodal metastases between contrast-enhanced PET/CT (61%) as compared with a contrast-enhanced CT without PET (41%) [14]. An additional study in 53 women who underwent preoperative imaging with both MRI and PET-CT showed equivalent accuracy (84% vs. 88%, respectively) in detecting nodal metastases between these 2 imaging modalities [15]. However, PET-CT has the additional advantage of simultaneously staging distant disease with high levels of sensitivity (100%), specificity (94%), and accuracy (93%) [15].

Which Adjuvant Therapies Optimize the Outcome in Patients With Stage IIIC Endometrial Cancer? What Data Support Modality Selection (Radiation Versus Systemic Therapy), Sequencing of Therapy, and Combination (Concurrent Versus Sequential) Therapy?

Adjuvant Treatment: Modality Selection

The management of stage IIIC endometrial cancer is controversial. Published prospective trials comparing the relative benefits of CT and RT alone as adjuvant management in this high-risk group have been unhelpful in ascertaining how to maximize outcomes with combinations of each modality while achieving manageable toxicity and the trials have shown conflicting results, possibly owing to differences in trial design and patient selection.

Three recent prospective trials in patients with intermediate-to-high-risk disease comparing adjuvant CT to RT have been reported [12,17,18]. In GOG-122, 396 patients with stage III and optimally debulked (defined as no single site of residual tumor greater than 2 cm) stage IV disease were randomized to RT (*n* = 202) or to doxorubicin–cisplatin CT every 3 weeks for 8 cycles (*n* = 194). All endometrial carcinoma histologies were eligible, including clear cell (RT/CT arms: 3.5%/5.2%) and papillary serous (RT/CT arms: 21.3%/20.6%). The RT was delivered with conventional techniques, prior to an era where more accurate CT-based 3-D treatment planning was routinely used, and delivered 30 Gy in 20 fractions to the whole abdomen (a dose not expected to control gross peritoneal disease up to 2 cm) with a pelvic boost of 15 Gy in 8 fractions ± a boost to the PALN. With a median follow up of 74 months, there was a significant improvement in progression-free survival (PFS) (50% vs. 38%, *p* = .007) and OS (55% vs. 42%, *p* = .004) in favor of the CT arm [17]. An analysis of the patterns of failure showed a lower rate of failure in the pelvis (13% vs. 18%, respectively) in patients receiving RT as compared with CT, and lower rates of distant failure in patients receiving CT as compared with RT (18% vs. 22, respectively). Acute grade 3 or higher hematologic toxicity was significantly worse in the CT arm compared with RT (88% vs. 14%, respectively), and grade 3 or higher gastrointestinal (GI) toxicity in the CT versus RT arms was 20% versus 13%. A trial from Japan randomized 385 patients with surgically staged (majority had PLN, without PALN sampling) endometrial carcinoma, stage IC–IIIC (greater than 50% myometrial invasion, 25% stage III) to either pelvic RT (45–50 Gy in 4–6 weeks) or cyclophosphamide, doxorubicin, and cisplatin CT every 4 weeks for a median of 3 cycles (range, 1–7) [18]. Patients with nonendometrioid histologies were excluded. At 5 years, there was no statistical difference in PFS or OS between the arms (RT vs. CT: PFS, 83.5% vs. 81.8%; OS, 85.3% vs. 86.7%). There were no significant differences between the arms in the incidence of grade 3 or higher overall toxicity percentages (RT vs. CT: 1.6% vs. 4.7%), which are markedly different with volume-directed RT and more limited use of CT than the GOG trial. Finally, a trial from the United Kingdom randomized 345 patients with surgically staged IC–II (greater than 50% myometrial invasion), grade 3, and stage III endometrial carcinoma to pelvic or extended-field RT (45–50 Gy) versus adjuvant CT (cisplatin 50 mg/m^2, doxorubicin 45 mg/m^2, and cyclophosphamide 600 mg/m^2 × 5 cycles) [12]. Importantly, similar to the Japanese trial and different from the GOG study, clear cell and papillary serous histologies were excluded. With a median follow up of 95.5 months, there was no difference in 3-, 5-, or 7-year OS between the arms (RT: 78%, 69%, and 62%; CT: 76%, 66%, 62%, respectively). PFS was also not statistically different between the arms. There was a nonsignificant reduction in initial local relapses in the patients receiving RT as compared with CT (7% vs. 11%, respectively) as well as a nonsignificant reduction in initial distant relapses in the patients receiving CT as compared with RT (16% vs. 21%, respectively). Late grade 3 or higher GI and genitourinary (GU) toxicity on the RT arm was 16% and 5%, respectively. The more moderate CT regimen chosen for this study (midway in aggressiveness between the GOG and Japanese trials), was reflected in the incidence of acute grade 3 or higher hematologic toxicity on the CT arm (41%).

Sequencing, Timing, and Optimization of Therapy

With a DFS of only 50% in the superior arm (CT) of the GOG-122 study, investigators sought to optimize an approach in this group of high-risk patients to include both RT and CT. However, owing to toxicity concerns, a sequential rather than concomitant regimen was selected. Thus, a randomized phase 3 trial was designed that included a treatment regimen of surgery followed by volume-directed RT, and then randomized 552 eligible patients to 6 cycles of cisplatin and doxorubicin, with and without paclitaxel [19]. At 36 months, recurrence free survival was 64% and 62% in the arms with and without paclitaxel. Two additional combined randomized trials and other single institutional retrospective series have reported results with sequential treatment for this high-risk group [11,20–22]. Hogberg et al. reported results in 534 patients with high risk International Federation of Gynecology and Oncology (FIGO) stage I–III endometrial cancer treated with surgery and adjuvant RT ± CT, with an improvement in PFS in the CT arm [22]. Alvarez-Secord et al. retrospectively reviewed 356 patients with stage III and IV disease treated adjuvantly with RT alone, CT alone, or sequential combination therapy [20]. The CT arm had significantly worse 3-year PFS and OS (19% and 33%, $p < .001$) in comparison with either the

RT alone arm (59% and 70%) or the combined therapy arm (62% and 79%). Similarly, Geller et al. found an excellent 5-year PFS and OS in 23 patients with high-risk endometrial cancer (78%, stage III) treated with sandwich CT and RT of 74% and 79%, respectively [21].

Concerns regarding toxicity have led to more investigations of sequential versus concurrent combined treatment approaches (chemoradiotherapy [CRT]) in patients with endometrial cancer. However, in patients requiring pelvic radiation delivered with CRT and receiving additional adjuvant CT, there are already several randomized cervical cancer trials demonstrating the feasibility of this approach [23,24]. One could argue that these are not comparable groups as patients with endometrial cancer have higher average ages at diagnosis and present with more frequent comorbid disease, rendering them a group that may not tolerate this increase in toxicity as well. It is thus heartening to know that the Radiation Therapy Oncology Group (RTOG) performed a phase 2 trial of CRT (cisplatin 50 mg/m^2 weeks 1, 4) concurrent with RT (45 Gy to pelvis followed by a vaginal brachytherapy cuff boost) followed by an additional 4 cycles of adjuvant CT with cisplatin and paclitaxel in 46 patients with stage IB–IIIC, with a resulting 4-year DFS and OS of 81% and 85%, respectively, and reasonable late grade 3 or higher overall toxicity of 21% [25]. An additional retrospective series from Japan in 76 women with stage III and IV endometrial cancer treated adjuvantly with CT alone, RT alone, or CRT with a median follow-up of 54 months, showed a statistically significant improvement in OS in the CRT group as compared with the CT arm ($p = .03$) and a trend toward improved OS in the CRT group compared with the RT arm ($p = .052$) [26]. Finally, the use of intensity-modulated radiation therapy (IMRT) to treat extended fields has been shown to reduce radiation doses to critical organs [27,28], and to be both safe and effective resulting in a 15% rate of grade 3 or higher toxicity when delivered in combination with concurrent cisplatin CT [29]. This approach of CRT followed by additional CT as compared with CT alone in patients with high-risk endometrial cancer is presently being studied in the cooperative group setting.

Recommendation

Further assessment of nodal and distant involvement would also be required in this patient. Based on sensitivity for nodal detection and utility in assessing distant disease, a PET-CT scan would provide the highest sensitivity for nodal involvement. It is important to consider that, at present, no imaging study has the sensitivity to assess microscopic disease. As the risk of para-aortic nodal involvement is as high as 50% in patients with known positive pelvic nodes, extended-field RT should be considered and weighed against the increased risk of bowel toxicity. This could potentially be mitigated by the use of extended-field IMRT. Prior to robust randomized, prospective data in endometrial cancer that suggest a benefit to concurrent radiation, and especially when considering extended-field CRT where toxicity is increased [10], a recommendation of sequential CT with 3 cycles of a platinum drug (either cisplatin or carboplatin) and paclitaxel, followed by an extended-field IMRT dose of 45 to 50.4 Gy in 25 to 28 fractions, followed by an additional 3 cycles of a platinum and paclitaxel would be appropriate.

ACADEMIC COMMENT

Jacob Estes

Endometrial cancer is the most common and, fortunately, most curable gynecologic malignancy owing to its frequent detection at an early stage. In many cases, the cancer is confined to the uterine corpus and potentially cured with hysterectomy and BSO. Unfortunately, clinical assessment inaccurately predicts spread of disease and, therefore, precludes appropriate stratification of an individual's risk of recurrence.

In 1987, the GOG published findings from protocol 33 demonstrating a significant incidence of pelvic and para-aortic nodal spread in patients with apparent clinical stage I/II disease [2]. At rates of 9% and 5%, respectively, these findings are used as a justification for the surgical staging of endometrial cancer. In addition, lymph node assessment allows appropriate risk stratification and aids in prescribing or withholding adjuvant therapy. A therapeutic benefit of LND has been reported in retrospective studies that have suggested an improvement in survival from removal of grossly positive lymph nodes, especially in the para-aortic chain [4,30,31]. However, the recently published ASTEC trial and Cochrane review of lymphadenectomy in endometrial cancer have not supported this observation [6,7,32,33].

All patients with endometrial cancer are surgically staged at our institution, if technically feasible. Patients undergo a systematic anatomical pelvic and para-aortic LND with node counts reported. There is controversy as to what represents an adequate dissection. Nodal counts of 8 to 12 have been reported [34,35] as being adequate, whereas the number of nodal zones/beds have served as a surrogate for adequacy. Increasing node counts and completeness of dissection have demonstrated increased positive node detection.

In this case, a 60-year-old female underwent limited surgical staging with final pathology revealing involvement of 1 of 5 PLN with no PALN removed. Rates of para-aortic nodal involvement are reported to be 38% to 50% [2,4] in the face of positive pelvic nodes and this incidence increases with the number of pelvic nodes involved as well as the presence of bilaterality. It is also known that patients with extrauterine pelvic disease have higher rates of PLN and PALN positivity [4].

Given the patient's stage III disease, she is at an extremely high risk for recurrence and needs treatment. An important consideration is whether this patient would benefit from further surgery. The answer to that question is based on her choice of adjuvant therapy. Classically, patients with node-positive endometrial cancer underwent pelvic RT. This was an effective regimen with excellent local control, but a high distant failure rate. If her practitioner were to choose this method, a more extensive lymph node assessment may allow tailoring of the radiation field or elimination of a potentially morbid para-aortic boost.

Given the distant failure rate, the GOG performed protocol 122. This study randomized patients to whole abdominal irradiation with a pelvic boost (total dose of 45 Gy) or systemic therapy with adriamycin and cispatin for 8 cycles. This trial demonstrated a significant difference in both PFS and OS (12% and 13%) favoring the CT arm [17]. These findings prompted the GOG to perform further CT studies in this patient population and established CT as the standard of care. In this case, if the practitioner decided on CT, the patient would not necessarily benefit from further surgery unless there was evidence of grossly positive para-aortic disease on imaging.

Owing to the excellent local control provided by whole pelvis radiation therapy (WPRT), as well as the demonstrated benefit of systemic therapy, some have advocated a combination therapy in a "sandwich" method. Geller et al. reported on their single-institution experience in high-risk endometrial cancer using 3 cycles of CT (a taxane and carboplatin) followed by WPRT, with an additional 3 cycles of CT after WPRT was complete. This multimodality regimen was well tolerated, with all patients completing their prescribed therapy. Kaplan–Meier estimates of 3- and 5-year survival were 88% and 79%, respectively [21]. This treatment modality represents a promising new treatment paradigm for patients with stage III disease.

In summary, surgical staging of endometrial cancer plays many important roles. It helps stratify risk, guide adjuvant therapy, and may be therapeutic. To date, there is no standard of nodal dissection adequacy; however, a multifocal anatomic dissection does appear to increase nodal counts and increase affected lymph node detection. For many gynecologic oncologists, CT is a mainstay of therapy for node-positive patients, but there appears to be an emerging role for combination therapy in individuals who can tolerate a potential increase in morbidity. Repeat surgical assessment should be reserved for patients with accessible, bulky para-aortic disease, or those patients with apparent stage I disease without lymph node assessment that may be spared unnecessary therapy.

In this clinical scenario, imaging to rule out bulky para-aortic disease and distant metastasis would be recommended. If available, enrollment in a clinical trial would be reasonable, as there are emerging data on the efficacy of multimodality therapy. Outside of this, 6 to 8 cycles of taxane- and platinum-based CT would adequately address her known lymph node disease and decrease her extrapelvic recurrence rate, which should result in improved DFS and OS as compared to locoregional RT.

COMMUNITY PRACTITIONER COMMENT

Elizabeth Falkenberg

As a community radiation oncologist, I base my treatment decision process on published randomized trials, when available, and the National Comprehensive Cancer Network (NCCN) Clinical Practice Guidelines, taking into consideration patient performance status, presence of comorbid diseases, and tolerability of approach. This patient is a 60-year-old obese female with vaginal bleeding and an endometrial biopsy consistent with an endometroid adenocarcinoma. She has a history of hypertension and adult onset diabetes mellitus. At the time of TAH/BSO, a total of 5 lymph nodes were removed and 1 was positive for metastatic disease. The tumor was a moderately differentiated endometrioid adenocarcinoma measuring 5 cm and invading more than half of the myometrial thickness with all margins negative. There was LVSI, but no cervical stromal invasion. Her final pathology is a stage IIIC because of the positive PLN. Ideally, this patient should be seen in consultation within 1 month of surgery in order to facilitate adjuvant therapy in a timely manner. Usually, a complete blood count (CBC) and comprehensive metabolic profile (CMP) have already been done at the time of surgery. A CT scan of the abdomen and pelvis with contrast and chest x-ray should be ordered to complete her staging and assess for distant metastases. Further studies such as CT/PET could then be ordered for equivocal findings. When considering treatment decisions, it is important to account for prognostic factors for recurrence that may influence treatment recommendations. In the Surveillance Epidemiology and End Results (SEER) database analysis of 41,120 cases of endometrial cancer from 1973 to 1987, FIGO stage, histology, histologic grade, lymph node status, age at diagnosis, and race were all prognostic factors of survival [36].

In patients who are obese, an extended LND can be surgically challenging and cause significant morbidity [7]. There has been no significant survival benefit seen for an extended LND, but surgical pathologic data from GOG 33 showed that 22% of clinical stage I patients had extrauterine disease (lymph node metastases, adnexal disease, intraperitoneal spread, and/or malignant cells in peritoneal washings) with extensive surgical staging [2]. Tumor grade, depth of invasion, and intraperitoneal disease significantly increased the risk of PLN and PALN metastases. Most of the data comparing no lymph node dissection versus pelvic and para-aortic dissection/sampling was not in the setting of a randomized trial [37]. Patients with clinical stage I/II endometrial cancer with TAH/BSO and no lymph node dissection were randomized to radiotherapy versus no radiotherapy resulting in equivalent OS [38,39]. In GOG 99 [40], patients were surgically staged with a lymph node dissection (surgical stage IB/C–IIA/B) and then randomized to pelvic radiotherapy versus no radiotherapy resulting in nonstatistically significant OS differences, but with a higher local recurrence of 12% (no radiotherapy) versus 1.2% (radiotherapy). The

Postoperative Radiation Therapy in Endometrial Carcinoma (PORTEC) study [38] and the randomized Norwegian trial [39] both showed that local recurrences were higher without pelvic radiotherapy, whether or not a patient had a full lymph node dissection. Since the publications of PORTEC 1 and the randomized Norwegian trials, there have been advances in surgical technique with both laparoscopic and robotically assisted surgery that have resulted in reductions in length of hospital stay, wound complications, and quality of life endpoints as compared with laparotomy [41–43]. However, as prospective data do not support a survival benefit from LND, further surgery would not be recommended for this patient [44].

After the patient has recovered from her surgery (approximately 4–6 weeks), recommended treatment would include external beam radiotherapy to the pelvis and high-dose-rate (HDR) brachytherapy to the vaginal cuff followed by CT in a sequential fashion. For advanced stage endometrial cancer, current national treatment guidelines through the NCCN recommend CT ± tumor-directed radiotherapy. Several trials have been performed to address the optimal adjuvant approach in stage III endometrial cancer patients. The GOG 122 trial randomized women with stage III/IV endometrial cancer with no distant metastasis to whole abdominal radiotherapy versus CT with cisplatin and doxorubicin every 3 weeks for 7 cycles [17]. The whole abdominal radiotherapy dose was limited to 30 Gy at 1.5 Gy/fx because of the potential for significant toxicity from whole abdominal radiotherapy, and there was a boost of 15 Gy given to the pelvis. The CT arm had a significant improvement in PFS and OS, but higher toxicity. In this high-risk population with a survival rate of 50% with 1 adjuvant modality of treatment, this study failed to answer how to optimally combine adjuvant CT and radiation. An open GOG randomized phase 3 trial is presently studying whether the addition of volume-directed RT to cisplatin CT followed by carboplatin and paclitaxel CT in optimally debulked stage III and IVA endometrial cancer is superior to CT alone and may ultimately answer this question. In addition, there have been European data to suggest that RT and CT is better than radiation alone. GOG 184 included stage III/IV patients (excluding distant metastasis) and treated all patients with pelvic radiotherapy ± para-aortic radiotherapy ± intravaginal brachytherapy and then randomized treatment between 2 different CT regimens [19].

Regimen I consisted of cisplatin, doxorubicin, and G-CSF every 3 weeks for 6 cycles (CD) while regimen II consisted of the same cisplatin, doxorubicin, and granulocyte colony-stimulating factor (G-CSF) with the addition of paclitaxel (CDP). The addition of paclitaxel to cisplatin and doxorubicin following surgery and RT did not improve relapse-free survival but was associated with higher toxicity.

For this particular patient, in the setting of radiographically negative PALN, recommendations would include delivery of external beam radiotherapy of 50.4 Gy at 1.8 Gy/fx in 28 fractions utilizing IMRT to minimize the dose to the normal tissue. The patient would undergo simulation in the supine position using intravenous (IV) contrast, a full bladder, and a vaginal marker. The clinical target volume (CTV) that would receive a dose of 50.4 Gy would be delineated on the basis of the published consensus guidelines for IMRT in postoperative endometrial cases and would include the common, external, and internal iliac lymph node regions along with the upper 3 cm of the vagina and the paravaginal soft tissue [45]. Then adding 7 mm to obtain the planning target volume (PTV) of 50.4 Gy, a treatment plan should be developed using 7 to 9 beams with 6 MV or 10 MV and 95% of the PTV should receive the prescription dose. Our dosimetrists use RTOG 0418 treatment planning guidelines to specify dose constraints to the bladder, small bowel, femoral heads, and rectum. IMRT should be used in this patient to reduce toxicity to the small bowel, bladder, and rectum. Dosimetric comparison between IMRT and 3-D conformal radiotherapy showed that IMRT was superior at all dose levels, with the largest reduction in normal tissue volume receiving greater than 30 to 40 Gy [46]. Several studies have shown that IMRT can optimize target coverage and reduce the volume of normal tissue irradiated, such as significantly reducing the small bowel volume receiving more than 45 Gy [47,48]. In addition, published retrospective studies suggest a reduction in acute and late GI toxicity with the use of IMRT [47,49]. Ideally, both IMRT and image-guided radiotherapy therapy (IGRT) would be utilized, but if not available, then delivering treatment with a 4-field box technique would be acceptable. Expected side effects possibly include loose stools, frequency of urination, and fatigue.

This patient had a moderately differentiated tumor invading the outer half of the myometrium with lymphovascular invasion. She has significant risk factors for vaginal recurrence, and vaginal brachytherapy can be delivered without significantly increasing toxicity. A vaginal cuff boost with HDR brachytherapy, using the largest diameter vaginal cylinder that is comfortable for the patient, would be planned near the completion of external beam radiotherapy. There should be no air gap between the vaginal cylinder and the vaginal wall mucosa on the treatment planning CT scan, and the treatment should encompass the upper 3 cm of the vagina. There are several appropriate HDR vaginal brachytherapy dose schemes after the completion of external beam radiotherapy, but 15 Gy in 3 fractions at 5 Gy per fraction prescribed to the vaginal surface delivered every third day is preferred.

After the completion of radiotherapy, it is reasonable to wait 4 weeks for the patient to recover from the acute side effects of treatment before initiating CT. When deciding which CT agents to deliver, performance status and comorbid diseases are important factors to consider. For patients with significant comorbidities, the combination of carboplatin and paclitaxel is a good alternative to the cisplatin, doxorubicin, and paclitaxel (CDP or TAP) regimen. GOG 184 did not show a benefit in relapse-free survival, but a subset analysis showed that CDP was associated with a 50% reduction in the risk of recurrence or death among patients with gross residual disease. This led to the current GOG 209 study that includes stage III/IV and recurrent disease comparing 2 CT regimens, doxorubicin/cisplatin/paclitaxel/G-CSF (every 21 days for 7 cycles) and carboplatin/paclitaxel (every 21 days for 7 cycles). This study is closed to patient accrual, but the results are not yet available. CT is beneficial in stage III disease, but the optimal regimen is not yet known. In a patient with hypertension and diabetes mellitus, it would be reasonable to give 4 to 6 cycles of carboplatin and paclitaxel (CP) as adjuvant treatment after external beam radiotherapy because of the potential for toxicity using the CDP regimen and no proven benefit over the CP regimen. Hopefully, in the near future, there will be targeted biologic agents with less toxicity and increased efficacy available for treatment in endometrial carcinoma.

In summary, for a 60-year-old obese female with hypertension and adult onset diabetes mellitus status-post TAH/BSO (all margins negative) with 1 of 5 pelvic nodes positive for metastatic carcinoma and a 5-cm moderately differentiated endometrioid adenocarcinoma invading greater than one-half of the myometrium with positive LVSI, recommendations would include external beam radiotherapy to the pelvis using IMRT followed by HDR brachytherapy to the vaginal cuff with sequential carboplatin/paclitaxel CT.

SECTION EDITOR'S NOTE

William Small, Jr.

All 3 opinions agree on the use of CT and radiotherapy. The opinions differ on the evaluation and exact radiotherapy regimens. I would favor cross-sectional imaging of the chest, abdomen, and pelvis with a PET/CT reserved for equivocal results. In the absence of abnormal imaging, I would deliver IMRT to a modified extended field (approximately L1/L2) possibly followed by a vaginal cuff boost. This would then be followed by 4 to 6 cycles of carboplatin/paclitaxel CT.

REFERENCES

1. Shah PH, Kudrimoti M, Feddock J, Randall M. Adjuvant treatment for stage IIIC endometrial cancer: Options and controversies. *Gynecol Oncol.* 2011 Sep;122(3):675–683.
2. Creasman WT, Morrow CP, Bundy BN, et al. Surgical pathologic spread patterns of endometrial cancer. A Gynecologic Oncology Group Study. *Cancer.* 1987 Oct 15;60(8 Suppl):2035–2041.
3. Mariani A, Dowdy SC, Cliby WA, et al. Prospective assessment of lymphatic dissemination in endometrial cancer: A paradigm shift in surgical staging. *Gynecol Oncol.* 2008 Apr;109(1):11–18.
4. McMeekin DS, Lashbrook D, Gold M, et al. Nodal distribution and its significance in FIGO stage IIIc endometrial cancer. *Gynecol Oncol.* 2001 Aug;82(2):375–379.
5. Benedetti Panici P, Basile S, Maneschi F, et al. Systematic pelvic lymphadenectomy vs. no lymphadenectomy in early-stage endometrial carcinoma: Randomized clinical trial. *J Natl Cancer Inst.* 2008 Dec 3;100(23):1707–1716.
6. Kitchener H, Swart AM, Qian Q, et al. Efficacy of systematic pelvic lymphadenectomy in endometrial cancer (MRC ASTEC trial): A randomised study. *Lancet.* 2009 Jan 10;373(9658):125–136.
7. May K, Bryant A, Dickinson HO, et al. Lymphadenectomy for the management of endometrial cancer. *Cochrane Database Syst Rev.* 2010 Jan 20;(1):CD007585.
8. Aalders JG, Thomas G. Endometrial cancer—revisiting the importance of pelvic and para aortic lymph nodes. *Gynecol Oncol.* 2007 Jan;104(1): 222–231.

9. Rotman M, Pajak TF, Choi K, et al. Prophylactic extended-field irradiation of para-aortic lymph nodes in stages IIB and bulky IB and IIA cervical carcinomas. Ten-year treatment results of RTOG 79-20. *JAMA*. 1995 Aug 2;274(5): 387–393.

10. Small W Jr, Winter K, Levenback C, et al. Extended-field irradiation and intracavitary brachytherapy combined with cisplatin chemotherapy for cervical cancer with positive para-aortic or high common iliac lymph nodes: Results of ARM 1 of RTOG 0116. *Int J Radiat Oncol Biol Phys*. 2007 Jul 15;68(4):1081–1087.

11. Nelson G, Randall M, Sutton G, et al. FIGO stage IIIC endometrial carcinoma with metastases confined to pelvic lymph nodes: Analysis of treatment outcomes, prognostic variables, and failure patterns following adjuvant radiation therapy. *Gynecol Oncol*. 1999 Nov;75(2): 211–214.

12. Maggi R, Lissoni A, Spina F, et al. Adjuvant chemotherapy vs radiotherapy in high-risk endometrial carcinoma: Results of a randomised trial. *Br J Cancer*. 2006 Aug 7;95(3):266–271.

13. Chao A, Chang TC, Ng KK, et al. 18F-FDG PET in the management of endometrial cancer. *Eur J Nucl Med Mol Imaging*. 2006 Jan;33(1): 36–44.

14. Kitajima K, Suzuki K, Senda M, et al. Preoperative nodal staging of uterine cancer: Is contrast-enhanced PET/CT more accurate than non-enhanced PET/CT or enhanced CT alone? *Ann Nucl Med*. 2011 Aug;25(7):511–519.

15. Park JY, Kim EN, Kim DY, et al. Comparison of the validity of magnetic resonance imaging and positron emission tomography/computed tomography in the preoperative evaluation of patients with uterine corpus cancer. *Gynecol Oncol*. 2008 Mar;108(3):486–492.

16. Signorelli M, Guerra L, Buda A, et al. Role of the integrated FDG PET/CT in the surgical management of patients with high risk clinical early stage endometrial cancer: Detection of pelvic nodal metastases. *Gynecol Oncol*. 2009 Nov;115(2):231–235.

17. Randall ME, Filiaci VL, Muss H, et al. Randomized phase III trial of whole-abdominal irradiation versus doxorubicin and cisplatin chemotherapy in advanced endometrial carcinoma: A Gynecologic Oncology Group Study. *J Clin Oncol*. 2006 Jan 1;24(1):36–44.

18. Susumu N, Sagae S, Udagawa Y, et al. Randomized phase III trial of pelvic radiotherapy versus cisplatin-based combined chemotherapy in patients with intermediate- and high-risk endometrial cancer: A Japanese Gynecologic Oncology Group study. *Gynecol Oncol*. 2008 Jan;108(1):226–233.

19. Homesley HD, Filiaci V, Gibbons SK, et al. A randomized phase III trial in advanced endometrial carcinoma of surgery and volume directed radiation followed by cisplatin and doxorubicin with or without paclitaxel: A Gynecologic Oncology Group study. *Gynecol Oncol*. 2009 Mar;112(3):543–552.

20. Alvarez Secord A, Havrilesky LJ, Bae-Jump V, et al. The role of multi-modality adjuvant chemotherapy and radiation in women with advanced stage endometrial cancer. *Gynecol Oncol*. 2007 Nov;107(2):285–291.

21. Geller MA, Ivy J, Dusenbery KE, et al. A single institution experience using sequential multi-modality adjuvant chemotherapy and radiation in the "sandwich" method for high risk endometrial carcinoma. *Gynecol Oncol*. 2010 Jul;118(1):19–23.

22. Hogberg T, Signorelli M, de Oliveira CF, et al. Sequential adjuvant chemotherapy and radiotherapy in endometrial cancer–results from two randomised studies. *Eur J Cancer*. 2010 Sep;46(13):2422–2431.

23. Duenas-Gonzalez A, Zarba JJ, Patel F, et al. Phase III, open-label, randomized study comparing concurrent gemcitabine plus cisplatin and radiation followed by adjuvant gemcitabine and cisplatin versus concurrent cisplatin and radiation in patients with stage IIB to IVA carcinoma of the cervix. *J Clin Oncol*. 2011 May 1;29(13):1678–1685.

24. Lorvidhaya V, Chitapanarux I, Sangruchi S, et al. Concurrent mitomycin C, 5-fluorouracil, and radiotherapy in the treatment of locally advanced carcinoma of the cervix: A randomized trial. *Int J Radiat Oncol Biol Phys*. 2003 Apr 1;55(5):1226–1232.

25. Greven K, Winter K, Underhill K, et al. Final analysis of RTOG 9708: Adjuvant postoperative irradiation combined with cisplatin/paclitaxel chemotherapy following surgery for patients with high-risk endometrial cancer. *Gynecol Oncol*. 2006 Oct;103(1):155–159.

26. Nakayama K, Nagai Y, Ishikawa M, et al. Concomitant postoperative radiation and chemotherapy following surgery was associated with improved overall survival in patients with FIGO stages III and IV endometrial cancer. *Int J Clin Oncol*. 2010 Oct;15(5):440–446.

27. Ahmed RS, Kim RY, Duan J, et al. IMRT dose escalation for positive para-aortic lymph nodes in patients with locally advanced cervical cancer while reducing dose to bone marrow and other organs at risk. *Int J Radiat Oncol Biol Phys*. 2004 Oct 1;60(2):505–512.

28. Portelance L, Chao KS, Grigsby PW, et al. Intensity-modulated radiation therapy (IMRT) reduces small bowel, rectum, and bladder doses in patients with cervical cancer receiving pelvic and para-aortic irradiation. *Int J Radiat Oncol Biol Phys*. 2001 Sep 1;51(1):261–266.

29. Salama JK, Mundt AJ, Roeske J, Mehta N. Preliminary outcome and toxicity report of extended-field, intensity-modulated radiation therapy for gynecologic malignances. *Int J Radiat Oncol Biol Phys*. 2006 Jul 15;65(4):1170–1176.

30. Havrilesky LJ, Cragun JM, Calingaert B, et al. Resection of lymph node metastases influences survival in stage IIIC endometrial cancer. *Gynecol Oncol*. 2005 Dec;99(3):689–695.

31. Fujimoto T, Nanjyo H, Nakamura A, et al. Para-aortic lymphadenectomy may improve disease-related survival in patients with multipositive pelvic lymph node stage IIIc endometrial cancer. *Gynecol Oncol*. 2007 Nov;107(2):253–259.

32. Kilgore LC, Partridge EE, Alvarez RD, et al. Adenocarcinoma of the endometrium: survival comparisons of patients with and without pelvic node sampling. *Gynecol Oncol*. 1995 Jan;56(1):29–33.

33. Todo Y, Kato H, Kaneuchi M, et al. Survival effect of para-aortic lymphadenectomy in endometrial cancer (SEPAL study): A retrospective cohort analysis. *Lancet*. 2010 Apr 3;375(9721): 1165–1172.

34. Huang M, Chadha M, Musa F, et al. Lymph nodes: Is total number or station number a better predictor of lymph node metastasis in endometrial cancer? *Gynecol Oncol*. 2010 Nov;119(2): 295–298.

35. Lutman CV, Havrilesky LJ, Cragun JM, et al. Pelvic lymph node count is an important prognostic variable for FIGO stage I and II endometrial carcinoma with high-risk histology. *Gynecol Oncol*. 2006 Jul;102(1):92–97.

36. Kosary CL. FIGO stage, histology, histologic grade, age and race as prognostic factors in determining survival for cancers of the female gynecological system: An analysis of 1973-87 SEER cases of cancers of the endometrium, cervix, ovary, vulva, and vagina. *Semin Surg Oncol*. 1994 Jan–Feb;10(1):31–46.

37. Resnick KE, Cohn DE, Fowler JM. Role of lymphadenectomy in the staging of endometrial cancer. *Nat Rev Clin Oncol*. 2009 Jul;6(7):382–384.

38. Creutzberg CL, van Putten WL, Koper PC, et al. Surgery and postoperative radiotherapy versus surgery alone for patients with stage-1 endometrial carcinoma: multicentre randomised trial. PORTEC Study Group. Post Operative Radiation Therapy in Endometrial Carcinoma. *Lancet*. 2000 Apr 22;355(9213):1404–1411.

39. Aalders J, Abeler V, Kolstad P, Onsrud M. Postoperative external irradiation and prognostic parameters in stage I endometrial carcinoma: Clinical and histopathologic study of 540 patients. *Obstet Gynecol*. 1980 Oct;56(4):419–427.

40. Keys HM, Roberts JA, Brunetto VL, et al. A phase III trial of surgery with or without adjunctive external pelvic radiation therapy in intermediate risk endometrial adenocarcinoma: A Gynecologic Oncology Group study. *Gynecol Oncol*. 2004 Mar;92(3):744–751.

41. Malzoni M, Tinelli R, Cosentino F, et al. Total laparoscopic hysterectomy versus abdominal hysterectomy with lymphadenectomy for early-stage endometrial cancer: A prospective randomized study. *Gynecol Oncol*. 2009 Jan;112(1):126–133.

42. Janda M, Gebski V, Brand A, et al. Quality of life after total laparoscopic hysterectomy versus total abdominal hysterectomy for stage I endometrial cancer (LACE): A randomised trial. *Lancet Oncol*. 2010 Aug;11(8):772–780.

43. Devaja O, Samara I, Papadopoulos AJ. Laparoscopically assisted vaginal hysterectomy (LAVH) versus total abdominal hysterectomy (TAH) in endometrial carcinoma: Prospective cohort study. *Int J Gynecol Cancer*. 2010 May;20(4):570–575.

44. Barton DP, Naik R, Herod J. Efficacy of systematic pelvic lymphadenectomy in endometrial cancer (MRC ASTEC Trial): A randomized study. *Int J Gynecol Cancer*. 2009 Nov;19(8):1465.

45. Small W, Jr., Mell LK, Anderson P, et al. Consensus guidelines for delineation of clinical target volume for intensity-modulated pelvic radiotherapy in postoperative treatment of endometrial and cervical cancer. *Int J Radiat Oncol Biol Phys*. 2008 Jun 1;71(2):428–434.

46. Heron DE, Gerszten K, Selvaraj RN, et al. Conventional 3D conformal versus intensity-modulated radiotherapy for the adjuvant treatment of gynecologic malignancies: A comparative dosimetric study of dose-volume histograms small star, filled. *Gynecol Oncol*. 2003 Oct;91(1):39–45.

47. Mundt AJ, Lujan AE, Rotmensch J, et al. Intensity-modulated whole pelvic radiotherapy in women with gynecologic malignancies. *Int J Radiat Oncol Biol Phys*. 2002 Apr 1;52(5):1330–1337.

48. Roeske JC, Lujan A, Rotmensch J, et al. Intensity-modulated whole pelvic radiation therapy in patients with gynecologic malignancies. *Int J Radiat Oncol Biol Phys*. 2000 Dec 1;48(5): 1613–1621.

49. Roeske JC, Bonta D, Mell LK, et al. A dosimetric analysis of acute gastrointestinal toxicity in women receiving intensity-modulated whole-pelvic radiation therapy. *Radiother Oncol*. 2003 Nov;69(2):201–207.

■ **CASE 3** ■

Use of Pelvic Radiotherapy in Intermediate-Risk Endometrial Cancer

CLINICAL PROBLEM

Given recent randomized trial results, the use of pelvic radiotherapy (RT) and lymph node dissection has fallen out of favor in "intermediate-risk" endometrial cancer patients. When, or whether, to use pelvic RT in intermediate-risk endometrial cancer is a common clinical dilemma.

CASE EXAMPLE

A 65-year-old female undergoes a total abdominal hysterectomy and bilateral salpingo-oophorectoomy (TAH/BSO) for a biopsy-proven grade 2, endometrial adenocarcinoma. The final pathology reveals a 2.5 cm, grade 3 endometrioid adenocarcinoma invading 15 of 18 mm of the myometrium with lymphovascular space invasion (LVSI).

Management Decisions

- What is the need for imaging?
- What is the role of a staging lymphadenectomy?
- What is the influence of tumor size, grade, depth of invasion, and age on risk for residual pelvic disease/lymph node metastasis and the need for pelvic RT?
- If used, what type of pelvic RT should be administered—intensity-modulated radiation therapy (IMRT) versus 3-D conformal therapy versus alternative techniques?

MAJOR OPINION

Loren Mell

This patient has high–intermediate-risk (HIR) disease as per Gynecologic Oncology Group (GOG) criteria and high-risk stage I disease by Postoperative Radiation Therapy for Endometrial Carcinoma (PORTEC) criteria. The first issue to address is regarding what other staging workup is necessary. Pelvic CT has a low specificity (57%) and positive predictive value (50%) [1] for pelvic nodal metastasis, and the pretest probability of distant metastatic disease, eg, to the liver or lung, is miniscule [2]. PET or PET/CT, while sensitive for nodal metastases when it is greater than about 1 cm, is probably more likely to yield a false-positive finding in this perioperative setting. MRI is useful to evaluate the extent of myometrial invasion and cervical invasion preoperatively, and may be superior to CT for evaluation of lymphadenopathy [3,4]. While pelvic MRI could be considered to assess for lymphadenopathy, its utility in the postoperative staging workup of uterine-confined disease is limited, and I would not recommend it in this case.

The likelihood of upstaging this patient on the basis of findings from lymphadenectomy is considerable. In the study by Creasman et al. [5], the probabilities of pelvic and para-aortic nodal spread in women with grade 3 deeply invasive tumors were 34% and 23%, respectively. Similarly, Chi et al. [6] found that the probability of pelvic nodal metastasis in clinical stage IB endometrial cancer was 28%. However, the randomized trials of lymphadenectomy discussed previously did not show evidence of a survival benefit to pelvic lymphadenectomy [7,8]. Both studies found similar treatment effect estimates, trending toward worse survival in the lymphadenectomy group. Both studies have also been criticized for failing to control completely for the delivery of adjuvant therapy, although A Study in the Treatment of Endometrial Cancer (ASTEC) trial controlled this partially by randomizing intermediate- and high-risk patients to pelvic RT, and the use of adjuvant therapy was well balanced across its 2 arms. These trials included many patients with a lower risk of nodal metastasis, and

98

neither was powered to detect a survival benefit in the high-risk subgroup. Still, neither study found a benefit of treatment even in high-risk subgroups; therefore, pelvic lymphadenectomy should not be advocated on the grounds of a therapeutic benefit. Interestingly, a large retrospective cohort study did find a survival benefit with para-aortic lymphadenectomy [9], but this hypothesis has not been tested in a randomized trial. In principle, tailoring adjuvant treatment according to pathologic stage should provide a therapeutic advantage to the patient. Because decisions such as whether to deliver adjuvant chemotherapy and whether to irradiate para-aortic lymph nodes in this patient hinge so critically on full pathologic staging, I would advocate for pelvic lymphadenectomy and para-aortic nodal sampling in order to optimally fashion her adjuvant therapy.

Irrespective of the findings after staging lymphadenectomy, for this patient I would recommend adjuvant RT if she were not to be treated in a clinical trial. In the absence of further therapy, this patient's 5-year risk of locoregional and distant recurrence are each approximately 30%. The majority of locoregional recurrences (LRRs) occur at the vaginal cuff [10,11], and therefore vaginal brachytherapy may be adequate for the majority of patients with intermediate-risk disease. However, the PORTEC-2 study, which concluded that vaginal brachytherapy is the treatment of choice for this subpopulation, excluded high-risk stage I patients such as the case presented here.

Pelvic RT has been shown to reduce the incidence of locoregional failure in early stage endometrial cancer by approximately twofold [10–13]. RT appears to be superior to chemotherapy alone for reducing LRR, while chemotherapy is superior to RT for reducing distant metastasis [14]. Therefore, it is likely that a combination of chemotherapy and RT would provide the best opportunity for long-term disease control. Interestingly, randomized trials have repeatedly failed to show survival benefits of either chemotherapy or RT in the treatment of high-risk early stage endometrial cancer [15–17]. Newer trials such as GOG-249 and PORTEC-3 [18] are seeking to test combined therapy regimens and would be applicable to this patient. GOG-249 is randomizing HIR patients to pelvic RT versus vaginal brachytherapy plus 3 cycles of carboplatin/paclitaxel, and would be the trial I would recommend for this patient if she were treated at my institution. If I could recommend any trial, I would choose PORTEC-3, which

would randomize her to pelvic RT (46.8 Gy in 26 fractions) versus pelvic RT with 2 cycles of concurrent cisplatin and 4 cycles of adjuvant carboplatin/paclitaxel.

Off-trial, if the lymphadenectomy were complete, extensive (ie, more than 12 nodes removed), and negative, then I would recommend vaginal brachytherapy 7 Gy × 3 to 0.5 cm, as the preponderance of failures in this setting are at the vaginal cuff, and there is some concern that pelvic RT could augment the risk of lymphedema. The absolute risk of lymphedema following hysterectomy with lymphadenectomy and external beam RT (EBRT), however, was low in both the ASTEC and GOG-99 trials. If the lymphadenectomy were incomplete, then I would recommend pelvic IMRT. If her nodal staging were positive, then I would recommend adjuvant chemotherapy and pelvic IMRT with para-aortic nodal field if either high common or para-aortic nodes were involved, according to the GOG 258 trial if the patient could not go on trial.

Many studies have indicated that IMRT can reduce gastrointestinal (GI) toxicity in patients who have endometrial cancer [19–23]. Multicenter randomized trials comparing pelvic IMRT to 4-field box techniques are under development, and IMRT techniques are currently allowed on postoperative endometrial cancer trials that are conducted through the GOG and the Radiation Therapy Oncology Group (RTOG). I would use a dose of 45 Gy in 25 daily fractions, with the clinical target volume (CTV) delineation per consensus guidelines [24]. I would simulate the patient with an empty bladder, and use planning margins of 5 mm around the nodal CTV, 15 mm around the vaginal cuff, and 10 mm elsewhere. I would use online cone beam CT to verify the position of the vaginal cuff with each treatment. Three recent studies have indicated that planning margins on the order of 15 to 20 mm are needed around the vaginal cuff to ensure adequate coverage during EBRT [25–27]. If daily image-guided RT is unavailable, I would recommend using either planning margins of 2 cm around the vaginal cuff or an internal target volume (per RTOG 0418).

ACADEMIC COMMENT

Catheryn Yashar

There have been 2 randomized studies that have attempted to evaluate whether pelvic lymph node dissection provides a survival advantage in endometrial carcinoma [7,8]. Neither study was able to demonstrate a survival advantage with lymphadenectomy, although some argue that the studies were flawed [28]. For many years, the Europeans have omitted lymphadenectomy, especially in low-risk patients. Recently, the PORTEC-2 study found that vaginal cuff brachytherapy was not statistically inferior to whole pelvic irradiation in reducing vaginal recurrence, although pelvic nodal failure rates did differ significantly (3.5% vs. 0.9%) [12]. Again, routine lymph node dissection was omitted in this study.

The population studied in PORTEC-2 was purportedly of higher risk than PORTEC-1, although the HIR population for PORTEC-2 is not as high risk as the HIR population identified by GOG 99. In PORTEC-1, stage IB grade 3 (AJCC 7th edition) patients were excluded from the randomization to pelvic RT versus observation. In POR-TEC-2, clear cell and papillary serous tumors were excluded as well. The HIR patient in PORTEC-1 was identified as having 2 of the following 3 characteristics: grade 3 tumor, outer half myometrial invasion (MMI), and age over 60 years. In GOG-99, HIR stage I disease was defined as either: (a) age 70 or more with 1 other risk factor, (b) age 50 or more with 2 risk factors, or (c) age 18 or more with 3 risk factors, where risk factors include grade 2–3, outer 33% MMI, and LVSI. In PORTEC-1, patients with HIR disease and no adjuvant pelvic irradiation had a recurrence rate of 23% versus 5% with pelvic irradiation ($p < .0001$), respectively (Figure 4.3.1). In GOG-99, patients with HIR disease and no adjuvant pelvic irradiation had a recurrence rate of 27% versus 13% with pelvic irradiation. Local recurrence rates for observation versus pelvic RT were 13% versus 5%. In both trials, vaginal disease represented 75% of the LRRs. In PORTEC-2, 80% were deeply invasive, but more than 90% were grades 1 or 2 (after review, 79% were grade 1), so it is not clear that the results from PORTEC-2 are applicable to the current patient.

The current patient is 65 years of age with a grade 3 deeply invasive cancer, 2.5 cm in size with LVSI. She fits both definitions of HIR disease, but does not fit into the PORTEC-2 study, which would suggest that vaginal cuff brachytherapy is sufficient. She fits more clearly into the nonrandomized PORTEC-1 study [30], where all patients with stage IC grade 3 were treated with pelvic irradiation and still had a locoregional failure rate of 14% at 5 years.

The best course of action in my opinion is to enroll the patient on the GOG 0249 trial, which randomizes HIR patients (GOG definition), regardless of nodal dissection, to vaginal cuff brachytherapy and 3 cycles of carboplatin/paclitaxel versus whole pelvic RT [31]. For pelvic RT, either 4-field, 3-D conformal, or IMRT techniques are allowed. For brachytherapy, either low-dose-rate (LDR) or high-dose-rate (HDR)

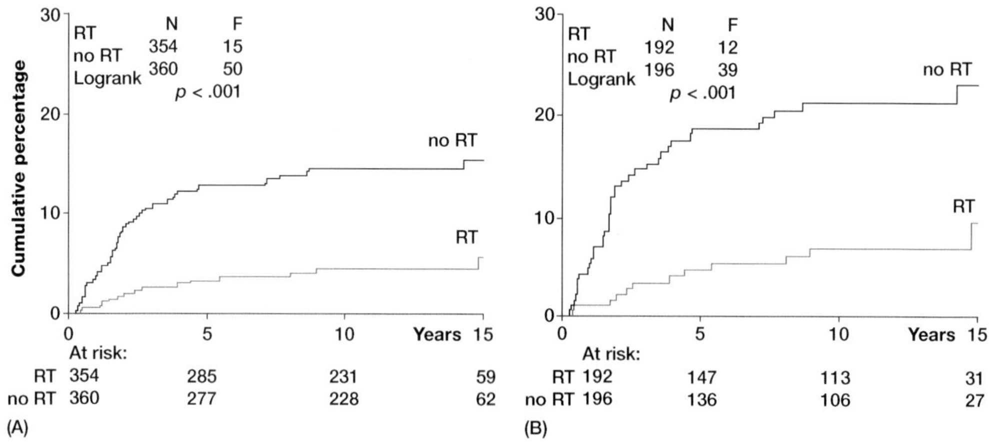

FIGURE 4.3.1 ■ Probability of locoregional (vaginal and/or pelvic) relapse for patients assigned to postoperative RT or no additional treatment (NAT) for the total group (A) and for patients with HIR features (B). *Source*: From Creutzberg et al. [29] used with permission.

techniques are acceptable. HDR brachytherapy is given as either 6 to 7 Gy × 3 fractions a week to 0.5 cm, 10 to 10.5 Gy × 3 fractions a week to the vaginal surface, or 6 Gy × 5 fractions 2 to 3 times a week to the surface. Off-protocol, I would propose pelvic RT using IMRT as the primary choice. If the patient were to refuse pelvic RT, then I would recommend a lymph node dissection, and if negative, I would recommend vaginal cuff brachytherapy and chemotherapy per the experimental arm of the GOG 0249 study. If she were found to have positive lymph nodes, then I would recommend she go on the GOG 0258 trial, which randomizes patients to 6 cycles of carboplatin/paclitaxel alone versus volume-directed RT with concurrent cisplatin and 4 cycles of adjuvant carboplatin/paclitaxel [32].

COMMUNITY PRACTITIONER COMMENT

Michael A. Nichols

Previous studies have identified several factors associated with increased risk of relapses in patients with stage I–IIA endometrial cancer [10,30,33–37]: advanced age, high grade, deep MMI, and LVSI. In the analysis of the PORTEC-1 study, grade 3 histology was the most significant predictor of relapse and death [30], with an increased hazard ratio (HR) for death and relapse compared to depth of MMI (HR 5.5 versus 2.1). LVSI has also been shown to predict for distant failure in patients who were not surgically staged and had disease believed to be confined to the uterus [10,34,35]. Age is a known adverse prognostic indicator [10,34,36,37]. While increased tumor size is generally considered a negative prognostic indicator, this has not been convincingly shown after controlling for factors such as grade and depth of invasion.

Patients with stage I–IIA endometrial cancer are categorized as HIR by the GOG as defined earlier. This patient would qualify as HIR, and actually has 3 adverse risk factors. She has stage IB grade 3 disease by the current (7th edition) AJCC staging system [38]. It is important to note, however, that there have been recent changes to the staging criteria and that patients previously considered to be stage IC are now stage IB. According to staging systems used in previous randomized controlled trials relevant to the discussion of her case, her stage is IC grade 3.

In this case, pelvic lymph node dissection was not performed, and we do not have any preoperative imaging. An appropriate question here is whether the patient would gain any therapeutic benefit from a pelvic lymph node dissection. This is a point of debate. The incidence of positive pelvic lymph nodes for patients with stage I disease ranges from 5% to 15% [5–8]. In this patient with 3 high-risk factors and age approaching 70, I would estimate her risk of positive nodes closer to 15%. Two recent randomized controlled trials from Europe suggest that the patient would not derive a survival benefit from lymphadenectomy [7,8]. However, older data from North America suggest that lymphadenectomy is beneficial [39,40]. In particular, Chan et al., in a retrospective study of over 27,000 women, observed a disease-free survival advantage to lymphadenectomy for patients with a stage IB grade 3 (AJCC 7th edition) disease [40]. For this patient, I would recommend a pelvic CT scan to assess whether she has any pathologically enlarged lymph nodes postoperatively. If bulky or necrotic nodes were seen, then I would recommend lymphadenectomy. If her imaging were negative, then I would not recommend lymphadenectomy, given its lack of clear therapeutic benefit.

The benefit of postoperative whole pelvic RT has been addressed in several randomized controlled trials. None, however, have adequately evaluated the role of whole pelvic irradiation versus observation in the specific subgroup of patients with stage IB grade 3 (AJCC 7th edition) disease. The trial by Aalders et al. [41] randomized women with stage I endometrial cancer to whole pelvic RT versus observation following TAH-BSO and vaginal brachytherapy. Their findings indicated a possible survival benefit in the subgroup with stage IB grade 3 (AJCC 7th edition) disease. The benefit of whole pelvic RT in the postoperative setting in patients who did not undergo staging lymphadenectomy was addressed in the PORTEC-1 trial [11]. This study, which randomized patients with stage I endometrial cancer to observation or whole pelvic irradiation, found that pelvic RT improved locoregional control, but not overall survival.

It is important to note, however, that stage IB grade 3 (AJCC 7th edition) patients were excluded from PORTEC-1 because it was thought to be unethical to randomize patients with deep MMI and high risk of occult pelvic nodal disease to observation [30]. Patients who were stage IB grade 3 (AJCC 7th edition) were registered and followed for outcome following whole pelvic irradiation [30].

Notably, these patients were more likely to have LVSI than other stage I patients (17% versus 2%–9%, $p < .001$). Following pelvic irradiation, the 5-year LRR was 14% for stage IB grade 3 (AJCC 7th edition) disease compared to 1% to 3% for other stage I patients on the PORTEC-1 trial. Pelvic-only failure was 8%. Overall survival was only 58% for stage IB grade 3 (AJCC 7th edition) compared to 74% for those with stage IA grade 3 (AJCC 7th edition) or 83% to 85% for others with grade 1–2 disease. Grade 3 GI complications were 3%. In a retrospective analysis of over 21,000 patients from the Surveillance Epidemiology and End Results (SEER) database, a survival benefit was observed specifically for patients with stage IB grade 3 (AJCC 7th edition) disease when treated with postoperative RT, regardless of whether patients had undergone lymph node dissection. This analysis included patients treated with either whole pelvic irradiation or brachytherapy [42].

In the PORTEC-2 trial [12], stage IB grade 3 (AJCC 7th edition) patients were again excluded. Routine lymphadenectomy was not performed, although clinically suspicious pelvic or para-aortic lymph nodes were sampled. Patients with stage I–IIA (other than stage IB grade 3) endometrial carcinoma were randomized to postoperative whole pelvic EBRT or vaginal brachytherapy. In this study, the risk of pelvic recurrence was 5.1% in patients treated with vaginal brachytherapy versus 2.1% for EBRT ($p = .17$). However, as noted earlier, in the PORTEC-1 trial, patients with stage IB grade 3 (AJCC 7th edition) disease had a failure rate of 14% following whole pelvic irradiation. When looking only at the risk of pelvic recurrence, the failure was reduced from 3.8% to 0.5% at 5 years ($p = .02$). If one assumes a magnitude of even a fivefold decrease, then the failure in patients from PORTEC-1 with stage IB grade 3 (AJCC 7th edition) would drop from 40% to 8%. This is consistent with data from Mundt et al. [43], which show a failure rate of 31% in the pelvis in patients with high risk of advanced endometrial carcinoma treated using adjuvant chemotherapy without pelvic irradiation.

In this patient, I would recommend whole pelvic RT, as opposed to vaginal cuff brachytherapy, and would recommend treating her with IMRT. Multiple reports have demonstrated improvement of rectal, small bowel, and bladder doses [44–48] using IMRT for pelvic irradiation. There is also evidence of reduction in both acute and chronic GI toxicity with resultant decrease in the need for antidiarrheal medication [19–21]. Importantly, IMRT may also improve target volume coverage when compared to a conventional 4-field plan [49].

As a guide for contouring, I recommend referring to the contouring atlas published on the RTOG website [50]. This atlas was based on consensus volumes generated by a panel of radiation oncologists [24]. These guidelines are used as a general guide and we modify volumes and expansions as appropriate depending on patient anatomy, operative note, and pathology. I recommend using any relevant preoperative and postoperative imaging in considering volumes, as well as findings on planning CT, when necessary. I use kV–kV matching and weekly cone beam CT to verify set-up accuracy. Typically, we are able to achieve coverage of over 95% of the PTV with over 95% of the prescription dose, but we attempt to treat more than 97% of the PTV of the prescription dose. We limit hot spots to less than 0.03 mL of PTV receiving more than 110% of the prescribed dose, and cold spots to less than 0.03 mL receiving lesser than 93% of the prescribed dose.

SECTION EDITOR'S NOTE

William Small, Jr.

I would recommend cross-sectional imaging with PET/CT for equivocal results. If there were no evidence for distant metastasis or lymphadenopathy, I would proceed with pelvic RT delivered with IMRT.

REFERENCES

1. Connor JP, Andrews JI, Anderson B, et al. Computed tomography in endometrial carcinoma. *Obstet Gynecol.* 2000;95:692–696.

2. Heyer H, Ohlinger R, Arndt D, et al. Selective pretreatment diagnostic imaging for detecting remote metastases in patients with endometrial cancer. *Onkologie.* 2006;29:85–89.

3. Lee JH, Dubinsky T, Andreotti RF, et al. ACR Appropriateness Criteria®: Pretreatment evaluation and follow-up of endometrial cancer of the uterus. *Ultrasound Q.* 2011;27:139–145.

4. Rockall AG, Meroni R, Sohaib SA, et al. Evaluation of endometrial carcinoma on magnetic resonance imaging. *Int J Gynecol Cancer.* 2007;17:188–196.

5. Creasman WT, Morrow CP, Bundy BN, et al. Surgical pathologic spread patterns of endometrial cancer. A Gynecologic Oncology Group Study. *Cancer.* 1987;60(8 Suppl):2035–2041.

6. Chi DS, Barakat RR, Palayekar MJ, et al. The incidence of pelvic lymph node metastasis by FIGO staging for patients with adequately surgically staged endometrial adenocarcinoma of endometrioid histology. *Int J Gynecol Cancer.* 2008;18:269–273.

7. Benedetti Panici P, Basile S, Maneschi F, et al. Systematic pelvic lymphadenectomy vs. no lymphadenectomy in early-stage endometrial carcinoma: randomized clinical trial. *J Natl Cancer Inst.* 2008;100:1707–1716.

8. ASTEC study group, Kitchener H, Swart AM, et al. Efficacy of systematic pelvic lymphadenectomy in endometrial cancer (MRC ASTEC trial): A randomised study. *Lancet.* 2009;373:125–136.

9. Todo Y, Kato H, Kaneuchi M, et al. Survival effect of para-aortic lymphadenectomy in endometrial cancer (SEPAL study): A retrospective cohort analysis. *Lancet.* 2010;375:1165–1172.

10. Keys HM, Roberts JA, Brunetto VL, et al. A phase III trial of surgery with or without adjunctive external pelvic radiation therapy in intermediate risk endometrial adenocarcinoma: A Gynecologic Oncology Group study. *Gynecol Oncol.* 2004;92:744–751.

11. Creutzberg CL, van Putten WL, Koper PC, et al. Surgery and postoperative radiotherapy versus surgery alone for patients with stage-1 endometrial carcinoma: Multicentre randomised trial. PORTEC Study Group. Post Operative Radiation Therapy in Endometrial Carcinoma. *Lancet.* 2000;355:1404–1411.

12. Nout RA, Smit VT, Putter H, et al. Vaginal brachytherapy versus pelvic external beam radiotherapy for patients with endometrial cancer of high-intermediate risk (PORTEC-2): An open-label, non-inferiority, randomised trial. *Lancet.* 2010;375:816–823.

13. ASTEC/EN.5 Study Group, Blake P, Swart AM, et al. Adjuvant external beam radiotherapy in the treatment of endometrial cancer (MRC ASTEC and NCIC CTG EN.5 randomised trials): Pooled trial results, systematic review, and meta-analysis. *Lancet.* 2009;373:137–146.

14. Maggi R, Lissoni A, Spina F, et al. Adjuvant chemotherapy vs radiotherapy in high-risk endometrial carcinoma: Results of a randomised trial. *Br J Cancer.* 2006;95:266–271.

15. Susumu N, Sagae S, Udagawa Y, et al. Randomized phase III trial of pelvic radiotherapy versus cisplatin-based combined chemotherapy in patients with intermediate- and high-risk endometrial cancer: A Japanese Gynecologic Oncology Group study. *Gynecol Oncol.* 2008;108:226–233.

16. Hogberg T. Adjuvant chemotherapy in endometrial carcinoma: overview of randomised trials. *Clin Oncol (R Coll Radiol).* 2008;20:463–469.

17. Hogberg T, Signorelli M, de Oliveira CF, et al. Sequential adjuvant chemotherapy and radiotherapy in endometrial cancer—results from two randomised studies. *Eur J Cancer.* 2010;46: 2422–2431.

18. http://www.trialregister.nl/trialreg/admin/rct view.asp?TC=729, Accessed July 9, 2011.

19. Mundt AJ, Lujan AE, Rotmensch J, et al. Intensity-modulated whole pelvic radiotherapy in women with gynecologic malignancies. *Int J Radiat Oncol Biol Phys.* 2002;52:1330–1337.

20. Mundt AJ, Mell LK, Roeske JC. Preliminary analysis of chronic gastrointestinal toxicity in gynaecologic patients treated with intensity-modulated whole pelvic radiation therapy. *Int J Radiat Oncol Biol Phys.* 2003;56:1354–1360.

21. Chen MF, Tseng CJ, Tseng CC, et al. Adjuvant concurrent chemoradiotherapy with intensity-modulated pelvic radiotherapy after surgery for high-risk, early stage cervical cancer patients. *Cancer J.* 2008;14:200–206.

22. Jhingran A, Winter K, Portelance L. A phase II study of intensity modulated radiation therapy (IMRT) to the pelvis for post-operative patients with endometrial carcinoma (RTOG 0418) (abstr.) *Int J Radiat Oncol Biol Phys.* 2008;72:S16–S17.

23. Roeske JC, Bonta D, Mell LK, et al. A dosimetric analysis of acute gastrointestinal toxicity in women receiving intensity-modulated whole-pelvic radiation therapy. *Radiother Oncol.* 2003;69:201–207.

24. Small W Jr, Mell LK, Anderson P, et al. Consensus guidelines for delineation of clinical target volume for intensity-modulated pelvic radiotherapy in postoperative treatment of endometrial and cervical cancer. *Int J Radiat Oncol Biol Phys.* 2008;71:428–434.

25. Jhingran A, Salehpour M, Sam M, et al. Vaginal motion and bladder and rectal volumes during pelvic intensity-modulated radiation therapy after hysterectomy. *Int J Radiat Oncol Biol Phys.* 2012;82(1):256–262.

26. Harris EE, Latifi K, Rusthoven C, et al. Assessment of organ motion in postoperative endometrial and cervical cancer patients treated with intensity-modulated radiation therapy. *Int J Radiat Oncol Biol Phys.* 2011;81(4):e645–e650.

27. Ma DJ, Michaletz-Lorenz M, Goddu SM, Grigsby PW. Magnitude of interfractional vaginal cuff movement: Implications for external irradiation. *Int J Radiat Oncol Biol Phys.* 2012;82(4):1439–1444.

28. Seamon LG, Fowler JM, Cohn DE. Lymphadenectomy for endometrial cancer: The controversy. *Gynecol Oncol.* 2010;117:6–8.

29. Creutzberg CL, Nout RA, Lybeert ML, et al. Fifteen-year radiotherapy outcomes of the randomized PORTEC-1 trial for endometrial carcinoma. *Int J Radiat Oncol Biol Phys.* 2011;81(4): e631–e638.

30. Creutzberg CL, van Putten WL, Wárlám-Rodenhuis CC, et al. Outcome of high-risk stage IC, grade 3, compared with stage I endometrial carcinoma patients: The Postoperative Radiation Therapy in Endometrial Carcinoma Trial. *J Clin Oncol.* 2004;22:1234–1241.

31. http://www.clinicaltrials.gov/ct2/show/NCT 00807768?term=GOG&rank=19, Accessed July 9, 2011

32. http://www.clinicaltrials.gov/ct2/show/NCT 00942357?term=GOG&rank=102, Accessed July 9, 2011

33. Morrow CP, Bundy BN, Kurman RJ, et al. Relationship between surgical-pathological risk factors and outcome in clinical stage I and II carcinoma of the endometrium: A Gynecologic Oncology Group study. *Gynecol Oncol.* 1991;40:55–65.

34. Greven KM, Corn BW, Case D, et al. Which prognostic factors influence the outcome of patients with surgically staged endometrial cancer treated with adjuvant radiation? *Int J Radiat Oncol Biol Phys.* 1997;39:413–418.

35. Nofech-Mozes S, Ackerman I, Ghorab Z, et al. Lymphovascular invasion is a significant predictor for distant recurrence in patients with early-stage endometrial endometrioid adenocarcinoma. *Am J Clin Pathol.* 2008;129:912–917.

36. Irwin C, Levin W, Fyles A, et al. The role of adjuvant radiotherapy in carcinoma of the endometrium-results in 550 patients with pathologic stage I disease. *Gynecol Oncol.* 1998;70: 247–254.

37. Alektiar KM, Venkatraman E, Abu-Rustum N, Barakat RR. Is endometrial carcinoma intrinsically more aggressive in elderly patients? *Cancer.* 2003;98:2368–2377.

38. Edge SB, Byrd DR, Compton CC, et al. Eds. AJCC Cancer Staging Manual. 7th ed. Springer; 2010.

39. Mariani A, Webb MJ, Galli L, Podratz KC. Potential therapeutic role of para-aortic lymphadenectomy in node-positive endometrial cancer. *Gynecol Oncol.* 2000;76:348–356.

40. Chan JK, Wu H, Cheung MK, et al. The outcomes of 27,063 women with unstaged endometrioid uterine cancer. *Gynecol Oncol.* 2007; 106:282–288.

41. Aalders J, Abeler V, Kolstad P, et al. Postoperative external irradiation and prognostic parameters in stage I endometrial carcinoma: Clinical and histopathologic study of 540 patients. *Obstet Gynecol.* 1980;56:419–427.

42. Lee CM, Szabo A, Shrieve DC, et al. Frequency and effect of adjuvant radiation therapy among women with stage I endometrial adenocarcinoma. *JAMA.* 2006;295:389–397.

43. Mundt AJ, Murphy KT, Rotmensch J, et al. Surgery and postoperative radiation therapy in FIGO Stage IIIC endometrial carcinoma. *Int J Radiat Oncol Biol Phys.* 2001;50:1154–1160.

44. Roeske JC, Lujan A, Rotmensch J, et al. Intensity-modulated whole pelvic radiation therapy in patients with gynecologic malignancies. *Int J Radiat Oncol Biol Phys.* 2000;48:1613–1621.

45. Portelance L, Chao KS, Grigsby PW, et al. Intensity-modulated radiation therapy (IMRT) reduces small bowel, rectum, and bladder doses in patients with cervical cancer receiving pelvic and para-aortic irradiation. *Int J Radiat Oncol Biol Phys.* 2001;51:261–266.

46. Ahmed RS, Kim RY, Duan J, et al. IMRT dose escalation for positive para-aortic lymph nodes in patients with locally advanced cervical cancer while reducing dose to bone marrow and other organs at risk. *Int J Radiat Oncol Biol Phys.* 2004;60:505–512.

47. Guo S, Ennis RD, Bhatia S, et al. Assessment of nodal target definition and dosimetry using three different techniques: Implications for re-defining the optimal pelvic field in endometrial cancer. *Radiat Oncol.* 2010;5:59.

48. Ahamad A, D'Souza W, Salehpour M, et al. Intensity-modulated radiation therapy after hysterectomy: Comparison with conventional treatment and sensitivity of the normal-tissue-sparing effect to margin size. *Int J Radiat Oncol Biol Phys.* 2005;62:1117–1124.

49. Bouchard M, Nadeau S, Gingras L, et al. Clinical outcome of adjuvant treatment of endometrial cancer using aperture-based intensity-modulated radiotherapy. *Int J Radiat Oncol Biol Phys.* 2008;71:1343–1350.

50. http://www.rtog.org/CoreLab/Contouring Atlases/GYN.aspx, accessed July 9, 2011.

Section 5

▪ **GENITOURINARY** ▪

Section Editor: Stanley L. Liauw

<h1 style="text-align:center">■ CASE 1 ■</h1>

Utilization of Hormonal Therapy With Dose-Escalated Radiation Therapy in the Management of Intermediate-Risk Prostate Cancer

CLINICAL PROBLEM

Men who are treated with external beam radiation therapy (EBRT) for prostate cancer are candidates to receive concurrent hormonal therapy if they present with intermediate-risk features (PSA 10–20, Gleason score 7, or clinical stage T2b-c). Dose-escalated radiation therapy is often favored over standard-dose radiation to improve the likelihood of biochemical control. It is unclear how to balance the use of hormonal therapy with higher radiation dose, as a higher dose could minimize the impact of hormonal therapy. In addition, in consideration of the risks of hormonal therapy, it has been proposed that medical comorbidity could help select the best candidates for concurrent hormonal therapy.

CASE EXAMPLE

A 68-year-old man is diagnosed with adenocarcinoma of the prostate on the basis of a first-time screening PSA of 12 ng/mL. Biopsy shows 7 of 12 cores involved (2 with Gleason 4 + 3, 2 with Gleason 3 + 4, and 3 with Gleason 3 + 3). He has clinical T1c disease. He has a history of well-controlled coronary artery disease with myocardial infarction over 5 years ago treated by percutaneous intervention. Treatment with EBRT is proposed.

Management Decisions

- Is dose-escalated radiation therapy always indicated for men with intermediate-risk disease?
- If dose-escalated radiation therapy is given, is concurrent hormonal therapy indicated?
- How does comorbidity influence the recommendation for hormonal therapy?

MAJOR OPINION

Paul L. Nguyen

Is Dose-Escalated Radiation Therapy Always Indicated for Men With Intermediate-Risk Disease?

If a man with intermediate-risk prostate cancer receives radiation alone, ie, without hormonal therapy, then dose escalation is generally indicated. This is based on 2 randomized trials of men with localized prostate cancer who received conventional dose (70 Gy) versus dose-escalated radiation without hormonal therapy. The MD Anderson Trial, first reported by Pollack et al. and then updated by Kuban et al., randomized 301 patients with cT1b to T3 prostate cancer to 70 Gy in 2.0 Gy per fraction versus 78 Gy in 2.0 Gy per fraction prescribed to the isocenter [1,2]. The distribution of patients by risk group was 20% low risk, 46% intermediate risk, and 34% high risk. Freedom from clinical or biochemical failure was significantly improved with dose escalation (78% vs. 59% at 8 years, $p = .004$). In the planned subgroup analysis, those with PSA higher than 10 appeared to have the greatest benefit (78% vs. 39% at 8 years, $p = <.001$). Interestingly, when a post-hoc analysis was performed by risk group, there did not appear to be a benefit among intermediate-risk patients ($p = .36$), although among those with intermediate risk and a PSA greater than 10, there was a trend toward a benefit (94% vs. 65% at 8 years, $p = .07$). Given that the overall trial was positive, that intermediate risk was the largest group represented, and that post-hoc analyses have their limitations, this trial is generally interpreted as providing support for dose escalation in intermediate risk, especially when no hormonal therapy is used.

One subtlety of this trial is that because the doses were prescribed to the isocenter, the equivalent doses in the modern convention of prescribing to planning target volumes (PTVs) may be closer to 75.6 Gy versus 66.6 Gy, and so some practitioners use the MD Anderson Trial to justify 75.6 Gy to the PTV as the minimum acceptable dose when patients receive radiation alone.

The second trial is the PROG 95-09 trial that was a collaboration between the Massachusetts General Hospital and Loma Linda University. Reported by Zietman et al. in 2005 and then updated in 2010, this trial randomized 393 men with cT1b to T2b prostate cancer and PSA of 15 or lesser to 70.2 Gy equivalents (GyE) versus 79.2 GyE in 1.8 Gy fractions prescribed to the PTV [3,4]. The term GyE is used because the first 50.4 Gy was delivered by 3-D conformal radiation and then patients received a boost of either 19.8 GyE or 28.8 GyE using protons. The risk group distribution was mainly low (58%) and intermediate (37%) risk. The 10-year American Society for Radiation Oncology (ASTRO) biochemical failure rate was 32.3% for conventional dose and only 16.7% for the dose-escalated arm ($p = .0001$). Similar to the MD Anderson Trial, an unplanned post-hoc analysis of the intermediate-risk group ($n = 144$) did not quite show a statistically significant benefit, but there was a very strong trend favoring dose escalation (42.1% vs. 30.4% failure at 10 years, $p = .06$). Given that the overall trial was positive, this trial can be reasonably interpreted as also providing support for dose escalation in intermediate-risk disease when hormonal therapy is not used.

When hormonal therapy is used, most practitioners will continue to use dose escalation although the data to support it are less clear. The British MRC R-01 trial reported by Dearnaley et al. randomized 843 men (24% low risk, 32% intermediate risk, 44% high risk) to 5–8 months of androgen deprivation plus either 64 Gy in 2 Gy fractions or 74 Gy in 2 Gy fractions, both prescribed to isocenter [5]. This trial found that the higher dose improved biochemical recurrence-free survival (71% vs. 60% at 5 years, $p = .007$), but given that the "high dose" regimen was equivalent to about 70 Gy to the PTV, this trial technically does not answer the question of whether doses above 70 Gy are needed when hormonal therapy is used. The Dutch trial reported by Peeters et al. randomized 669 patients (27% intermediate risk) to 68 Gy versus 78 Gy, both prescribed to isocenter [6]. Dose escalation improved the freedom-from-failure rate from 54% to 64% at

5 years ($p = .02$). In this trial, hormones were given to 22% at the discretion of the treating center. A test for interaction between dose arm and hormonal therapy use was not significant ($p = .6$), suggesting that the benefit of dose escalation did not vary whether or not hormones were given. However, because only 22% of the patients were given hormonal therapy, it is not possible to firmly conclude that dose escalation is needed when hormonal therapy is being used. Nevertheless, a reanalysis of the PROG 95-09 trial found that there was no difference in long-term bowel-related quality of life between the conventional dose and dose-escalated arms [7], and so with modern image-guided techniques there is little reason not to use dose-escalated radiation with hormones as long as normal tissue metrics can be met, although conventional dose with hormones could be considered for patients with a high risk of bleeding due to anticoagulant use [8] or other medical conditions.

If Dose-Escalated Radiation Therapy Is Given, Is Concurrent Hormonal Therapy Indicated?

There are no randomized data currently available to answer this question because the 2 trials showing survival benefits to the addition of short-course (4–6 months) hormonal therapy to radiation for intermediate- and high-risk prostate cancer used conventional dose radiation. Specifically, the DFCI 95-096 trial reported by D'Amico et al. used 70 Gy to the isocenter and found that 6 months of hormones improved overall survival from 61% to 74% at 8 years ($p = .01$) [9]. A post-hoc analysis found that those with specifically intermediate-risk disease also had a survival benefit with hormonal therapy if they had only minimal comorbidities (91% vs. 85% overall survival at 7 years [$p = .009$]). The RTOG 94-08, reported by Jones et al., randomized 1979 (54% intermediate risk) men to 66.6 Gy to the isocenter plus-or-minus 4 months of hormonal therapy [10]. Overall, hormonal therapy improved overall survival from 57% to 62% at 10 years ($p = .03$). Interestingly, when a post-hoc analysis was done by risk group, only patients in intermediate risk appeared to have a significant survival benefit (61% vs. 54% by 10 years, $p = .03$). It remains unclear whether 4 months was too short to benefit patients in the high-risk group or whether the high-risk subgroup was too small to detect a statistically significant difference.

A trial specifically designed to determine the need for hormones with dose escalation is the RTOG 08-15 that is randomizing men to high dose radiation [external beam radiation to 79.2 Gy or external beam plus brachytherapy (BRT) boost] plus-or-minus 6 months of hormones. It aims to enroll 1520 patients with the endpoint of overall survival.

How Does Comorbidity Influence the Recommendation for Hormonal Therapy?

There is evolving evidence that a patient's comorbidities can impact whether a patient is likely to benefit from the addition of hormonal therapy. A post-hoc reanalysis of the DFCI 95-096 trial found that men with no or minimal comorbidity on the ACE-27 scale experienced a very large survival benefit from the addition of 6 months of hormonal therapy to 70 Gy of radiation (90% vs. 64% at 8 years, $p < .001$), while those with moderate or severe comorbidity (mainly cardiac) experienced a near-significant worsening of survival with hormonal therapy (25% vs. 54% at 8 years, $p = .08$) [9]. These data suggest that for men with significant underlying comorbidity, the adverse metabolic and cardiovascular effects of hormonal therapy may outweigh its benefits. A large retrospective study attempted to identify which specific comorbidities placed a man at highest risk of harm from hormonal therapy, and found that hormonal therapy was associated with an increased risk of death only in men with a history of prior myocardial infarction or congestive heart failure [11]. However, these men accounted for only 5% of the total prostate cancer study population, suggesting that the proportion of patients at risk for harm due to hormonal therapy may be small. In 2011, a meta-analysis of 4,141 men in 8 randomized trials of hormonal therapy versus no hormonal therapy in unfavorable-risk prostate cancer could not find any difference in the incidence of cardiovascular death in the 2 arms (11.0% vs. 11.2%, respectively), but found that hormonal therapy was associated with a significant reduction in prostate-cancer specific mortality (RR = 0.69, $p < .001$) and all-cause mortality (RR = 0.86, $p < .001$) [12]. However, patients who enroll in randomized trials tend to be healthier than the general population, and this meta-analysis could not stratify patients by comorbidities. Taken together, the data suggest that the majority of men with unfavorable-risk

prostate cancer will benefit from hormonal therapy, but there may be a small subgroup of men with significant underlying cardiac comorbidity, particularly a prior myocardial infarction or congestive heart failure, who can be harmed by hormonal therapy. In this population of men, caution should be taken to weigh the potential risks and benefits, and potentially refer to a cardiologist for further evaluation. To examine this issue more definitively, the RTOG 08-15 trial discussed earlier is stratifying men by their ACE-27 comorbidity status, and will be able to provide further information about how comorbidity impacts the benefits derived from hormonal therapy.

Case Discussion and Recommendations

"Intermediate risk" encompasses a very wide range of patients with variable risk of harboring micrometastatic disease. While some patients with favorable intermediate-risk disease (eg, T1c, PSA 4.2, Gl $3 + 4 = 7$ in 10% of 1/12 cores) will have purely localized disease and will do well with dose-escalated radiation alone, it has been well established that intermediate-risk patients with multiple intermediate risk factors, such as this patient (ie, with Gleason 7 and PSA 10–20), have a substantially higher risk of dying of prostate cancer [13,14] and thus would be good candidates for dose-escalated radiation to 75.6 to 79.2 Gy plus 4 to 6 months of hormonal therapy to address any micrometastatic disease. In addition, he has Gleason $4 + 3$, which places him at higher risk of death than if he had Gleason $3 + 4$ [15]. The 1 complicating factor is his cardiac history. He had a myocardial infarction 5 years ago, which places him automatically into the moderate to severe comorbidity group on the ACE-27 scale (minimal = MI by ECG only, age undetermined; moderate = MI more than 6 months ago; severe = MI 6 months ago or less), and the reanalysis of the DFCI 95-096 trial suggests that he may not benefit from the use of hormonal therapy. The patient has been revascularized, and retrospective data suggest that revascularization can help reduce the adverse cardiovascular impact of hormonal therapy in this vulnerable population, but does not completely eliminate the increased risk [16]. Ultimately, because the data raising concern for hormonal therapy in this patient are either based on post-hoc or retrospective analyses, and because 2 randomized trials have demonstrated a survival benefit for hormonal therapy in intermediate risk, the best recommendation for this patient is probably to proceed with hormonal therapy, but with caution. He should ideally be "medically optimized" with the input of a cardiologist and be encouraged to exercise and diet as needed to minimize the metabolic effects of hormonal therapy. I would treat this patient with 75.6 Gy at 1.8 Gy per fraction to the prostate and seminal vesicles [17,18], along with 6 months of hormonal therapy.

ACADEMIC COMMENT

Michael J. Zelefsky

Intermediate-risk prostate cancer represents a unique cohort of patients. Such patients often have significant volume disease although the cancer is clinically confined to the gland. The higher density of tumor clonogens within the prostate would likely require escalated radiation doses to achieve local tumor control. At the same time, the risk of micrometastatic disease may still be low. Thus, more aggressive local therapy would be warranted for this patient subgroup.

There is ample evidence demonstrating a benefit for dose escalation in patients with clinically localized prostate cancer. Indeed, the available phase 3 trials have clearly shown the importance of using higher radiation dose levels in the range of 78 to 80 Gy for all prognostic risk groups. However, among the various risk groups, intermediate-risk prostate cancer patients appear to benefit the most from the application of escalated radiation doses, and therefore this should be considered the standard of care. Our recently published retrospective data [19] have shown that among patients with intermediate-risk disease, the 10 year biochemical control outcomes for patients treated to dose levels of 81 Gy versus lower doses were 76% and 57% ($p < .001$).

At the present time, it remains unclear what is the most optimal or most effective mode of treatment delivery for dose escalation. While there have been no randomized controlled trials comparing outcomes of patients treated with EBRT versus BRT, there are retrospective reports that have demonstrated improved tumor control outcomes for favorable and intermediate risk treated with a combination of BRT and or supplemental EBRT compared to high-dose intensity modulated radiotherapy alone [20,21]. In 1 study [20],

among 160 patients treated with high-dose-rate (HDR) BRT followed by supplemental intensity modulated radiation therapy (IMRT), the 7 year PSA relapse-free survival rate was 100% compared to 84% for patients treated with 86.4 Gy of IMRT alone ($p < .001$). Other reports have also suggested higher tumor control outcomes for intermediate-risk patients treated with BRT regimens compared to EBRT alone [21,22]. The improved biochemical control outcomes for more intense dose escalation associated with BRT may be explained by its greater potential to more effectively ablate the prostatic epithelium resulting in lower PSA nadir values after treatment compared to EBRT [21,23]. Nevertheless, there are no published data demonstrating clearly that this improved biochemical control outcome translates consistently into a reduced incidence of distant metastases.

The role of androgen deprivation therapy (ADT) for the intermediate-risk cohort is controversial, especially in the setting of patients who receive high-dose radiotherapy. The recently published RTOG 94-08 has demonstrated a survival benefit for patients with intermediate-risk disease treated with short-course ADT compared to EBRT alone [10]. The radiation dose used in that study was only 66 Gy, and with the dose being prescribed to a point within the prostate, the periphery of the gland (which, in general, harbors the bulk of the cancer) probably received doses in the range of only 60 Gy. In a smaller phase 3 trial ($n = 206$), D'Amico et al. demonstrated similar findings when using 70 Gy and short-course ADT compared to EBRT alone [9]. Some have claimed that when such suboptimal dose levels are delivered, ADT is necessary and critical to improve outcomes and compensate for the low doses received by the tumor [24].

Despite these theoretical considerations, our experience from Memorial Sloan-Kettering Cancer Center has shown that ADT actually further improved outcomes for intermediate-risk patients who received dose levels of 81 Gy [19]. Among 1074 patients with intermediate-risk disease treated with a 6 month course of ADT, the 10 year PSA-relapse-free survival was 80% compared to 59% among patients treated with IMRT alone ($p < .001$). Taken together, these data indicate: (a) intermediate-risk patients require dose-escalation therapy, and (b) ADT is likely beneficial for these patients even in the setting of escalated radiation dose levels. Future prospective randomized trials such as RTOG-0815 will hopefully shed light on the role of ADT in the setting of escalated doses of radiation for patients with intermediate-risk disease.

It is interesting to note that while there are no phase 3 data currently available, most retrospective reports have been unable to demonstrate any evidence of a benefit for ADT among patients treated with BRT. Several reports using low-dose-rate (LDR) BRT with or without supplemental EBRT and the use of HDR BRT in combination with EBRT have not demonstrated improved outcomes with the use of ADT [25–27]. It is possible to speculate that as a mode of ultra-dose escalation, combined modality BRT and supplemental EBRT may obviate the need for ADT in intermediate-risk patients. However, among those treated with EBRT alone where safe dose escalation is given in the range of 81 to 86.4 Gy, ADT may confer a continued outcome benefit. The above-mentioned RTOG 08-15 is, in fact, testing this hypothesis.

So, in conclusion, I would agree in the case presented that if EBRT is offered to the patient, the addition of ADT would be appropriate; however, the duration of ADT need not be longer than 6 months. In my clinical practice for such patients with intermediate-risk disease I would not routinely treat the pelvic lymph nodes but rather would limit the treatment to the prostate and seminal vesicles only. In my opinion, if the patient were a candidate for BRT (prostate size less than 50 g, International Prostate Symptom score less than 15, and without significant medical comorbidities), he would not require ADT and may choose this approach if he wanted to avoid the anticipated side effects of androgen deprivation and the increased risk of sexual dysfunction. From the quality of life perspective of the patient, this in fact may be the more desirable form of therapy to avoid the androgen deprivation side effects in an individual who is described as having prior cardiac comorbidities. Some studies have shown increased cardiac-related morbidity even with short-course ADT among patients with 2 or more risk factors, such as a prior myocardial infarction or a prior stroke [12]. This patient has 2 risk factors and even a short course of ADT may be associated with an increased cardiac risk. Nevertheless, the morbidity of ADT in terms of cardiac complications especially for short course duration has not been consistently observed [28]. I would discuss these issues with the patient and present the uncertainties of benefit using ADT especially at this time without the guidance of randomized data.

COMMUNITY PRACTITIONER COMMENT

Alan T. Monroe

Intermediate-risk prostate cancer covers a relatively broad spectrum of clinical risk. The classic D'Amico criteria [29] worked fairly well to stratify patients on the basis of T-stage (2b or 2c), Gleason score [7], and PSA (10–20 ng/mL). However, as additional prognostic variables were appreciated, it has become clear that risk could be further stratified within the traditional definition of intermediate risk [30]. PSA velocity, PSA doubling time, percent positive biopsy cores, and predominant pattern comprising the Gleason 7 total score (4 + 3 vs. 3 + 4) all contribute to risk assessment. While the NCCN guidelines still rely on the basic 3 categories proposed by D'Amico, there is provision to upstage patients to high risk if multiple adverse factors are present [31].

Numerous radiation treatment options exist for a patient with intermediate-risk prostate cancer, including the option of active surveillance in select cases. In our practice, active surveillance based on the Epstein criteria [32] is utilized predominantly for those with low-risk prostate cancer or the occasional low-intermediate-risk patient with considerable comorbidities. Thus, assessing an individual's risk of competing morbidity and mortality between prostate cancer and other medical conditions becomes vital in individualizing treatment. On a population basis, actuarial tables of expected survival for a 68-year-old male would point to a 15 year life expectancy. The presence of cardiovascular disease in this patient likely reduces his survival to some degree, but probably not below the 10 year expectation that we use to decide on active treatment. Based on this patient's multiple adverse features (PSA higher than 10 ng/mL, Gleason 4 + 3, and percent positive cores higher than 50%) and reasonable life expectancy with well-controlled cardiovascular disease, we would recommend dose-escalated radiation with short-term hormonal therapy.

Dose escalation in intermediate-risk prostate cancer has been extensively studied, and a few recent studies warrant attention. The MD

Anderson experience that first supported dose escalation has been updated with a median of 9.5 years of follow-up [1]. When the data were first presented [2], intermediate-risk patients with PSA higher than 10 ng/mL demonstrated improvement in freedom from biochemical or clinical failure when treated with 78 Gy versus 70 Gy in the absence of hormonal therapy. With additional follow-up, the intermediate-risk group as a whole failed to show benefit; however, the subset of patients with PSA higher than 10 ng/mL continued to show a trend toward significantly improved biochemical control (94% vs. 65%)—albeit at the expense of greater gastrointestinal toxicity. Conversely, the recent Dutch study showed benefit for the intermediate risk population as a whole [33]. The MRC RT01 trial showed a benefit to dose escalation for intermediate-risk patients in the setting of neoadjuvant hormonal therapy [5]. Improved biochemical control may translate into a clinical survival advantage with longer follow up. Additional study is clearly needed to determine which subsets of intermediate-risk patients benefit from dose escalation. In practice, we continue to offer dose escalation to everyone with intermediate-risk disease because toxicity has been low in our experience and potential disease control benefits are viewed as sufficiently worthy.

Our institutional preference is to treat intermediate risk patients with image-guided radiation therapy (IGRT) to a dose of 45 Gy to the prostate with a 5–8 mm margin followed by a single implant incorporating HDR BRT (9.5 Gy × 2 fractions) as a boost. When external beam radiation alone is selected, our total dose is 78 Gy in 2 Gy fractions with IGRT techniques. Highly selected patients with low–intermediate risk are treated with Cyberknife stereotactic body radiotherapy, exclusively on a clinical trial that mimics HDR dosimetry. HDR boost is our preferred form of dose escalation because of a comfort level that comes with experience (more than 600 cases in 8 years), more forgiving dosimetry compared with permanent seeds, and emerging data suggesting a potential clinical benefit to BRT over external beam radiation alone [34,35]. HDR BRT may also be performed without hormonal downsizing in glands up to 90 mL, thereby eliminating the need for hormones in select low–intermediate clinical risk patients [36].

The case in question raises another controversy regarding the use of anti-androgen therapy in the setting of dose escalation. RTOG 94-06 was a phase 1/2 dose escalation trial that incorporated 2 to 6 months of neoadjuvant hormonal therapy in selected patients. Although not specifically designed to test the addition of hormones to high dose radiation, subsequent analysis failed to demonstrate a clinical benefit despite an increased risk of genitourinary complications [37]. Conversely, data from D'Amico published in 2008 demonstrated an overall survival advantage with 6 months of hormonal therapy added to conventional doses of radiation [9]. There is no consensus as to which intermediate-risk patients need both dose escalation and hormonal therapy. Until the debate is settled with randomized data, we find the D'Amico survival benefit difficult to ignore and typically offer a 6 month course of anti-androgen therapy for those on the higher end of the intermediate risk scale (Gleason 4 + 3 or more than 50% positive cores). In those with cardiovascular morbidity and a lower risk profile within the intermediate-risk subgroup, we feel comfortable with dose-escalated radiation alone.

SECTION EDITOR'S NOTE

Stanley L. Liauw

All 3 opinions agree on the use of dose-escalated radiation therapy for this case with intermediate-risk prostate cancer. The concurrent use of hormonal therapy is a more difficult decision because the patient's medical comorbidity may alter the risk/benefit ratio, and the role of hormonal therapy with dose-escalated radiation has not been prospectively proven. Despite this uncertainty, all authors feel most comfortable offering hormonal therapy with RT. Two authors would consider BRT, either as monotherapy or as a boost after EBRT, to potentially obviate the need for hormonal therapy. Although the use of BRT as a means to eliminate the need for concurrent hormonal therapy in intermediate-risk disease has not been proven, it is a compelling consideration. It is possible that for this patient, progression after therapy would predominantly be the result of local, rather than distant, failure. Because BRT can deliver much higher doses compared to external beam radiation, local control could be improved with this modality, and the role of a radiation sensitizer would therefore be minimized. In this case, I would discuss the role for hormonal therapy with this gentleman. His preference to prioritize the optimization of biochemical control versus quality of life would have a bearing on the final recommendation. In the absence of any preference or lack of an available clinical trial, I would offer dose-escalated RT (78 Gy to the prostate and proximal seminal vesicles, with daily image guidance and intensity-modulated radiation therapy) with 6 months of combined androgen blockade.

REFERENCES

1. Kuban DA, Tucker SL, Dong L, et al. Long-term results of the M. D. Anderson randomized dose-escalation trial for prostate cancer. *Int J Radiat Oncol Biol Phys.* 2008;70:67–74.

2. Pollack A, Zagars GK, Smith LG, et al. Preliminary results of a randomized radiotherapy dose-escalation study comparing 70 Gy with 78 Gy for prostate cancer. *J Clin Oncol.* 2000;18:3904–3911.

3. Zietman AL, DeSilvio ML, Slater JD, et al. Comparison of conventional-dose vs high-dose conformal radiation therapy in clinically localized adenocarcinoma of the prostate: A randomized controlled trial. *JAMA.* 2005;294:1233–1239.

4. Zietman AL, Bae K, Slater JD, et al. Randomized trial comparing conventional-dose with high-dose conformal radiation therapy in early-stage adenocarcinoma of the prostate: Long-term results from Proton Radiation Oncology Group/American College of Radiology 95-09. *J Clin Oncol.* 2010;28:1106–1111.

5. Dearnaley DP, Sydes MR, Graham JD, et al. Escalated-dose versus standard-dose conformal radiotherapy in prostate cancer: First results from the MRC RT01 randomised controlled trial. *Lancet Oncol.* 2007;8:475–487.

6. Peeters ST, Heemsbergen WD, Koper PC, et al. Dose-response in radiotherapy for localized prostate cancer: Results of the Dutch multicenter randomized phase III trial comparing 68 Gy of radiotherapy with 78 Gy. *J Clin Oncol.* 2006;24:1990–1996.

7. Talcott JA, Rossi C, Shipley WU, et al. Patient-reported long-term outcomes after conventional and high-dose combined proton and photon radiation for early prostate cancer. *JAMA.* 2010;303:1046–1053.

8. Choe KS, Jani AB, Liauw SL. External beam radiotherapy for prostate cancer patients on anticoagulation therapy: How significant is the bleeding toxicity? *Int J Radiat Oncol Biol Phys.* 2010;76:755–760.

9. D'Amico AV, Chen MH, Renshaw AA, et al. Androgen suppression and radiation vs radiation alone for prostate cancer: A randomized trial. *JAMA.* 2008;299:289–295.

10. Jones CU, Hunt D, McGowan DG, et al. Radiotherapy and short-term androgen deprivation for localized prostate cancer. *N Engl J Med.* 2011;365:107–118.

11. Nanda A, Chen MH, Braccioforte MH, et al. Hormonal therapy use for prostate cancer and mortality in men with coronary artery disease-induced congestive heart failure or myocardial infarction. *JAMA.* 2009;302:866–873.

12. Nguyen PL, Je Y, Schutz FA, et al. Association of androgen deprivation therapy with cardiovascular death in patients with prostate cancer: A meta-analysis of randomized trials. *JAMA.* 2011;306:2359–2366.

13. Zelefsky MJ, Leibel SA, Gaudin PB, et al. Dose escalation with three-dimensional conformal radiation therapy affects the outcome in prostate cancer. *Int J Radiat Oncol Biol Phys.* 1998;41:491–500.

14. Tsai HK, Chen MH, McLeod DG, et al. Cancer-specific mortality after radiation therapy with short-course hormonal therapy or radical prostatectomy in men with localized, intermediate-risk to high-risk prostate cancer. *Cancer.* 2006;107:2597–2603.

15. Stark JR, Perner S, Stampfer MJ, et al. Gleason score and lethal prostate cancer: Does 3 + 4 = 4 + 3? *J Clin Oncol.* 2009;27:3459–3464.

16. Nguyen PL, Chen MH, Goldhaber SZ, et al. Coronary revascularization and mortality in men with congestive heart failure or prior myocardial infarction who receive androgen deprivation. *Cancer.* 2011;117:406–413.

17. Lawton CA, Desilvio M, Roach M 3rd, et al. An update of the phase III trial comparing whole pelvic to prostate only radiotherapy and neoadjuvant to adjuvant total androgen suppression: Updated analysis of RTOG 94-13, with emphasis on unexpected hormone/radiation interactions. *Int J Radiat Oncol Biol Phys.* 2007;69(3):646–655.

18. Pommier P, Chabaud S, Lagrange JL, et al. Is there a role for pelvic irradiation in localized prostate adenocarcinoma? Preliminary results of GETUG-01. *J Clin Oncol.* 2007;25:5366–5373.

19. Zelefsky MJ, Pei X, Chou JF, et al. Dose escalation for prostate cancer radiotherapy: Predictors of long-term biochemical tumor control and distant metastases-free survival outcomes. *Eur Urol.* 2011;60:1133–1139.

20. Deutsch I, Zelefsky MJ, Zhang Z et al. Comparison of PSA relapse-free survival in patient treated with ultra-high dose IMRT versus combination HDR brachytherapy and IMRT. *Brachytherapy.* 2010;9:313–318.

21. Zelefsky MJ, Yamada Y, Pei X, et al. Comparison of tumor control and toxicity outcomes of high dose intensity modulated radiotherapy and brachytherapy for patients with favorable risk prostate cancer. *Urology.* 2011;77:986–990.

22. Wong WW, Vora SA, Schild SE, et al. Radiation dose escalation for localized prostate cancer: Intensity-modulated radiotherapy versus permanent transperineal brachytherapy. *Cancer.* 2009;115:5596–5606.

23. Zelefsky MJ, Kuban DA, Levy LB, et al. Multi-institutional analysis of long-term outcome for stages T1-T2 prostate cancer treated with permanent seed implantation. *Int J Radiat Oncol Biol Phys.* 2007;67:327–333.

24. Zumsteg ZS, Zelefsy MJ. Short-term androgren deprivation therapy for patients with intermediate-risk prostate cancer undergoing dose-escalated radiotherapy: The standard of care. *Lancet.* 2012;13:e259–e269.

25. Merrick GS, Butler WM, Wallner KE, et al. Androgen-deprivation therapy does not impact cause-specific or overall survival after permanent prostate brachytherapy. *Int J Radiat Oncol Biol Phys.* 2006;65:669–677.

26. Lee LN, Stock RG, Stone NN. Role of hormonal therapy in the management of intermediate- to high-risk prostate cancer treated with permanent radioactive seed implantation. *Int J Radiat Oncol Biol Phys.* 2002;52:444–452.

27. Zelefsky MJ, Chou JF, Pei X, et al. Predicting biochemical tumor control after brachytherapy for clinically localized prostate cancer: The Memorial Sloan-Kettering Cancer Center experience. *Brachytherapy.* 2011 Sep 17. [Epub ahead of print]

28. Bolla M, Van Tienhoven G, Warde P, et al. External irradiation with or without long-term androgen suppression for prostate cancer with high metastatic risk: 10-year results of an EORTC randomised study. *Lancet Oncol.* 2010;11:1066–1073.

29. D'Amico AV, Moul J, Carroll P, et al. Cancer specific mortality after surgery or radiation for patients with clinically localized prostate cancer managed during the prostate-specific antigen era. *J Clin Oncol.* 2003;21:2163–2172.

30. D'Amico AV, Keshaviah A, Manola J, et al. Clinical utility of the percentage of positive prostate biopsies in predicting prostate cancer-specific and overall survival after radiotherapy for patients with localized prostate cancer. *Int J Radiat Oncol Biol Phys.* 2002;53(3):581–587.

31. Mohler JL, Armstrong AJ, Bahnson RR, et al. Prostate cancer, version 3.2012 featured updates to the NCCN guidelines. *J Natl Compr Canc Netw.* 2012;10:1081–1087.

32. Epstein JI, Srigely J, Grignon D, et al. Recommendations for the reporting of prostate cancer. *Hum Pathol.* 2007;38:1305–1309.

33. Al-Mamgani A, Heemsbergen WD, Levendag PC, et al. Subgroup analysis of patients with localized prostate cancer treated within the Dutch-randomized dose escalation trial. *Radiother Oncol.* 2010;96(1):13–18.

34. Hostkin PJ, Motohashi K, Bownes P, et al. High dose rate brachytherapy in combination with external beam radiotherapy in the radical treatment of prostate cancer: Initial results of a randomized phase three trial. *Radiother Oncol.* 2007;84(2):114–120.

35. Guix B, Bartrina J, Henriquez I, et al. Combined treatment 3D-conformal radiotherapy plus HDR brachytherapy as treatment for intermediate or high risk prostate cancer: Early toxicity and biochemical outcome of a dose-escalation prospective randomized trial. *Int J Radiat Oncol Biol Phys.* 2007;69(3):S85.

36. Monroe AT, Faricy PO, Jennings SB, et al. High dose rate brachytherapy for large prostate volumes (> or = 50 cc)- Uncompromised dosimetric coverage and acceptable toxicity. *Brachytherapy.* 2008;7(1):7–11.

37. Valicenti RK, Kwounghwa B, Michalski J, et al. Does hormone therapy reduce disease recurrence in prostate cancer patients receiving dose-escalated radiation therapy? An analysis of radiation therapy oncology group 94-06. *Int J Radiot Oncol Biol Phys.* 2011;79(5):1323–1329.

*Radiation and Hormonal Decision Points in the Treatment of Biochemical Failure
After Radical Prostatectomy*

CLINICAL PROBLEM

Certain patients who undergo radical prostatectomy for prostate cancer are at high risk for biochemical relapse. Although adjuvant radiation therapy (ART) can help reduce the risk of recurrence, salvage radiation therapy (SRT) (waiting for a detectable, but very low prostate-specific antigen [PSA]) may be similarly effective, and might help prevent some men from being overtreated. Meanwhile, the inclusion of pelvic lymph nodes in the radiation volume and the use of concurrent hormonal therapy are controversial, given the lack of prospective evidence to prove that benefits outweigh risks.

CASE EXAMPLE

A 62-year-old man undergoes a robotic-assisted radical prostatectomy for adenocarcinoma of the prostate that was diagnosed after a screening PSA of 14. The disease is of pathologic stage T3aN0, with 12 lymph nodes (LNs) dissected, negative surgical margins, and Gleason 4 + 3 disease involving 20% of the gland. His PSA initially falls to undetectable (less than 0.05 ng/mL), but 1 year later it is 0.11 ng/mL, and now, 1½ years after his prostatectomy, it is 0.22 ng/mL.

Management Decisions

- Which patients are the best candidates for ART compared to early SRT (eSRT)?
- When treating with SRT, should the radiation volume include pelvic nodes at risk?
- When treating with SRT, is concurrent hormonal therapy recommended?

MAJOR OPINION

Matthew C. Abramowitz and Alan Pollack

Which Patients Are the Best Candidates for ART Compared to eSRT?

This remains a controversial question. Three randomized studies have evaluated adjuvant radiation versus observation in men with high-risk pathologic features, such as extracapsular extension, positive margins, or seminal vesicle (SV) involvement, and have shown improved clinical and biochemical outcomes. However, 50% to 60% of these patients might not have experienced biochemical failure at 5 to 10 years when treated with prostatectomy alone and hence might have received unnecessary treatment. The risk of biochemical failure at 5 to 10 years is 40% to 50% [1–5]. The caveat is that a longer follow-up may yield even more failures.

The European Organization for Research and Treatment of Cancer (EORTC) trial 22911 [6] randomized 1,005 patients to prostate bed irradiation of a dose of 60 Gy or "wait and see." Freedom from biochemical failure was significantly greater with adjuvant radiotherapy (74% vs. 52.6%; hazard ratio [HR] 0.48, 98% CI 0.37–0.62). Local–regional (15.4% vs. 5.4%; $p < .0001$) and any clinical failure (19.0% vs. 8.8%; $p < .0001$) were lower when adjuvant radiotherapy was administered. There was a small but significant increase in late grade 2 or 3 complications with radiotherapy. SRT was administered to only 23% of patients in the observation group.

The Southwestern Oncology Group (SWOG) trial reported by Thompson et al. randomized 425 men to prostate bed irradiation to a dose of 60 to 64 Gy versus "usual care plus observation" [7].

The primary endpoint was distant metastasis-free survival (DMFS). One-third of patients went on to receive SRT (70 of 211). The study showed an improvement in DMFS with a HR 0.71 (p = .016). Survival improved significantly with adjuvant radiation HR 0.72 (p = .023) [8].

A group from Germany published the results of another multi-institutional postoperative adjuvant radiotherapy trial (ARO96-02/AUO AP 09/95) [9]. Patients (n = 385) were randomized prior to achieving an undetectable PSA as radiation was started within 6 to 12 weeks of surgery. Patients with persistently elevated PSA after randomization were excluded. At 4 years, 81% of patients who received radiation were free from biochemical failure compared to 60% of the patients who were under observation (p < .0001; HR 0.4). Late grade 2 rectal bleeding was 3%.

These 3 studies show that postoperative radiation therapy (RT), when given adjuvantly, reduces the risk of recurrence and, in the SWOG trial, mortality. However, as SRT was not uniformly given and no set threshold for triggering salvage treatment was utilized, it is difficult to say whether ART would be better than early salvage treatment.

It is quite clear that the early initiation of SRT with a PSA as low as possible has a direct correlation with the outcome. In a large pooled multi-institutional analysis, 48% of men who received SRT without androgen deprivation (AD) when the PSA was 0.50 ng/mL or less maintained a posttreatment PSA of lesser than 0.2 ng/mL at 6 years compared with 40%, 28%, and 18% of those treated at PSA levels of 0.51 to 1.00 ng/mL, 1.01 to 1.50 ng/mL, and greater than 1.50 ng/mL, respectively [10]. Similar relationships of the preradiotherapy PSA to eventual failure have been reported by King [11] and Ohri et al. [12]. If we assume that 50% of the patients in the randomized studies would not have failed, a 20% to 25% reduction in failure rate is similar to that seen with early salvage treatment. When the potential for significant overtreatment and concerns regarding morbidity of treatment without clear impact in overall survival are combined with the opinions of the surgeons, early salvage treatment is preferred. This requires a patient who can commit to close PSA follow-up.

When Treating With SRT, Should the Radiation Volume Include Pelvic Nodes at Risk?

The potential benefit of nodal irradiation therapy in the management of prostate cancer is an area of active debate. There are no phase 3 data to guide us in this situation and I do not treat LNs if they were negative pathologically and there is no evidence of disease on pelvic imaging. There are, however, patients who might benefit from LN treatment. Extrapolating from the intact prostate literature is also difficult. The largest study to attempt to answer this question is RTOG 9413. This 2 × 2 study was completely negative, showing that in the population tested, which had a 15% or greater risk of LN involvement using the Roach formula, there was no difference between pelvic irradiation versus prostate-only irradiation [13]. Despite the lack of data, consideration is given to those who have SV involvement or few or no LNs removed at prostatectomy. Patients should be encouraged to participate in the RTOG 0534 (discussed subsequently) trial and in our practice, the LNs are not treated if a patient is a candidate for this trial and refuses. We treat the pelvic LNs when pelvic lymph node involvement is documented.

When Treating With SRT, Is Concurrent Hormonal Therapy Recommended?

This is a question where some phase 3 data exist. In RTOG 9601, 771 men with elevated PSA levels after radical prostatectomy received a dose of 64.8 Gy to the prostate bed alone or an additional 2 years of bicalutamide (150 mg/day). PSA values up to 4 ng/mL were included. An improvement in freedom from PSA progression from 40% to 57% at 7 years was seen with the addition of bicalutamide [14]. The degree of benefit was dependent on the prostatectomy Gleason score. Of patients with Gleason score lesser than 7 disease, the rates were 63% versus 50%; for Gleason 7 patients it was 55% versus 39%; and for Gleason score 8 to 10 the rate was 56% versus 26%. However, this study used a nonstandard antiandrogen treatment, for which some data indicate increased risks of significant gynecomastia and gynecodynia and possibly increased mortality [15]. Whether a similar degree of benefit would be obtained within luteinizing hormone releasing hormone (LHRH) agonist is unknown. Furthermore, this study included a broad spectrum of patients and whether this benefit was seen across all pretreatment PSA levels remains to be determined. The primary endpoint is survival and not enough events have occurred to sufficiently analyze the data.

There are at least 2 current studies attempting to answer this question, RTOG 0534 and the Radicals study. In the Radicals study, patients are randomized after surgery to early or delayed radiation. Delayed radiation is given when there are 2 consecutive rises with a PSA greater than 0.1 ng/mL or 3 consecutive rises. This study incorporates a second randomization for all patients receiving radiation to either no androgen deprivation therapy (ADT), 6 months of ADT, or 2 years of ADT. The endpoint is cause-specific survival [16]. RTOG 0534 is a 3-arm study that hopes to answer two questions: (a) Is neoadjuvant and concurrent short-term AD (NC-STAD) plus prostate bed radiotherapy (PBRT) superior to PBRT alone, and (b) is NC-STAD plus pelvic lymph node RT (PLNRT) superior to NC-STAD plus PBRT?

With these data in mind and with the generally low salvage rates for men with a PSA of more than 1 ng/mL after radical prostatectomy, a course of ADT concurrent with SRT could be considered for those with Gleason score 8 to 10 disease, SV involvement, or a PSA of higher than 1 ng/mL at the time of SRT. We routinely recommend that ADT be added to SRT for men with a preradiotherapy PSA of more than 2 ng/mL (not a candidate for RTOG 0534), palpable mass on digital rectal exam (not a candidate for RTOG 0534), or when the SVs are involved (and other factors preclude enrollment in RTOG 0534). Enrollment on RTOG 0534 is strongly encouraged.

Recommendations for the Clinical Case

In the case of this 62-year-old man with postoperative PSA of 0.22 ng/mL and stage pT3aN0 disease, at the University of Miami we would recommend SRT to the prostate bed alone to a dose of 68 Gy at 2 Gy/fraction. We would not recommend AD or nodal treatment. A staging bone scan can be considered but may be of little utility with PSA values this low. We use dynamic contrast-enhanced (DCE) MRI for treatment planning and, if a patient has an identifiable lesion consistent with recurrent disease, he is offered enrollment on randomized study where the DCE-MRI abnormality is treated at a dose of 2.25 Gy/day to 76.5 Gy, the remaining prostate bed is treated to a dose of 68 Gy.

ACADEMIC COMMENT

Christopher R. King

In this section I will address: (a) the primary and more general clinical dilemma of whether one needs to treat patients with high-risk pathology (pT3 or positive margin) in the setting of an undetectable PSA, and (b) when given, how to best deliver postoperative radiotherapy.

ART Versus eSRT?

Radiotherapy in the absence of measurable disease is defined as ART. With incomplete randomized trials that only compared ART to "observation" and not to SRT (ie, EORTC 22911 [6], ARO 9602 [9], and SWOG 8794 [7]), and ongoing open trials comparing ART to eSRT (RADICALS [17], Groupe d'Etude des Tumeurs Uro-Génitales (GETUG)-17 [18], and RAVES [19]), we are often left to proceed on intuition, motivated by not wanting to miss an opportunity for cure. Even the survival benefit seen in the SWOG trial is unconvincing as the comparison to ART was management with either ADT alone or late SRT when PSA was hopelessly high. In the process of delivering ART, we overtreat many who are cancer-free, leave some with unnecessary toxicity, add cost without value to health care, and, most importantly, overlook the possibility that eSRT may indeed be as effective as ART.

Clearly, postoperative RT can potentially eradicate microscopic residual disease, and in the setting of ART it is implied that this microscopic disease burden is actually present but insufficient to produce a detectable PSA. If one proposes that ART is superior to SRT, it can only be because it is preferable to deliver RT at a lower microscopic disease burden. While this fundamental radiation biology premise is certainly reasonable, the next logical question is how much is actually at stake when this microscopic disease burden increases? A recent systematic review and meta-analysis of SRT quantified the answer to this question [20]. Pooling together 41 published series, this study showed that PSA level prior to SRT was independently associated with PSA relapse-free survival (RFS) ($p < .0001$) and that there was an approximate 2.6% loss of RFS for each incremental PSA of 0.1 ng/mL prior to SRT (Figure 5.2.1).

A simple radiobiological model based on Poisson statistics and the assumption that PSA is proportional to disease burden fits the data

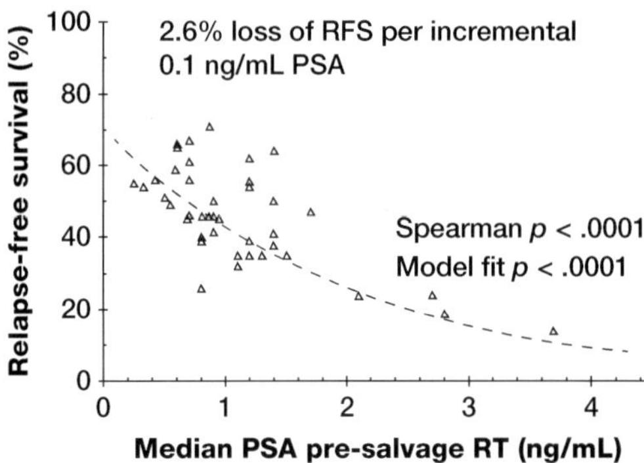

FIGURE 5.2.1 ■ Relapse-free survival as a function of PSA level at time of SRT. Each symbol represents an individual published series of SRT. The dashed curve is a fit to the data with a simple radiobiological model of Poisson statistics tumor control probability and where PSA is proportional to disease burden, yielding the relationship RFS ~ e – PSA. The data suggest that there is an average approximate 2.6% loss of RFS for each incremental 0.1 ng/mL PSA prior to SRT.

very well. At a PSA of 0.2 ng/mL or lower, SRT achieved a 64% rate of RFS. Therefore, when providing SRT, it should be desirable to initiate it at the lowest possible PSA level in order to achieve the best outcomes.

Thus, the difference between ART (with an undetectable ultrasensitive PSA of less than 0.01 ng/mL) and eSRT with a PSA = 0.1 ng/mL would only be about 2.5% at best in favor of ART. Initiating SRT even earlier, say at an ultrasensitive PSA of 0.02 ng/mL, would reduce this difference to an approximate 0.5%. It is evident that there are assumptions underlying these arguments and the most meaningful one is whether high-risk pathology itself is actually an indicator of systemic disease. If so, then examining ART versus SRT becomes moot. Nevertheless, even high-risk patients can sometimes be successfully treated. Even in the best case scenario, whether one considers these small differences of 0.5% to 2.5% in RFS clinically meaningful or relevant is certainly debatable, but this small gain needs to be placed in context with the toxicities, costs, and, most importantly, the necessity of offering ART.

This brings us to the next question: How often do patients with high-risk pathology actually have residual microscopic disease? In the 3 similar randomized trials, EORTC 22911, ARO 9602, and SWOG 8794, a comparison between ART with an "observation" group was made for patients at high

risk. The randomized observation arm from these trials provides the proportion of patients who did not fail despite having high-risk pathology. The 5 year biochemical relapse free survival (bRFS) rates were 53% in the EORTC trial, 54% in the ARO trial, and 44% in the SWOG trial. Despite some differences in PSA entry criteria and pathology, results from these trials were remarkably similar. Perhaps the ARO study provides the best estimate as its entry criteria were stricter in that all patients had an undetectable postoperative PSA of less than 0.1 ng/mL. Therefore, one can conclude that about one-half of patients would not demonstrate a PSA relapse at 5 years despite having high-risk features. Given this remarkable fact, it becomes even more debatable whether to offer ART or to wait for a detectable PSA before offering eSRT.

In the ultrasensitive PSA era with assay thresholds of 0.01 ng/mL, the distinction between what was once considered adjuvant and salvage becomes blurred. In the EORTC trial, 9% of patients had a PSA greater than 0.2 ng/mL; in the SWOG trial, 35% had a PSA greater than 0.2 ng/mL; and in the ARO trial (which had access to assays with lower threshold), 20% of patients had a PSA greater than 0.05 to 0.1 ng/mL, and 59% of patients had a PSA greater than 0.03 to 0.1 ng/mL. Determining the relevance of these trials to current practice is challenging because many of the patients enrolled did have measurable PSA levels.

Postoperative RT: Prostate Bed or Pelvic Nodes—With or Without Hormones—and to What Dose?

The definitive answer to these questions should be given by current, open randomized trials; for example, the multiarm RTOG 05-34 compares RT to PB ± ADT versus RT to LN with ADT for pT3 or positive margin with bPFS as an outcome measure (RT given as a dose of 64.8 to 70.2 Gy to PB, 45 Gy to LN and ADT given as 4 to 6 months LHRH + bicalutamide).

The value of treating pelvic nodes in any prostate cancer patient is the subject of passionate debate for many. Certainly, in the definitive setting, randomized trials have failed to provide a clear answer. The conclusions of RTOG 94-13 [13] were so inconclusive that even the principal investigators are planning for another trial comparing prostate only versus prostate + pelvic node RT. The negative results of GETUG-01, however, comparing prostate versus whole pelvic RT do not provide much encouragement for any measurable benefit [21]. Therefore, on the surface there appears to be little reason to expect any benefit in the postoperative setting. Nevertheless, enough positive retrospective data exist to have warranted the above-mentioned trial (RTOG 05-34). For example, in a study from Stanford of patients receiving postoperative RT, an approximately 25% improvement in 5 year bRFS ($p = .008$) was observed for high-risk patients who got whole pelvic RT as compared to those getting prostate bed only [22]. Furthermore, this benefit was present only among patients who received concurrent ADT as well, a provocative result somewhat analogous to the effect seen in RTOG 94-13.

Recently, several retrospective studies have suggested the potential beneficial role that concurrent ADT may have in the setting of postoperative RT. For example, in a study of patients receiving SRT, King et al. [23] have shown that the addition of a short course of neoadjuvant and concurrent total androgen blockade was an independent factor ($p = .002$) conferring a bRFS advantage and an overall survival advantage as compared to RT alone. In another study of patients receiving ART with a dose of 69.1 Gy or more to the prostate bed only, Ost et al. [24] showed an improved bRFS for those getting concurrent LHRH (HR 0.4, $p = .02$).

Finally, the answer to the question of dose required to eradicate microscopic disease in the prostate bed rests on retrospective data. A recent systematic review [25] shows that there is a fairly steep dose response for postoperative RT within the 60 to 70 Gy range that parallels the dose response known for primary prostate RT. With an approximately 2.5% improvement in 5 year bRFS for each additional Gray of radiation, a substantial gain is expected in escalating the dose from the conservative and conventional dose of 64.8 Gy to a dose more than 70 Gy. With careful techniques that include measures to stabilize rectal distension and constant bladder filling throughout the course of therapy, such dose escalation should be very safe.

Recommendations

Given these considerations and until results of randomized trials become available, I have 2 recommendations: (a) Observe all prostate cancer patients postoperatively, even the high-risk ones, but to proceed with SRT at the earliest possible time when an ultrasensitive PSA is clearly evident (in general I proceed with SRT when PSA is ~0.04 ng/mL or more and preferably ~0.1 ng/mL or lesser). The benefits of the eSRT strategy would be to avoid unnecessary treatments for up to one-half of high-risk patients, avoid the added cost and toxicities, and have a measurable tumor marker to assess the effectiveness of postoperative RT. (b) Once having decided to proceed with postoperative RT, deliver 72 Gy in 40 fractions to the prostate bed anatomy (inclusive of SV remnants) for low-risk patients [ie, pT2, and positive margins, and pathologic Gleason score (pGS) of 7 or less] or include pelvic nodes (50.4 Gy in 28 fractions) in addition to the prostate bed and concurrent with a short course of ADT (4–6 months LHRH + bicalutamide) for high-risk patients [ie, pT3a/b, or pGS 8–10, or negative margins, or PSA doubling time (PSADT) lesser than 6 months]. Imaging prior to initiating eSRT can, of course, always be considered depending on clinical and pathologic indicators available (eg, high Gleason score, SV invasion, short PSADT). However, at a PSA level of approximately 0.1 to 0.2 ng/mL, none of the currently available modalities (bone scan, CT scan, MRI, or FDG-PET scan) have the capabilities to detect such a small disease burden. Even newer modalities such as C-11 acetate PET scans have a sensitivity threshold of higher than 1 ng/mL.

COMMUNITY PRACTITIONER COMMENT

Brian Robert Knab

In the era of the robotic-assisted radical prostatectomy, many men with clinical early stage disease and low-/intermediate-risk factors often select surgery. Despite the use of predictive nomograms [26,27] and improved imaging modalities, many men are found to have more advanced disease and/or higher risk features when their pathology is examined postoperatively. These adverse findings place clinicians in a challenging role in terms of determining who benefits from adjuvant therapy, which type of treatment(s) to offer, and the optimal timing to initiate these therapies.

Initial results from EORTC trial 22911 and SWOG trial 8794 suggested a benefit for immediate postprostatectomy radiotherapy with an undetectable postoperative PSA for men with high-risk features, including extraprostatic extension, SV involvement, or positive surgical margins [6–8]. However, subset analysis of EORTC 22911 indicates that men with positive surgical margins derived the greatest benefit from immediate postprostatectomy radiotherapy [28]. Men with negative surgical margins, such as the patient presented here, are often surveilled postoperatively, delaying the discussion of ART or SRT until the time of clinical or biochemical failure.

A rising postprostatectomy PSA in an asymptomatic man in the absence of identifiable locoregional recurrence or distant metastatic disease presents a difficult clinical challenge. There is considerable variability in the clinical course of men with biochemical-only failure following prostatectomy. A minority of men will ultimately die of disease progression [29], while others will follow an indolent, though ultimately terminal, course [30]. Along this spectrum, there is a group of men with localized disease that can be potentially salvaged with radiotherapy, and who, if left untreated, would potentially develop clinical symptoms or die of disease progression [31].

The decision to initiate salvage therapy following a rising PSA is influenced by clinical and pathological features of the disease, competing medical comorbidities, and patient age. Multiple retrospective studies indicate that the most influential factors in discriminating between potentially salvageable patients versus those with widespread disease include the posttreatment PSA velocity/doubling time, absolute PSA level at the time of recurrence, time to PSA recurrence, as well as the stage, grade, and PSA level at diagnosis [32–34]. Overall life expectancy should also factor into the decision to offer salvage therapy, and predictive tables for life expectancy can be utilized to aid in determining the benefit of the treatment [35].

Several retrospective series have demonstrated a local control and PFS benefit with SRT following biochemical failure [10]. However, retrospective series are conflicting as to whether or not SRT prolongs overall survival [36]. The option of salvage therapy should be discussed when life expectancy exceeds 5 years with a reasonable chance of disease control following RT. Utilizing the predictive nomogram developed by Stephenson et al., this patient would be expected to have a 4-year PFS of 69% following SRT [10]. The absolute low PSA level at the time of failure and a PSADT of greater than 10 months places him in a group more likely to derive benefit from radiotherapy.

Once the decision to proceed with SRT has been made, many more clinical decisions emerge, and most of these questions do not have clearly defined answers. Currently, there is no randomized data indicating the optimal radiation dose to be used in the salvage setting. The immediate postoperative trials (EORTC 22911 and SWOG 8794) utilized doses between 60 Gy and 64 Gy to the prostate bed, and ASTRO consensus guidelines last published in 1999 [37] recommend a minimum salvage dose of 64 Gy. However, retrospective data indicate that higher doses, ie, 66 to 70 Gy, are associated with higher rates of biochemical control [38,39]. The use of image-guided radiotherapy techniques and intensity-modulated radiotherapy (IMRT) enables higher doses to be delivered in the postprostatectomy setting without a considerable increase in either the acute or long-term gastrointestinal or urinary toxicity [40].

The optimal treatment volume in the salvage setting remains an area of active investigation. Foremost, delineation of the prostate bed is a technically difficult task given the considerable changes in normal anatomy following surgery. The RTOG has published consensus guidelines for the definition of the clinical target volume in the postoperative setting. These guidelines include a corresponding online CT atlas (www.rtog.org /CoreLab/ContouringAtlases/ProstatePostOp .aspx), allowing greater uniformity in treatment volumes, with the intent of minimizing the morbidity of therapy while increasing the efficacy of treatment through improved target delineation [41]. Positive or close margins are often located at the apex of the prostate bed, involving the bladder neck or the vesicourethral anastomosis [42]. It is crucial to ensure proper coverage of this region, which is often at highest risk for residual/recurrent disease. The use of endorectal coil MRI [43] and/or the use of a urethrogram at the time of CT simulation greatly aids in the identification of this region. In addition, the patient's initial pathology report, operative findings from the prostatectomy procedure, and surgeon's input should also be taken into account when delineating the treatment volume.

The routine inclusion of the pelvic lymph nodes in the treatment volume remains debatable. For the treatment of intact prostate cancer, 2 large randomized trials, RTOG 9413 [13] and GETUG -01 [21], failed to show a long-term survival benefit with the addition of pelvic lymph node irradiation. In the immediate postoperative setting, neither EORTC 22911 nor SWOG 8794 included pelvic lymph nodes in the treatment volume.

However, the results from these trials might not be directly applicable to the salvage setting. The RTOG is currently conducting a 3-arm trial, RTOG 0534, to evaluate the benefit of including pelvic lymph node irradiation in the treatment volume. In the absence of prospective randomized data supporting a significant benefit to more comprehensive treatment fields, routine elective pelvic lymph node remains investigational and is not routinely recommended.

Improved imaging modalities such as MR spectroscopy and radioimmunoscintigraphy is likely to influence treatment volume delineation in the future. New MRI techniques such as lymphotropic superparamagnetic nanoparticles also show promise in the identification of pelvic lymph node metastases in the treatment of prostate cancer [44]. High magnetic field strength MRI (3 Tesla magnet) improves spatial resolution and the potential for improved visualization of the prostate bed and bladder neck following prostatectomy, which may even obviate the need for the use of the endorectal coil [45]. Ideally, once these newer techniques are standardized and routinely available, they will enable the clinician to determine the need for more or less comprehensive treatment fields, tailoring treatment to the individual clinical situation.

There are mounting data to support the use of concurrent and/or neoadjuvant ADT with SRT. RTOG 9601, thus far reported only in abstract form, compares SRT alone to radiation plus bicalutamide. Initial results support the use of concurrent AD, with a significant improvement in freedom from PSA progression, and a trend for improved survival in men with high-risk features [46]. Retrospective data also support the early initiation of hormonal therapy in men who underwent prostatectomy with high-risk features (GS greater than 7, PSADT less than 12 months) in delaying the development of symptomatic metastases after biochemical failure [47]. It remains unknown whether there is a synergistic effect among SRT and the concurrent administration of ADT, the optimal length of ADT, and the type of ADT. It also remains unknown whether men with lower risk features also benefit from ADT. Results from RTOG 0534 will shed light on the role of concurrent hormonal therapy in this scenario.

The use of ADT comes with risks. Multiple retrospective and population-based studies support a link between ADT and increased risk of cardiovascular disease, myocardial infarction, disruption in lipid profiles, diabetes, stroke, and possibly all-cause mortality [48]. However, more recently published data suggest that the risk of cardiovascular disease from ADT may be overestimated [49], or the increased risk of ADT may be more detrimental to men with cardiovascular risk factors at baseline [50,51]. ADT does have other well-known health risks (weight gain, loss of bone and muscle mass) and a significant detriment in quality of life measures resulting from diminished libido and erectile dysfunction [52]. Treatment with ADT should be individualized and take into consideration patient preferences and concerns, quality of life, preexisting health conditions, as well as clinical and pathological factors.

For the gentleman discussed in this case, his treatment would entail SRT to the prostate bed to a dose of 66 Gy utilizing conventional fractionation and IMRT technique. MRI of the pelvis using a high field strength magnet (3T) would be obtained to aid in target volume delineation. The decision to initiate immediate concurrent hormonal therapy would be discussed with the patient, but would not be strongly recommended for this gentleman, in light of his lower risk features. ADT would be recommended only if the patient had a persistently detectable and/or rising PSA following the completion of radiotherapy to avoid the potentially unnecessary toxicity of ADT. Entry into a clinical trial is strongly encouraged.

SECTION EDITOR'S NOTE

Stanley L. Liauw

Men with biochemical recurrence after radical prostatectomy with a life expectancy of over 10 years are typically offered SRT. All authors agree to treat this gentleman with SRT, as progression could compromise the quality of life or life expectancy of a healthy man who is 62 years old at initial recurrence. There is some variation in the authors' use of hormonal therapy and pelvic RT, and in the total dose prescription, which ranged from 66 to 72 Gy. In the absence of enrollment in a clinical trial such as RTOG 0534, 2 authors recommend treatment to the prostate bed alone without ADT, while 1 author recommends whole pelvic RT with short course ADT owing to the high-risk features (pT3a, negative margins). I would not require a pretreatment bone scan, but would order an endorectal MRI to evaluate the bed for local recurrence. Off protocol, I would recommend SRT to the pelvic lymph nodes (50.4 Gy at 1.8 Gy/fx) and the prostate bed (68.4 Gy at 1.8 Gy/fx), along with short course hormonal therapy. If the MRI demonstrated local disease, I would consider a boost of any suspicious area to approximately 72 Gy. In younger men with higher risk features, pelvic nodal RT and concurrent hormonal therapy are reasonable to discuss with patients who are willing to assume more risk with treatment. Ultimately, we await randomized data to guide this decision.

REFERENCES

1. Dahl DM, He W, Lazarus R, et al. Pathologic outcome of laparoscopic and open radical prostatectomy. *Urology.* 2006;68(6):1253–1256.
2. Vis AN, Schroder FH, van der Kwast TH. The actual value of the surgical margin status as a predictor of disease progression in men with early prostate cancer. *Eur Urol.* 2006;50(2):258–265.
3. Katz MS, Zelefsky MJ, Venkatraman ES, et al. Predictors of biochemical outcome with salvage conformal radiotherapy after radical prostatectomy for prostate cancer. *J Clin Oncol.* 2003;21(3):483–489.
4. Roehl KA, Han M, Ramos CG, et al. Cancer progression and survival rates following anatomical radical retropubic prostatectomy in 3,478 consecutive patients: Long-term results. *J Urol.* 2004;172(3):910–914.
5. Swanson GP, Riggs M, Hermans M. Pathologic findings at radical prostatectomy: Risk factors for failure and death. *Urol Oncol.* 2007;25(2):110–114.
6. Bolla M, van Poppel H, Collette L, et al. Postoperative radiotherapy after radical prostatectomy: A randomised controlled trial (EORTC trial 22911). *Lancet.* 2005;366(9485):572–578.
7. Thompson IM Jr, Tangen CM, Paradelo J, et al. Adjuvant radiotherapy for pathologically advanced prostate cancer: A randomized clinical trial. *JAMA.* 2006;296(19):2329–2335.
8. Thompson IM, Tangen CM, Paradelo J, et al. Adjuvant radiotherapy for pathological T3N0M0 prostate cancer significantly reduces risk of metastases and improves survival: Long-term followup of a randomized clinical trial. *J Urol.* 2009;181(3):956–962.
9. Wiegel T, Bottke D, Steiner U, et al. Phase III postoperative adjuvant radiotherapy after radical prostatectomy compared with radical prostatectomy alone in pT3 prostate cancer with postoperative undetectable prostate-specific antigen: ARO 96-02/AUO AP 09/95. *J Clin Oncol.* 2009;27(18):2924–2930.
10. Stephenson AJ, Scardino PT, Kattan MW, et al. Predicting the outcome of salvage radiation therapy for recurrent prostate cancer after radical prostatectomy. *J Clin Oncol.* 2007;25(15):2035–2041.
11. King CR. Adjuvant radiotherapy after prostatectomy: Does waiting for a detectable prostate-specific antigen level make sense? *Int J Radiat Oncol Biol Phys.* 2011;80(1):1–3.
12. Ohri N, Dicker AP, Trabulsi EJ, Showalter TN. Can early implementation of salvage radiotherapy for prostate cancer improve the therapeutic ratio? A systematic review and regression meta-analysis with radiobiological modelling. *Eur J Cancer.* 2012;48(6):837–844.
13. Lawton CA, Desilvio M, Roach M 3rd, et al. An update of the phase III trial comparing whole pelvic to prostate only radiotherapy and neoadjuvant to adjuvant total androgen suppression: Updated analysis of RTOG 94-13, with emphasis on unexpected hormone/radiation interactions. *Int J Radiat Oncol Biol Phys.* 2007;69(3):646–655.
14. Shipley WU, Hunt H, Lukka P, et al. Initial Report of RTOG 9601: A phase III trial in prostate cancer: Anti-androgen therapy (AAT) with bicalutamide during and after radiation therapy (RT) improves freedom from progression and reduces the incidence of metastatic disease in patients following radical prostatectomy (RP) with pT2-3, N0 disease and elevated PSA levels. *Int J Rad Onc Biol Phys.* 2010;78:S27.
15. McLeod DG, Iversen P, See WA, et al. Bicalutamide 150 mg plus standard care vs standard care alone for early prostate cancer. *BJU International.* 2006;97(2):247–254.
16. Parker C, Sydes MR, Catton C, et al. Radiotherapy and androgen deprivation in combination after local surgery (RADICALS): A new Medical Research Council/National Cancer Institute of Canada phase III trial of adjuvant treatment after radical prostatectomy. *BJU Int.* 2007;99(6):1376–1379.
17. Parker C, Clarke N, Logue J, et al. RADICALS (Radiotherapy and Androgen Deprivation in Combination after Local Surgery). *Clin Oncol (R Coll Radiol).* 2007;19:167–171.
18. Richaud P, Sargos P, Henriques de Figueiredo B, et al. Postoperative radiotherapy of prostate cancer (GETUG-17). *Cancer Radiother.* 2010;14:500–503.
19. Trans Tasman Radiation Oncology Group (TROG 08-03) RAVES trial: Radiotherapy – Adjuvant Versus Early Salvage.
20. King CR. The timing of salvage radiotherapy following radical prostatectomy: A meta-analysis. *Int J Radiat Oncol Biol Phys.* 2012;84:104–111.
21. Pommier P, Chabaud S, Lagrange JL, et al. Is there a role for pelvic irradiation in localized

prostate adenocarcinoma? Preliminary results of GETUG-01. *J Clin Oncol.* 2007;25:5366–5373.

22. Spiotto MT, Hancock SL, King CR. Radiotherapy after prostatectomy: Improved biochemical relapse-free survival with whole pelvic compared with prostate bed only for high-risk patients. *Int J Radiat Oncol Biol Phys.* 2007;69:54–61.

23. King CR, Presti JC Jr, Gill H, et al. Radiotherapy after radical prostatectomy: Does transient androgen suppression improve outcomes? *Int J Radiat Oncol Biol Phys.* 2004;59:341–347.

24. Ost P, Cozzarini C, De Meerleer G, et al. High-dose adjuvant radiotherapy after radical prostatectomy with or without androgen deprivation therapy. *Int J Radiat Oncol Biol Phys.* 2012;83(3):960–965.

25. King CR, Kapp DS. Radiotherapy after prostatectomy: Is the evidence for dose escalation out there? *Int J Radiat Oncol Biol Phys.* 2008;71:346–350.

26. Shariat SF, Karakiewicz PI, Suardi N, Kattan MW. Comparison of nomograms with other methods for predicting outcomes in prostate cancer: A critical analysis of the literature. *Clin Cancer Res.* 2008 Jul 15;14(14):4400–4407.

27. Makarov DV, Trock BJ, Humphreys EB, et al. Updated nomogram to predict pathologic stage of prostate cancer given prostate-specific antigen level, clinical stage, and biopsy Gleason score (Partin tables) based on cases from 2000 to 2005. *Urology.* 2007 Jun;69(6):1095–1101.

28. Van der Kwast TH, Bolla M, Van Poppel H, et al. Identification of patients with prostate cancer who benefit from immediate postoperative radiotherapy: EORTC 22911. *J Clin Oncol.* 2007 Sep 20;25(27):4178–4186.

29. Freedland SJ, Humphreys EB, Mangold LA, et al. Death in patients with recurrent prostate cancer after radical prostatectomy: Prostate-specific antigen doubling time subgroups and their associated contributions to all-cause mortality. *J Clin Oncol.* 2007 May 1;25(13):1765–1771.

30. Pound CR, Partin AW, Eisenberger MA, et al. Natural history of progression after PSA elevation following radical prostatectomy. *JAMA.* 1999 May 5;281(17):1591–1597.

31. Freedland SJ, Humphreys EB, Mangold LA, et al. Risk of prostate cancer-specific mortality following biochemical recurrence after radical prostatectomy. *JAMA.* 2005 Jul 27;294(4):433–439.

32. D'Amico AV, Chen MH, Sun L, et al. Adjuvant versus salvage radiation therapy for prostate cancer and the risk of death. *BJU Int.* 2010 Dec;106(11):1618–1622.

33. D'Amico AV, Moul JW, Carroll PR, et al. Surrogate end point for prostate cancer-specific mortality after radical prostatectomy or radiation therapy. *J Natl Cancer Inst.* 2003 Sep 17;95(18):1376–1383.

34. Zhou P, Chen MH, McLeod D, et al. Predictors of prostate cancer-specific mortality after radical prostatectomy or radiation therapy. *J Clin Oncol.* 2005 Oct 1;23(28):6992–6998.

35. Mohler JL, Armstrong AJ, Bahnson RR, et al. Prostate cancer, version 3.2012 featured updates to the NCCN guidelines. *J Natl Comp Canc Netw.* 2012 Sep 10:1081–1087.

36. Boorjian SA, Karnes RJ, Crispen PL, et al. Radiation therapy after radical prostatectomy: Impact on metastasis and survival. *J Urol.* 2009 Dec;182(6):2708–2714.

37. Cox JD, Gallagher MJ, Hammond EH, et al. Consensus statements on radiation therapy of prostate cancer: Guidelines for prostate re-biopsy after radiation and for radiation therapy with rising prostate-specific antigen levels after radical prostatectomy. American Society for Therapeutic Radiology and Oncology Consensus Panel. *J Clin Oncol.* 1999 Apr;17(4):1155.

38. King CR, Spiotto MT. Improved outcomes with higher doses for salvage radiotherapy after prostatectomy. *Int J Radiat Oncol Biol Phys.* 2008 May 1;71(1):23–27.

39. Bernard JR Jr, Buskirk SJ, Heckman MG, et al. Salvage radiotherapy for rising prostate-specific antigen levels after radical prostatectomy for prostate cancer: dose-response analysis. *Int J Radiat Oncol Biol Phys.* 2010 Mar 1;76(3):735–740.

40. Nath SK, Sandhu AP, Rose BS, et al. Toxicity analysis of postoperative image-guided intensity-modulated radiotherapy for prostate cancer. *Int J Radiat Oncol Biol Phys.* 2010 Oct 1;78(2):435–441.

41. Michalski JM, Lawton C, El Naqa I, et al. Development of RTOG consensus guidelines for the definition of the clinical target volume for postoperative conformal radiation therapy for prostate cancer. *Int J Radiat Oncol Biol Phys.* 2010 Feb 1;76(2):361–368.

42. Connolly JA, Shinohara K, Presti JC Jr, Carroll PR. Local recurrence after radical prostatectomy: Characteristics in size, location, and relationship to prostate-specific antigen and surgical margins. *Urology.* 1996 Feb;47(2):225-31

43. Silverman JM, Krebs TL. MR imaging evaluation with a transrectal surface coil of local recurrence of prostatic cancer in men who have undergone radical prostatectomy. *AJR Am J Roentgenol.* 1997 Feb;168(2):379–385.

44. Harisinghani MG, Barentsz J, Hahn PF, et al. Noninvasive detection of clinically occult lymph-node metastases in prostate cancer. *N Engl J Med.* 2003 Jun 19;348(25):2491–2499.

45. Sosna J, Pedrosa I, Dewolf WC, et al. MR imaging of the prostate at 3 Tesla: Comparison of an external phased-array coil to imaging with an endorectal coil at 1.5 Tesla. *Acad Radiol.* 2004;11:857–862.

46. Shipley WU, Hunt D, Lukka HR, et al. Initial report of RTOG 9601, a phase III trial in prostate cancer: Effect of anti-androgen therapy (AAT) with bicalutamide during and after radiation therapy (RT) on freedom from progression and incidence of metastatic disease in patients following radical prostatectomy (RP) with pT2-3,N0 disease and elevated PSA levels. *J Clin Oncol.* 2011;29(Suppl 7):abstract #1.

47. Moul JW, Wu H, Sun L, et al. Early versus delayed hormonal therapy for prostate specific antigen only recurrence of prostate cancer after radical prostatectomy. *J Urol.* 2008 May; 179 (5 Suppl):S53–S59.

48. Levine GN, D'Amico AV, Berger P, et al. Androgen-deprivation therapy in prostate cancer and cardiovascular risk: A science advisory from the American Heart Association, American Cancer Society, and American Urological Association: Endorsed by the American Society for Radiation Oncology. *CA Cancer J Clin.* 2010 Feb 16; 21(6):833–840.

49. Nguyen PL, Je Y, Schutz FA, et al. Association of androgen deprivation therapy with cardiovascular death in patients with prostate cancer: A meta-analysis of randomized trials. *JAMA.* 2011 Dec 7;306(21):2359–2366.

50. Nguyen PL, Chen MH, Beckman JA, et al. Influence of androgen deprivation therapy on all-cause mortality in men with high-risk prostate cancer and a history of congestive heart failure or myocardial infarction. *Int J Radiat Oncol Biol Phys.* 2012 Mar 15;82(4):1411–1416.

51. Nanda A, Chen MH, Braccioforte MH, et al. Hormonal therapy use for prostate cancer and mortality in men with coronary artery disease-induced congestive heart failure or myocardial infarction. *JAMA.* 2009 Aug 26;302(8): 866–873.

52. Saylor PJ, Smith MR. Metabolic complications of androgen deprivation therapy for prostate cancer. *J Urol.* 2009 May;181(5):1998–2006; discussion 2007-8.

■ CASE 3 ■

Treatment Options in the Management of High-Risk Prostate Cancer

CLINICAL PROBLEM

Some men with nonmetastatic, high-risk prostate cancer (PSA of more than 20, clinical stage higher than T3, Gleason score of 8 or higher) are considered candidates for either radiation therapy (RT) (with long-term hormonal therapy [HT]) or radical prostatectomy (RP) (with possible postoperative RT to follow). It is debatable whether surgery or RT offers the best risk–benefit ratio in this high-risk group. For men who are treated with primary RT, a brachytherapy boost is sometimes proposed to maximize local control. It is unclear whether a combined approach of external beam radiation therapy (EBRT) and implant is preferred over dose-escalated EBRT alone because of the higher risk of distant failure in the high-risk population, and the potential for additional morbidity with more aggressive local therapy. The optimal duration of HT for men who receive a brachytherapy boost is also unknown.

CASE EXAMPLE

A 58-year-old man with a PSA level of 22 ng/mL undergoes a prostate biopsy, showing adenocarcinoma of the prostate, Gleason score 4 + 4, involving 6 of 12 cores. His clinical exam shows stage T2c disease. He has no other medical problems, and has excellent urinary and sexual function. CT shows no suspicious lymphadenopathy, and bone scan is negative for metastasis.

Management Decisions

- What are the advantages of primary radiotherapy versus primary surgery for high-risk disease?
- When high-risk prostate cancer is treated with RT, which patients, if any, should receive a brachytherapy boost?
- What is the role of HT for patients getting a brachytherapy boost?

MAJOR OPINION

Richard G. Stock

What Are the Advantages of Primary Radiotherapy Versus Primary Surgery for High-Risk Disease?

This case is a classic presentation of high-risk, high-volume prostate cancer. Assuming that the patient has had a negative metastatic work-up with a total body bone scan and a CT scan of the abdomen and pelvis, the significantly elevated PSA correlates with a high local tumor burden. My primary approach to this type of cancer would be with trimodality therapy (HT, external beam irradiation, and permanent seed prostate brachytherapy). This approach is optimal because it uses 2 current advances in the radiotherapeutic management of prostate cancer: dose escalation and adjuvant androgen deprivation. In addition, it differs from a surgical approach in that it does not risk the inadvertent cutting through of areas involved with the tumor and provides much better coverage of extraprostatic disease spread.

The surgical approach to high-risk, high-grade prostate cancer has resulted in suboptimal biochemical control rates. For RP, findings of positive margins on the pathologic specimen or non-organ confined disease can be seen as surrogates for inadequate local control. In one large series, the likelihood of obtaining negative margins and finding organ-confined disease was only 21% for patients with Gleason scores of 8 to 10 [1]. Biochemical failure rates, especially for Gleason scores of 8 to 10, have unexpectedly been high following RP. Outcomes from the Henri Mondor University Hospital in France on 180 patients with Gleason scores of 8 to 10 show a 7 year progression-free survival of only 37% [2]. The Mayo Clinic's

125

experience with patients with Gleason scores of 8 to 10 demonstrates a 10-year progression-free survival rate of 36% [3]. Reports from 2 experienced and high-volume centers, Memorial Sloan Kettering Cancer Center (MSKCC) and Washington University in St. Louis, reveal biochemical control rates for patients with Gleason scores of 8 to 10 following RP at 10 years of 39% and 37%, respectively [4,5]. In a large retrospective study by Walz et al., 4760 patients from 3 institutions underwent RP for high-risk prostate cancer. At 10 years, the actuarial biochemical freedom from failure rate for patients with biopsy Gleason scores of 8 to 10 was 20% [6]. These high biochemical failure rates are most likely a result of local failure due to the inability of the surgical procedure to remove all local disease. Confirming this finding was a recent analysis in Southwestern Oncology Group (SWOG) trial 8794, which examined the role of postoperative RT following RP in high-risk disease. One of the conclusions of the study, referring to surgical treatment, was "the pattern of treatment failure in high-risk patients is predominantly local with a surprisingly low incidence of metastatic failure" [7].

When High-Risk Prostate Cancer Is Treated With RT, Which Patients, if Any, Should Receive a Brachytherapy Boost?

Another approach to high-risk disease is external beam irradiation. Unfortunately, the dose delivered by this treatment is probably too low to adequately control a large tumor burden with aggressive histology that is typically found in high-risk disease. For conventional external beam irradiation, the best method for assessing local control is posttreatment prostate biopsy. Positive postirradiation prostate biopsies have ranged from 18% to 62% [8–11]. In a series by Dugan et al., the positive posttreatment prostate biopsy rate for high-grade cancers was 64% [9]. The addition of androgen deprivation to external beam therapy has been shown to improve treatment outcomes, but the overall likelihood of biochemical control still remains low. In Radiation Therapy Oncology Group (RTOG) 92-02, the treatment arm consisting of long-term HT (2 years) and external beam irradiation to a dose of 70 Gy EBRT only resulted in a 40% disease-free survival rate at 8 years [12]. Even in the European Organisation for Research and Treatment of Cancer (EORTC) trial, which had the arm with the longest duration of androgen

suppression (3 years), the progression-free survival at 10 years was still slightly less than 50% [13].

The combination of brachytherapy and external beam therapy results in the highest delivered radiation dose. The importance of radiation dose has been shown many times in both randomized and nonrandomized RT trials. In addition, it delivers higher doses of radiation than either brachytherapy alone or external beam therapy alone [14]. For example, a combination of a Pd-103 implant with a prescription dose of 100 Gy in combination with an external beam dose of 45 Gy is typically associated with a biologically effective dose (BED) of more than 200 Gy using an alpha/beta ratio of 2 [14]. This is significantly greater than the typical high dose of intensity-modulated radiation therapy (IMRT) of 81 Gy, which has a BED of 155 Gy using the same formulation. Published outcomes using combined low-dose-rate brachytherapy and external beam irradiation, with or without HT, reveal that this approach appears to yield the best outcomes for high-risk disease. Stock showed a biochemical control rate of 83% at 7 years for 360 high-risk patients treated using HT, brachytherapy, and external beam irradiation [15]. Dattoli et al. found a 70% biochemical control rate at 10 years for 124 high-risk patients [16]. Sylvester et al. found a 68% control rate at 15 years for high-risk patients [17]. Potters et al. reported on 418 high-risk patients (173 patients received combined implant and external beam therapy) and found a 12-year biochemical control rate of 63% [18]. Merrick et al. reported on 204 high-risk patients treated using combination therapy, with and without HT, and found a 10-year biochemical control rate of 86% [19]. In a multi-institutional pooled analysis, Stone et al., reporting on 522 high-risk patients, showed a 90% freedom from biochemical failure at 5 years for patients with BED more than 200 Gy (doses typically achieved with combination therapy) [20]. In addition, in the subset of high-risk patients with Gleason scores of 8 to 10, the results have been excellent as well. Merrick et al. showed a 10-year freedom from PSA failure rates of 80% and 89% (without and with HT) for patients with Gleason scores higher than 8 [19]. Stock et al., in a study of 181 patients with Gleason scores of 8 to 10-treated with combination therapy, found that at 8 years the actuarial freedom from biochemical failure, freedom from distant metastases, prostate cancer-specific survival, and overall survival were 73%, 80%, 87%, and 79%, respectively [21]. Sylvester et al. found a 61% rate at 12 years [17]. Dattoli et al. demonstrated a 58% rate for patients with a Gleason score of 9 and an 80% rate for those with a Gleason 8 at 10 years [16]. Results for another subgroup of high-risk patients, those with PSA higher than 20 ng/mL, have also been good. Rise in biochemical control rates from 66% to 72% has been reported [15–17]. This apparent improvement seen in biochemical control rates over RP stem from improvements in local control. Stock et al. found a negative posttreatment biopsy rate of 97% in 70 high-risk patients undergoing posttreatment prostate biopsies [15]. A recent analysis from the Surveillance Epidemiology and End Results (SEER) database found that the inclusion of brachytherapy in the radiotherapeutic management of high-grade prostate cancer improved prostate cancer-specific survival over external beam therapy without brachytherapy. The 10-year prostate cancer-specific mortality was at 21.1% when treating with external beam therapy, at 11.3% when treating with brachytherapy, and at 13.4% when treating with a combination of brachytherapy and external beam therapy [22].

What Is the Role of HT for Patients Getting a Brachytherapy Boost?

As a combination of brachytherapy and external beam therapy results in extremely high prostate doses, the question concerning the need for additional hormonal manipulation arises in this setting. Clearly, HT has been shown to decrease the likelihood of obtaining a positive biopsy post-RT [11,23]. This suggests that one of the key roles HT plays when used in combination therapy is to increase local control. If high enough doses are delivered, is this enhancement really needed? Stock et al. examined this question in intermediate-risk patients and found that HT did not improve biochemical control when added to combined brachytherapy and external beam irradiation [24]. There may be a different type of benefit to using HT in high-risk patients. HT in this setting may provide a benefit, not in primarily increasing local control, but in suppressing microscopic systemic disease. In a retrospective analysis of 1342 patients treated using brachytherapy from multiple community-based centers, D'Amico found that trimodality therapy (HT, brachytherapy, and external beam therapy) reduced prostate cancer-specific mortality over brachytherapy with HT or brachytherapy combined with external beam therapy alone [25].

Treatment Recommendation

At Mount Sinai Medical Center, this high-risk patient would be treated with 3 months of HT followed by a brachytherapy implant to the prostate and seminal vesicles using Pd-103 seeds to a prescription dose of 100 Gy. Two months following implantation, IMRT would be delivered to the prostate and seminal vesicles to a dose of 45 Gy in 25 fractions. The total duration of HT would be 9 months. The exact duration of HT to be used in this setting is not known. In the setting of external beam therapy alone, both short-term hormonal therapies (4–6 months) as well as long-term HT (2–3 years) have been tested in randomized trials. For high-grade disease (Gleason score 8–10), there appears to be a benefit to using long-term HT. How much of this benefit is derived from increased local versus distant control of disease is not known. Our institution has used 9 months of HT since 1994 with combination brachytherapy and external beam irradiation and results for Gleason scores of 8 to 10 have been impressive. This suggests that long-term HT may not be needed with higher radiation dose.

ACADEMIC COMMENT

Andrew K. Lee

Regardless of the definition used, this patient would be considered at high risk of failing local monotherapy. While clinical T2c disease alone may be considered a high-risk factor in some risk stratification schema, the presence of Gleason 4 + 4 disease and a presenting PSA of more than 20 ng/mL represent an even higher risk situation. Despite a negative CT and bone scan, this patient is at high risk of failing local monotherapy as well as at substantial risk for having occult disease outside the prostate.

Choosing the optimal therapy in this case depends on addressing the local disease and the systemic components of failure. Essentially, 2 possible scenarios exist: either this patient has distant metastatic disease at presentation or the disease is still relatively localized to the prostate and periprostatic regions. If the patient still has local-only disease, maximizing local therapy is paramount for a local cure and also to minimize the chances for subsequent systemic seeding from the primary tumor. If the patient has microscopic distant disease, then the role of local therapy is still important as evidenced from randomized trials showing a survival advantage to patients receiving local therapy and HT versus HT alone [26,27]. Furthermore, addressing the local primary tumor may yield some advantage in patients who are receiving systemic therapy for distant disease [28,29]. The exact mechanism for this clinical benefit is unknown, but it may involve minimization of subsequent androgen-independent cells where the bulk of disease is greatest.

Surgical monotherapy (ie, RP) would offer less than a 65% chance of durable cure for this patient and therefore should be reserved for those patients enrolled in a clinical trial or if there is a clear understanding that subsequent adjuvant therapy will likely be needed. Surgical extirpation would not be considered a primary, stand-alone recommendation, but it would offer the advantage of obtaining pathologic information on the status of the pelvic lymph nodes and the extent of the local disease. Furthermore, postoperative RT has offered reasonable clinical outcomes in patients with unfavorable pathologic features (ie, positive surgical margins and pathologic T3 disease) [13,30], which this patient would likely have. In the setting of pathologically node-positive patients following prostatectomy, early adjuvant HT is one option based on the Eastern Cooperative Oncology Group (ECOG) randomized study [31]. The benefit of adjuvant pelvic radiation in these particular node-positive patients is uncertain. Any theoretical advantages of surgery would need to be weighed against the potential morbidity of the surgery and postoperative side effects.

Another reasonable therapeutic option would be a combination of long-term HT (ie, at least 28 months) and dose-escalated EBRT. Based on randomized data, we know the following: (a) Combination HT with local RT is better than HT alone [26,27]. (b) Longer term HT is better than shorter term HT especially for men with higher Gleason scores [32,33]. (c) Higher radiation doses improve clinical outcomes but not necessarily overall survival [34,35].

In the RTOG 92-02 trial, 1554 men with high-risk and locally advanced prostate cancer were randomized to either 4 months of neoadjuvant and concurrent total androgen blockade and RT (45 Gy to pelvic lymph nodes and 65–70 Gy to prostate) or the same treatment with an additional 24 months of adjuvant goserelin alone. After a median follow-up of over 11 years, there was a significant advantage in all clinical endpoints (ie, local progression, distant metastasis, biochemical failure) to the long-term HT arm. No difference in overall survival was noted except in those patients

with Gleason scores of 8 to 10 with 10 year overall survival rates of 31.9% versus 45.1% ($p = .0061$) in favor of the long-term HT arm. Absolute rates of local progression for the long-term HT arm were relatively low at 12.3% despite using relatively low doses of radiation [32]. Data from dose-escalation series suggest even lower rates of clinical local progression (less than 5%) with higher radiation doses [34,36,37]. However, despite the improvement in local control, no randomized study has shown an improvement in overall survival for higher radiation doses in prostate cancer.

Using a brachytherapy boost following a lower dose of external beam radiation is a valid method to escalate the total radiation dose, and this technique does permit a relatively high BED to the prostate gland. Single institution and pooled series have shown good results with this technique with shorter duration HT (eg, less than 1 year) even in patients with high-risk features [21,23,38]. However, few patients (less than 10%) in those high-risk series contained this particular patient's constellation of high-risk features (ie, T2c, Gleason 8, *and* PSA 22). Furthermore, the biochemical failure rates for these patients was still on the order of 30% or higher. While these results may be better than older prospective results in patients with more advanced disease using lower radiation doses, they seem to be reasonably equivalent to more modern series using higher external beam doses (ie, higher than 76 Gy) [34,39,40]. Improvements in external beam radiation planning and delivery and image guidance have allowed safe escalation of radiation doses with relatively low side-effect profiles. Modern techniques would deliver a high radiation dose to not only the prostate but also to the periprostatic tissues (risk of extracapsular extension of approximately 35%) and seminal vesicles [risk of seminal vesicle involvement (SVI) of approximately 30%] for this patient.

The possibility of using trimodality therapy (ie, external beam therapy, brachytherapy, and HT) should not be dismissed, but one should be cautious about its clinical superiority over modern high-dose EBRT and HT. Randomized data from the EORTC trials have shown superior prostate cancer-specific survival with the combination of 3 years of HT versus 6 months of HT with RT. In the absence of randomized (or prospective) data comparing longer term HT (greater than 28 months) versus intermediate regimens (eg, 9–12 months), recommending less than 2 to 3 years of HT for patients with this level of disease should be done with extreme care. While shorter course HT may be appropriate for carefully selected patients with high-risk prostate cancer, this particular patient has several unfavorable features and 2 to 3 years of adjuvant HT would be considered standard. While the morbidity of 2 to 3 years of adjuvant HT should not be dismissed, it is likely less morbid than receiving indefinite HT, whether continuous or intermittent, in the salvage setting.

Furthermore, the potential morbidity of combination EBRT and brachytherapy has been shown to be significant in prospective RTOG studies [41]. Other factors to consider include the patient's current urinary function, prostate size and anatomy, possible SVI, and the patient's preference.

I would ask this patient to consider one of the following options for treatment: (a) Combination long-term HT for at least 28 months beginning at least 2 months prior to external beam radiation, and radiation to the prostate and seminal vesicles, with a cumulative dose of at least 78 Gy. (b) The same hormone regimen with 45 to 50 Gy of external beam radiation to the prostate and seminal vesicles followed by a brachytherapy boost (endorectal coil MRI may be helpful in assessing the extent of extracapsular extension and SVI). (c) Participation in a clinical trial with more intensive systemic therapy that also contains a local therapy component.

COMMUNITY PRACTITIONER COMMENT

Robert K. Takamiya

The patient described in the case study has high-risk prostate cancer. In fact, his prognosis is especially serious given the presence of 2 out of 3 high-risk features, namely Gleason score 8 and PSA higher than 20 [42]. Most would agree that this high-risk patient has resilient/aggressive local disease, regional disease, or early metastatic disease. The Partin tables [43] describe this patient as carrying a 12% probability of prostate confined disease, a 33% chance of extra prostatic extension (EPE), a 28% chance of SVI, and a 26% chance of lymph node involvement (LNI). Although controversial [44], the Mack Roach Formula [45] similarly estimates a locally advanced disease in this case (83% risk of ECE, 42% risk of SVI, and 34% risk of LNI). Given this prognostic profile, aggressive brachytherapy-based treatment has the best chance of rendering the patient disease-free.

For high-risk patients, there is a growing body of literature that supports superior cure rates with brachytherapy-based treatment over surgery [1,3,21,46–49]. The Johns Hopkins surgical series [1] showed 21% of the patients with a Gleason score of 8 to 10 had negative margins and prostate-confined disease after surgery, of which only 50% achieved biochemical-free survival at 10 years. By contrast, supplemental external beam radiation can treat at-risk periprostatic tissues. The addition of a permanent prostate implant (PPI) boost allows for escalation of BED to the prostate, which has shown excellent outcomes in intermediate- and high-risk patients, as recently demonstrated by a multicenter study [46,47]. The Mount Sinai group published their Gleason 8 to 10 experience with trimodality therapy including a total of 8 to 9 months of neoadjuvant, concurrent, and adjuvant androgen deprivation therapy (ADT) with a dose of 45 Gy external beam radiation and PPI boost with a freedom-from-biochemical failure rate of 73% at 8 years [21]. The group from West Virginia confirmed these results with a similar treatment plan [10,11].

One could consider an additional workup for this patient. If biopsies were positive at the "base" of the prostate, seminal vesicle biopsies could be considered. This may alter the radiation dose relationship between the brachytherapy and the external beam therapy components. MRI may aid in decision making. If seemingly involved or suspicious, inclusion of the proximal 1.0 to 1.5 cm of seminal vesicles within the planning target volume (PTV) of the implant would be reasonable. Furthermore, a patient with a PSA level of 22 and a Gleason score 8 disease has significant risk for LNI. Although controversial [50–52] and the subject of an open randomized trial (RTOG 0924) [53], treatment of the pelvic lymph nodes with external beam therapy is reasonable. The use of IMRT with image guidance will aid in minimizing toxicity [54–56].

This patient should undergo a brachytherapy planning transrectal ultrasound (TRUS) volume study in the office by the treating radiation oncologist. Owing to androgen suppression, timing the TRUS close in proximity to the implant and at least 2 months postinitiation of ADT is important to ensure proper correlation of prostate gland geometry at the time of the actual implant. Consecutive 5-mm transverse (axial) images are taken through the prostate gland. The prostate gland is contoured on each image to generate the prostate volume. Images are exported to the brachytherapy planning system. Margins are added to the gross target volume (prostate) to generate the PTV, including a margin to account for potential microscopic disease and dose delivery uncertainty. The prostate volume is enhanced on the order of 3 to 5 mm in every dimension, with generous margins (approximately 10 mm) added in the lateral and posterolateral aspect based on pathologic studies identifying this as a high-risk region [56]. Planning ensues following Seattle Prostate Institute's technique that was described earlier [57]. Typically, stranded Pd-103 radioactive seeds are utilized to a prescription dose of 90 to 100 Gy (NIST-99). The 100% isodose line typically covers more than 99% of the PTV, often with additional margin beyond the PTV. PTV V150% and V100%, measurements of heterogeneity and the "hot spot" are on the order of 50% to 60% and 10% to 20%, respectively. Rectal volume receiving 100% of the prescription dose (RV100%) is kept at less than 1 mL to ensure minimal toxicity. Urethral doses are estimated, keeping the central prostate at less than 120% of the prescription dose. Seed activity varies with geometry; usually 1.2 mCi (range 1.1–1.3 mCi) per seed is utilized.

During the procedure, adjustments to the preplan are made to the periurethral needles and the posterior row [57]. Visualizing the urethra with aerated KY jelly is extremely helpful in minimizing urethral dose, especially at the apex. Careful assessment of the posterior row is equally important to minimize rectal complications [58]. After the PPI, electromagnetic beacon transponders are placed at the right base, left base, and apex of the prostate to provide real-time fiducial localization during external beam therapy. Fluoroscopic imaging is helpful to ensure proper separation between the transponders. A cystoscopy is performed to assess the urethra for strands and to remove blood clots to prevent retention. A Foley catheter is subsequently placed and connected for the purpose of saline irrigation. The patient is then taken to recovery. After postanesthesia criteria are met, and if the urine is clear, the Foley catheter is removed. Postoperatively, a 5 day course of antibiotics is given. A selective alpha blocker is prescribed prophylactically. Narcotic medication or over-the-counter (OTC) NSAIDs are used for pain control and to fight inflammation. Radiation safety precautions, activity restrictions, and diet recommendations are given on discharge.

Day 0 CT-based dosimetry is performed to ensure proper dose benchmarks are met. This represents the worst-case scenario in terms of target-dose coverage because of prostate edema. Generally speaking, criteria for a satisfactory implant include a prostate V100 of 85% to 90%, D90 greater than 90%, and V150 less than 30%. Optimally, the RV100 is below 1 mL, indicating a minimal risk of grade 2 proctitis [59]. If variations are detected, the external beam therapy component can be adjusted.

External beam simulation takes place 6 weeks postimplant, and treatment commences 8 weeks afterward. A "vacuum-lock" bag is used for patient immobilization. Margins are minimal in the posterior aspect (1–2 mm expansion beyond the prostate). Again, generous margins in the lateral aspect are included (an approximate 10 mm). Seminal vesicles are included in the target volume. In this case, the pelvic lymph nodes would be included as well. "Point and shoot" IMRT with 7 to 9 gantry angles and 6x photons are utilized. Two-arc vesicular monoamine transporter (VMAT) plans also demonstrate excellent conformality, often with a shorter treatment time. Dosimetric goals include having the 98% isodose line covering 98% of the volume, with the typical hot spot running 4% to 6% above the prescription dose of 45 Gy in 25 fractions. Three percent hot spots are qualitatively superior and anterior within the prostate PTV. Dose constraints to the proximal femurs, bladder, and rectum are defined by RTOG 0126 [60] scaled to 45 Gy. Patients are given a low-fiber diet and instructed to drink water prior to treatment. Treatments are delivered with the goal of an empty rectum and full bladder. Real-time electromagnetic localization takes place with a window of 3 mm.

Side effects from external beam include irritable urinary symptoms, bowel irregularity, and mild fatigue. NSAIDs, alpha blockers, and OTCs such as imodium are useful in managing side effects. ADT is initiated 2 to 3 months prior to radiation, continuing during the PPI and external beam therapy component, and for 3 to 4 months afterward, for a total of 8 to 9 months. Clinical follow-up and PSA monitoring ensue.

To summarize, recommendations include neoadjuvant, concurrent, and adjuvant ADT on the order of 9 months, PPI boost, and supplemental EBRT for the case study presented. Although not addressed, it would be reasonable to consider a high-dose-rate (HDR) boost instead of PPI. And despite the controversy, whole pelvic radiotherapy may be beneficial given the high-risk prognostic features present in this case.

SECTION EDITOR'S NOTE

Stanley L. Liauw

Men with high-risk prostate cancer treated with primary RT are at risk for failing both locally and systemically. All authors agree with offering dose-escalated RT and concurrent HT, but there is no consensus on the role for brachytherapy and the length of HT. All are open to the possibility of a brachytherapy boost. Two authors are comfortable with only 9 months of ADT in the setting of a brachytherapy boost, while 1 author recommends 28 months of ADT. In this case, I would favor a brachytherapy boost after an initial course of EBRT inclusive of the pelvic lymph nodes to optimize local control. While EBRT along with brachytherapy may result in more local morbidity compared to EBRT alone, a high-risk patient who is younger, has good urinary function, and does not have a very high risk of distant failure may derive the most benefit from aggressive local therapy. In addition, although not formally proven, EBRT along with brachytherapy could minimize the gains of long-term HT and allow for greater flexibility to reduce the duration of ADT, and minimize hormonal related toxicity. Unfortunately, there are no data that adequately address the risk–benefit ratio regarding the length of ADT after brachytherapy. Given the patient's young age, lack of medical comorbidity, and risk for systemic recurrence, I would favor 28 total months of ADT.

REFERENCES

1. Bastian PJ, Gonzalgo ML, Aronson WJ, et al. Clinical and pathologic outcome after radical prostatectomy for prostate cancer patients with a preoperative Gleason sum of 8 to 10. *Cancer.* 2008;107:1265–1272.

2. Rodrigues-Covarrubias F, Larre S, De La Taille A, et al. The outcome of patients with pathological Gleason score > or =8 prostate cancer after radical prostatectomy. *BJU Int.* 2008;101:305–307.

3. Lau WK, Bergstralh EJ, Blute ML, et al. Radical prostatectomy for pathological Gleason 8 or greater prostate cancer: Influence of concomitant pathological variables. *J Urol.* 2002;167:117–122.

4. Donohue JF, Bianco FJ, Kuroiwa K, et al. Poorly differentiated prostate cancer treated with radical prostatectomy: Long-term outcome and incidence of pathological downgrading. *J Urol.* 2006;176:991–995.

5. Desireddi NV, Roehl KA, Loeb S, et al. Improved stage and grade-specific progression-free survival rates after radical prostatectomy in the PSA era. *Urology.* 2007;70:950–955.

6. Walz J, Joniau S, Chun FK, et al. Pathological results and rates of treatment failure in high-risk prostate cancer patients after radical prostatectomy. *BJU Int.* 2011;107:765–770.

7. Swanson GP, Hussey MA, Tangen CM, et al. Predominant treatment failure in post-prostatectomy patients is local: Analysis of patterns of treatment failure in SWOG 8794. *J Clin Oncol.* 2007;25:2225–2229.

8. Crook J, Robertson S, Collin G, et al. Clinical relevance of trans-rectal ultrasound, biopsy and serum prostate-specific antigen following external beam radiotherapy for carcinoma of the prostate. *Int J Radiat Oncol Biol Phys.* 1993;27:31–37.

9. Dugan TC, Shipley WU, Young RM, et al. Biopsy after external beam radiation therapy for adenocarcinoma of the prostate: Correlation with original histological grade and current prostate specific antigen levels. *J Urol.* 1991;146:1313–1316.

10. Kuban DA, El-Mahdi AM, Schellhammer P. The significance of post-irradiation prostate biopsy with with long-term follow-up. *Int J Radiat Oncol Biol Phys.* 1992;24:409–414.

11. Laverdiere J, Gomez, Jl, Cusan L, et al. Beneficial effect of combination therapy administered prior and following external beam radiation therapy in localized prostate cancer. *Int J Radiat Oncol Biol Phys.* 1997;37:247–252.

12. Hanks GE, Pajak TF, Porter A, et al. Phase III trial of long-term adjuvant androgen deprivation after neoadjuvant hormonal cytoreduction and radiotherapy in locally advanced carcinoma of the prostate: The Radiation Therapy Oncology Group Protocol 92-02. *J Clin Oncol.* 2003;21:3972–3978.

13. Bolla M, Van Tienhoven G, Warde P, et al. External irradiation with or without long-term androgen suppression for prostate cancer with high metastatic risk: 10-year results of an EORTC randomised study. *Lancet Oncol.* 2010;11: 1066–1073.

14. Stock RG, Stone NN, Cesaretti JA, et al. Biologically effective dose values for prostate brachytherapy: Effects on PSA failure and post-treatment biopsy results. *Int J Radiat Oncol Biol Phys.* 2006;64:527–533.

15. Stock RG, Ho A, Cesaretti JA, et al. Changing the patterns of failure for high-risk prostate cancer patients by optimizing local control. *Int J Radiat Oncol Biol Phys.* 2006;66:389–394.

16. Dattoli M, Wallner K, True L, et al. Long-term outcomes after treatment with brachytherapy and supplemental conformal radiation for prostate

cancer patients having intermediate and high-risk features. *Cancer.* 2007;110:551–555.

17. Sylvester JE, Grimm PD, Blasko JC, et al. 15-year biochemical relapse free survival in clinical stage T1-T3 prostate cancer following combined external beam radiotherapy and brachytherapy; Seattle experience. *Int J Radiat Oncol Biol Phys.* 2007;67:57–64.

18. Potters L, Morgenstern C, Calugaru E, et al. 12-year outcomes following permanent prostate brachytherapy in patients with clinically localized prostate cancer. *J Urol.* 2005;173:1562–1566.

19. Merrick GS, Butler WM, Wallner KE, et al. Androgen deprivation therapy does not impact cause specific survival or overall survival in high-risk prostate cancer managed with brachytherapy and supplemental external beam. *Int J Radiat Oncol Biol Phys.* 2007;68:34–40.

20. Stone NN, Potters L, Davis BJ, et al. Customized dose prescription for permanent prostate brachytherapy: Insights from a multicenter analysis of dosimetry outcomes. *Int J Radiat Oncol Biol Phys.* 2007;69:1472–1477.

21. Stock RG, Cesaretti JA, Hall SJ, Stone NN. Outcomes for patients with high-grade prostate cancer treated with a combination of brachytherapy, external beam radiotherapy and hormonal therapy. *BJU Int.* 2009 Dec;104(11):1631–1636.

22. Shen X, Keith SW, Mishra MV, et al. The impact of brachytherapy on prostate cancer-specific mortality for definitive radiation therapy of high-grade prostate cancer: A population-based analysis. *Int J Radiat Oncol Biol Phys.* 2012 Jul 15;83(4):1154–1159.

23. Stone NN, Stock RG, Cesaretti JA, Unger P. Local control following permanent prostate brachytherapy: Effect of high biologically effective dose on biopsy results and oncologic outcomes. *Int J Radiat Oncol Biol Phys.* 2010;76:355–360.

24. Stock RG, Yalamanchi S, Hall SJ, Stone NN. Impact of hormonal therapy on intermediate risk prostate cancer treated with combination brachytherapy and external beam irradiation. *J Urol.* 2010;183:546–550.

25. D'Amico AV, Moran BJ, Braccioforte et al. Risk of death from prostate cancer after brachytherapy alone or with radiation, androgen suppression therapy, or both in men with high-risk disease. *J Clin Oncol.* 2009;27:3923–3928.

26. Widmark A, Klepp O, Solberg A, et al. Endocrine treatment, with or without radiotherapy, in locally advanced prostate cancer (SPCG-7/SFUO-3): An open randomised phase III trial. *Lancet.* 2009;373:301–308.

27. Warde P, Mason M, Ding K, et al. Combined androgen deprivation therapy and radiation therapy for locally advanced prostate cancer: A randomised phase 3 trial. *Lancet.* 2011;378:2104–2111.

28. Zagars GK, Pollack A, von Eschenbach AC. Addition of radiation therapy to androgen ablation improves outcome for subclinically node-positive prostate cancer. *Urology.* 2001;58:233–239.

29. Tzelepi V, Efstathiou E, Wen S, et al. Persistent, biologically meaningful prostate cancer after 1 year of androgen ablation and docetaxel treatment. *J Clin Oncol.* 2011;29:2574–2581.

30. Thompson IM, Tangen CM, Paradelo J, et al. Adjuvant radiotherapy for pathological T3N0M0 prostate cancer significantly reduces risk of metastases and improves survival: Long-term followup of a randomized clinical trial. *J Urol.* 2009;181:956–962.

31. Messing EM, Manola J, Yao J, et al. Immediate versus deferred androgen deprivation treatment in patients with node-positive prostate cancer after radical prostatectomy and pelvic lymphadenectomy. *Lancet Oncol.* 2006;7:472–479.

32. Horwitz EM, Bae K, Hanks GE, et al. Ten-year follow-up of radiation therapy oncology group protocol 92-02: A phase III trial of the duration of elective androgen deprivation in locally advanced prostate cancer. *J Clin Oncol.* 2008;26:2497–2504.

33. Bolla M, de Reijke TM, Van Tienhoven G, et al. Duration of androgen suppression in the treatment of prostate cancer. *N Engl J Med.* 2009;360:2516–2527.

34. Kuban DA, Levy LB, Cheung MR, et al. Long-term failure patterns and survival in a randomized dose-escalation trial for prostate cancer. Who dies of disease? *Int J Radiat Oncol Biol Phys.* 2011;79:1310–1317.

35. Peeters ST, Heemsbergen WD, Koper PC, et al. Dose-response in radiotherapy for localized prostate cancer: Results of the Dutch multicenter randomized phase III trial comparing 68 Gy of radiotherapy with 78 Gy. *J Clin Oncol.* 2006;24:1990–1996.

36. Eade TN, Hanlon AL, Horwitz EM, et al. What dose of external-beam radiation is high enough for prostate cancer? *Int J Radiat Oncol Biol Phys.* 2007;68:682–689.

37. Pahlajani N, Ruth KJ, Buyyounouski MK, et al. Radiotherapy doses of 80 Gy and higher are associated with lower mortality in men with Gleason score 8 to 10 prostate cancer. *Int J Radiat Oncol Biol Phys.* 2012 Apr 1;82(5):1949–1956.

38. Martinez AA, Gonzalez J, Ye H, et al. Dose escalation improves cancer-related events at 10 years for intermediate- and high-risk prostate cancer patients treated with hypofractionated high-dose-rate boost and external

beam radiotherapy. *Int J Radiat Oncol Biol Phys.* 2011;79(2):363–370.

39. Jacob R, Hanlon AL, Horwitz EM, et al. Role of prostate dose escalation in patients with greater than 15% risk of pelvic lymph node involvement. *Int J Radiat Oncol Biol Phys.* 2005;61:695–701.

40. Zelefsky MJ, Eastham JA, Cronin AM, et al. Metastasis after radical prostatectomy or external beam radiotherapy for patients with clinically localized prostate cancer: a comparison of clinical cohorts adjusted for case mix. *J Clin Oncol.* 2010;28(10):1508–1513.

41. Lee WR, Bae K, Lawton C, et al. Late toxicity and biochemical recurrence after external-beam radiotherapy combined with permanent-source prostate brachytherapy: Analysis of Radiation Therapy Oncology Group study 0019. *Cancer.* 2007;109:1506–1512.

42. Stenmark MH, Blas K, Halverson S, et al. Continued benefit of androgen deprivation therapy for prostate cancer patients treated with dose-escalated radiation therapy across multiple definitions of high risk disease. *Int J Radiat Oncol Biol Phys.* 2011;81:e335–e344.

43. Makarov DV, Trock BJ, Humphreys EB, et al. Updated nomogram to predict pathologic stage of prostate cancer given prostate-specific antigen level, clinical stage, and biopsy Gleason score (Partin tables) based on cases from 2000 to 2005. *Urology.* 2007;59:1095–1101.

44. Yu JB, Makarov DV, Gross C. A new formula for prostate cancer lymph node risk. *Int J Radiat Oncol Biol Phys.* 2011;80(1):69–75.

45. Roach M, Marquez C, You HS, et al. Predicting the risk of lymph node involvement using the pretreatment prostate specific antigen and Gleason score in me with clinically localized prostate cancer. *Int J Radiat Oncol Biol Phys.* 1994;28:33–37.

46. Stone NN, Potters L, Davis BJ, et al. Customized dose prescription for permanent prostate brachytherapy: Insights from a multicenter analysis of dosimetric outcomes. *Int J Radiat Oncol Biol Phys.* 2007;69:1472–1477.

47. Stone NN, Potters L, Davis BJ, et al. Multicenter analysis of effect of high biologic effective dose on biochemical failure and survival outcomes in patients with Gleason score 7-10 prostate cancer treated with permanent prostate brachytherapy. *Int J Radiat Oncol Biol Phys.* 2009;73:341–346.

48. Taira AV, Merrick GS, Butler WM, et al. Long term outcome for clinically localized prostate cancer treated with permanent interstitial brachytherapy. *Int J Radiat Oncol Biol Phys.* 2011;79:1336–1342.

49. Fang LC, Merrick GS, Butler WM, et al. High risk prostate cancer with Gleason score 8-10 and PSA level <$/$=15 ng/ml treated with permanent interstitial brachytherapy. *Int J Radiat Oncol Biol Phys.* 2011;81:992–996.

50. Nguyen PL, D'Amico AV. Targeting pelvic lymph nodes in men with intermediate and high-risk prostate cancer despite two negative randomized trials. *J Clin Oncol.* 2008;26:2055–2056.

51. Nguyen PL, Chen MH, Hoffman KE, et al. Predicting the risk of pelvic node involvement among men with prostate cancer in the contemporary era. *Int J Radiat Oncol Biol Phys.* 2009;74:104–109.

52. Aizer AA, Yu JB, McKeon AM, et al. Whole pelvic radiotherapy versus prostate only radiotherapy in the management of locally advanced or aggressive prostate adenocarcinoma. *Int J Radiat Oncol Biol Phys.* 2009;75:1344–1349.

53. http://www.rtog.org/ClinicalTrials/Protocol Table/StudyDetails.aspx?study=0924

54. Chan LW, Xia P, Gottschalk AR, et al. Proposed rectal dose constraints for patients undergoing definitive whole pelvic radiotherapy for clinically localized prostate cancer. *Int J Radiat Oncol Biol Phys.* 2008;72:69–77.

55. Chung HT, Xia P, Chan LW, et al. Does image guided radiotherapy improve toxicity profile in whole pelvic-treated high-risk prostate cancer? Comparison between IG-IMRT and IMRT. *Int J Radiat Oncol Biol Phys.* 2009;73:53–60.

56. Chao KK, Goldstein NS, Yan D, et al. Clinicopathologic analysis of extracapsular extension in prostate cancer: Should the clinical target volume be expanded posterolaterally to account for microscopic extension? *Int J Radiat Oncol Biol Phys.* 2006;65:999–1007.

57. Sylvester JE, Grimm PD, Eulau SE, et al. Permanent prostate brachytherapy pre-planned technique: The modern Seattle method step by step and dosimetric outcomes. *Brachytherapy.* 2009;8:197–206.

58. Pinkawa M, Asadpour B, Piroth MD, et al. Rectal dosimetry following prostate brachytherapy with stranded seeds – Comparison of transrectal ultrasound intra-operative planning (day 0) and computed tomography-postplanning (day 1 vs. day 30) with special focus on sources placed close to the rectal wall. *Radiother Oncol.* 2009;91:91–207.

59. Snyder KM, Stock RG, Hong SM, et al. Defining the risk of grade 2 proctitis following 125I prostate brachytherapy using a rectal dose-volume histogram analysis. *Int J Radiat Oncol Biol Phys.* 2001;50:335–341.

60. http://www.rtog.org/ClinicalTrials/Protocol Table/StudyDetails.aspx?study=0126

■ **CASE 1** ■

Laryngeal Preservation in the Treatment of Bulky Laryngeal Carcinoma

CLINICAL PROBLEM

Several randomized phase 3 trials help guide management of patients with laryngeal squamous cell carcinoma. Although voice preservation is typically favored by patients and physicians, total laryngectomy is still a valid treatment option. In the Radiation Therapy Oncology Group (RTOG) phase 3 trial 99-11, patients were ineligible if they had more than a minimal T4 disease.

CASE EXAMPLE

A 58-year-old salesman with chronic obstructive pulmonary disease (COPD) and a 35-pack-year smoking history presents with gradual, but progressive hoarseness and dyspnea on exertion. He is referred to an otolaryngologist after unsuccessful treatment for a COPD exacerbation. Office laryngoscopy reveals a bulky supraglottic mass with a paralyzed left vocal cord and extension to the base of the tongue. The airway was narrowed, but urgent tracheostomy was not felt to be necessary. Multiple, 2- to 3-cm mobile lymph nodes were palpated bilaterally in levels II and III. CT and PET/CT scans confirmed a bulky supraglottic mass with bilateral lymphadenopathy without distant metastatic disease. The tumor destroyed and invaded through much of the left thyroid cartilage and involved some of the left thyroid gland. The superior extent of the tumor just involved the base of tongue (see Figures 6.1.1 and 6.1.2). The surgeon recommended total laryngectomy, bilateral neck dissection, and likely postoperative radiation therapy and chemotherapy. The patient's lung function was poor, but judged adequate for surgery. The patient was cleared for surgery, but hears about nonsurgical therapy from a family member. He subsequently refuses surgical intervention and is referred to radiation oncology.

Management Decisions

- How does one advise a patient with a bulky but operable T4 laryngeal tumor who wishes to avoid surgery?
- What data are there for laryngeal preservation in patients presenting with bulky disease?
- What role does chemotherapy play in improving organ preservation outcomes?

MAJOR OPINION

Shyam S. Rao and Nancy Y. Lee

The central role of the larynx in speech, swallowing, and breathing has driven decades of research into laryngeal preservation in head and neck cancers. The current management of advanced laryngeal cancer is largely framed by 2 landmark studies. The first was initiated in 1985 by the Department of Veterans Affairs (VA) Laryngeal Cancer Study Group as a multi-institutional, randomized controlled study that compared a strategy for laryngeal preservation with induction chemotherapy followed by radiation therapy to total laryngectomy followed by postoperative radiation therapy [1]. Three hundred thirty-two patients with stage III or IV squamous cell carcinoma of the larynx were randomized to either surgery and postoperative radiation or induction chemotherapy with cisplatin and 5-fluorouracil (5-FU) given every 3 weeks. After 2 cycles of induction chemotherapy, if the primary site showed greater than a 50% reduction in size and there was no progression of neck disease, patients continued with a third cycle of chemotherapy and then definitive radiation therapy. However, patients with any lesser response underwent laryngectomy and postoperative radiation. Those with later recurrence underwent salvage laryngectomy.

137

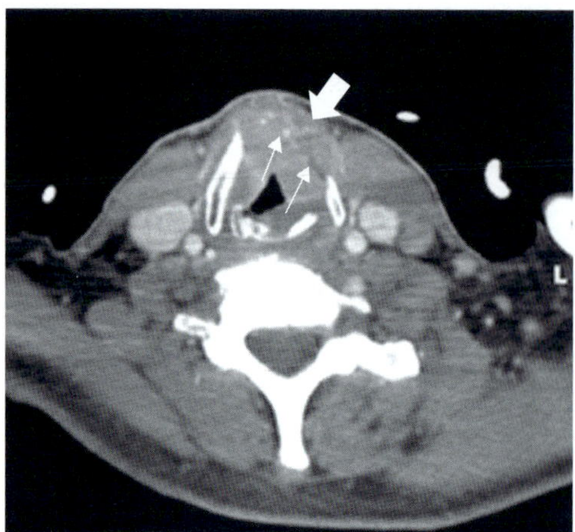

FIGURE 6.1.1 ■ CT scan shows destruction of the left and part of the anterior thyroid cartilage (thin arrows) and tumor extension into the soft tissues of the neck (thick arrow).

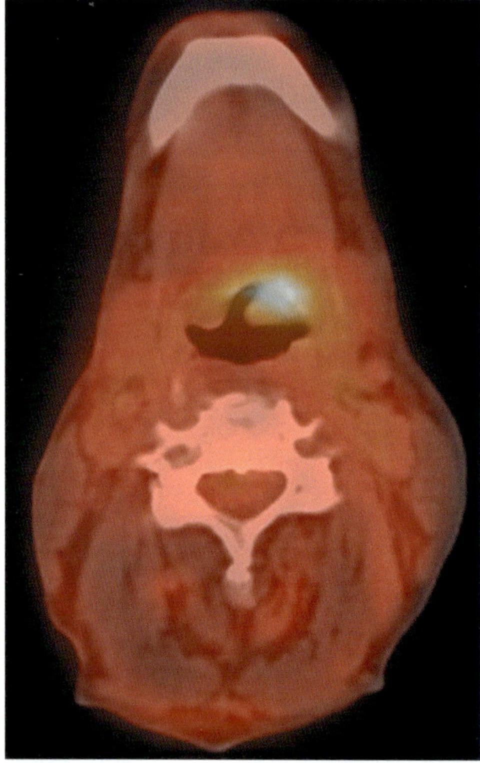

FIGURE 6.1.2 ■ PET/CT scan depicts the most superior part of the tumor extending to the inferior base of the tongue on the left. The tongue base involvement was not appreciated with CT images, physical examination, or endoscopic evaluation.

The 2-year overall survival was not statistically different between the 2 groups (68%) and the majority of patients in the sequential chemotherapy then radiation arm were able to avoid laryngectomy (64%). Patients in the induction chemotherapy arm had higher rates of primary recurrence but lower rates of distant metastases. Rates of regional lymph node recurrences were the same in both arms. Salvage laryngectomy was required more often in patients with glottic rather than supraglottic tumors, fixed rather than mobile vocal cords, and gross invasion of cartilage rather than no invasion, though these differences were not statistically significant. Follow-up analyses found significantly better patient-reported quality of life outcomes for those undergoing laryngeal preservation with respect to pain and emotional well-being, but not speech [2]. This trial established laryngeal preservation as a reasonable approach to managing advanced laryngeal cancer.

The second landmark study was based on the success of the VA Larynx trial. In 1992, the RTOG and the Head and Neck Intergroup launched RTOG 91-11 to compare 3 approaches to laryngeal preservation with radiation therapy [3]. Patients were randomly assigned to receive induction cisplatin and 5-FU followed by radiation therapy, radiation therapy with concurrent cisplatin, or radiation therapy alone. Five hundred forty-seven patients with stage III–IV squamous cell carcinoma of the glottic or supraglottic larynx were enrolled. Of note, patients with T1 primaries or large volume T4 lesions, defined as tumor penetrating through cartilage or extending more than 1 cm into the base of tongue, were excluded. Similar to the VA trial, patients who had less than a partial response underwent laryngectomy, while those with a partial response continued for a third cycle of induction chemotherapy and then definitive radiation therapy. The dose of radiation was the same in all 3 groups (70 Gy in 35 fractions over a 7-week period).

At 2 years, while overall survival was similar in all 3 groups, the rates of laryngeal preservation were significantly better in patients who were treated using radiation and concurrent cisplatin compared to patients who were treated using induction chemotherapy followed by radiation, or those treated using radiation alone (88%, 75%, and 70%, respectively). Also, the rate of local control was significantly better in the concurrently treated patients than in those treated with induction or radiation alone (78%, 61%, and 56%, respectively). Both chemotherapy groups had better disease-free survival and lower distant metastases rates, but higher toxicity rates. This trial established concurrent chemoradiation as a standard for laryngeal preservation in advanced laryngeal cancer. Overall survival between the 3 groups was not different, though a statistically non-significant trend for worse survival with concurrent chemoradiation reported with long-term follow-up raises the suggestion that late toxicity may be under-appreciated [3].

For this patient, with a T4aN2c supraglottic cancer, treatment options could include surgery followed by postoperative radiation therapy with or without chemotherapy, definitive radiation therapy with chemotherapy, or induction chemotherapy followed by radiation therapy with chemotherapy. Although laryngeal preservation is desirable, there are several factors that could limit the effectiveness of this approach. As discussed, RTOG 91-11 excluded patients with T4 lesions that penetrated through cartilage because of concerns that these patients had a worse prognosis. Indeed, in the VA larynx trial, T4 patients with invasion through cartilage showed a trend of more often requiring salvage laryngectomy and having poorer overall survival [5]. Other series have reported decreased overall survival for T4 lesions treated with definitive radiation therapy rather than surgery, and inferior local control in patients with invasion through cartilage [6–8]. Based on such concerns, and consistent with current American Society of Clinical Oncology (ASCO) practice recommendations and National Comprehensive Cancer Network (NCCN) guidelines for patients with T4 disease invading through cartilage, we advise total laryngectomy followed by postoperative radiation therapy with possible chemotherapy for this patient [9].

Given the significance of invasion through cartilage, imaging studies have grown to play a more pivotal role in treatment decision making. Recent studies suggest low positive predictive values for CT determination of cartilage invasion [10,11]. This has prompted some to raise the concern that overestimation of invasion through cartilage could dissuade patients from laryngeal preservation approaches.

In addition to his locally advanced disease with gross cartilage invasion and thyroid involvement, our patient has other issues of concern. As with penetration through cartilage, patients with supraglottic tumors and immobile vocal cords showed a nonsignificant trend to require salvage laryngectomy in the VA Larynx trial. Furthermore, patients who continue to smoke following treatment have decreased rates of laryngeal preservation and overall survival [12]. Given the patient's history, this message should be made clear to him.

Finally, the patient's history of COPD and, in particular, presentation with COPD exacerbation is of concern. Patients with laryngeal tumors are at risk for aspiration, and radiation therapy may increase that risk [13]. Aspiration events can be fatal, particularly for patients with underlying respiratory disease. For these patients, laryngectomy is the only treatment that can prevent aspiration by eliminating the connection between the gastrointestinal and respiratory tracts.

Clearly, there are multiple reasons to recommend laryngectomy, rather than laryngeal preservation, for this patient. Nevertheless, laryngectomy is a procedure with major quality-of-life consequences that some patients refuse to accept. If our patient still declined surgery after a thorough discussion of these risks, other options remain. One potential approach involves using induction chemotherapy to determine whether his tumor may be responsive and then proceeding with radiation therapy and concurrent chemotherapy if a partial response is seen, or else choosing laryngectomy. Note that this approach differs from RTOG 91-11 in giving chemoradiation rather than radiation alone following response to induction chemotherapy. This alternate strategy has demonstrated good success in a phase 2 study, as well as retrospective series of patients specifically with T4 laryngeal cancer with cartilage invasion [14,15].

A new variation of induction therapy—adding docetaxel to cisplatin and 5-FU prior to chemoradiation—has now taken root with studies showing increased locoregional control, survival, and laryngeal preservation rates compared to induction with the traditional course of cisplatin and 5-FU [16,17]. The rapid response often seen with induction chemotherapy may also have the benefit of potentially addressing impending airway issues from a bulky tumor before tracheostomy is necessary. Although this new induction regimen allows for potentially improved "chemo-selection" of responsive tumors, there will be increased toxicity. Finally, chemoradiation or radiation alone remain as treatment options. It should be noted again, however, that these laryngeal preservation approaches would not address the long-term risk of aspiration.

In conclusion, this patient with a T4aN2c supraglottic laryngeal cancer has multiple features that complicate pursuing a laryngeal preservation treatment strategy. While we believe that total laryngectomy may provide the best overall survival in terms of local control and airway protection from aspiration, induction chemotherapy followed by chemoradiation, if partial response is seen, would be a reasonable alternative.

ACADEMIC COMMENT

Andrew J. Hope, John N. Waldron, Laura A. Dawson, and Brian O'Sullivan

In the case in discussion, the patient is a salesman who relies on his voice and has declined surgery. The "Major Opinion" section endorses total laryngectomy for this patient on the basis of both airway protection and local control with larynx-sparing treatment offered as a secondary reasonable alternative. Total laryngectomy for advanced larynx cancer is a profound surgical alteration associated with significant impairment in quality of life when compared to larynx-sparing approaches [2,18]. To justify such an impact on this patient's life, it is important to demonstrate a benefit to primary surgical therapy. If such a benefit cannot be conclusively shown, organ-sparing regimens are the preferred treatment if good posttreatment laryngeal functions (swallowing, breathing, and speech) are expected.

The "Majority Opinion" illustrates a regional preference in treatment approach for patients with advanced larynx cancer. Besides disease extent, specialty and practice location largely determine one's bias toward surgical or nonsurgical management [19]. Notably, population-based comparisons between the Surveillance Epidemiology and End Results (SEER) areas of the United States and Ontario, Canada, show wide variation in management of advanced supraglottic and glottic malignancy with a substantial bias toward surgery in the United States [20–22]. Most relevant for the case in discussion, at 3 years, 66% of patients in the SEER data with T4 supraglottic disease had laryngectomy, whereas only 33% of patients in Ontario underwent laryngectomy. However, despite this management difference, overall survival at 5 years was the same (29.1% vs. 28.5%) [22].

In the VA Larynx trial, there was no significant difference in overall survival between the patients assigned to organ-sparing induction chemotherapy followed by radiation and those who received primary surgery [1]. Most of these patients had supraglottic tumors (63%), fixed vocal cord(s) (57%), and a portion had cartilage invasion (9%) similar to the case in discussion. As this was a VA study, many patients continued to smoke [1] (more on the larynx-sparing arm) and had increased risk of local failure [23]. Despite this, a majority of patients assigned to organ-sparing treatment had their larynx preserved (64%) with sequential radiation.

RTOG 91-11 demonstrated that further improvements can be made in larynx preservation rates with concurrent chemoradiation treatment compared to induction chemotherapy followed by radiation (88% vs. 75%) [4]. Although RTOG 91-11 did not include patients with base of tongue involvement as in the case in discussion, induction chemotherapy followed by concurrent chemoradiation has been delivered to similar patients with supraglottic tumors and base of tongue extension in trial settings with no difference in overall survival and a high larynx preservation rate (61%) [14]. Similar rates of larynx sparing (68%) were obtained in another randomized comparison of surgery to organ-sparing chemoradiation [24]. Using even more aggressive concurrent chemotherapy (paclitaxel, 5-FU, hydroxyurea) and a dose of 1.5 Gy twice a day, week on/week off radiation to 73 Gy, laryngectomy-free rates of 85% have been reported [25]. Recently, induction chemotherapy (docetaxel/cisplatin) followed by modern chemo- or bioradiotherapy showed similar (82–86%) larynx preservation rates at 18 months [26].

If organ-sparing approaches are to be the primary modality, it is important to consider the role and results of salvage laryngectomy compared to primary laryngectomy. In the VA Larynx trial, patients with T4 tumors or cartilage invasion showed a trend to more often require salvage laryngectomy; however, patients with supraglottic primary tumors were less likely to require laryngectomy [1]. Retrospective series comparing salvage laryngectomy following chemotherapy and radiation to primary laryngectomy suggests lightly increased rates of complications for both fistula formation and voice prostheses with the salvage approach [27,28]. However, even with the increased risks associated with salvage laryngectomy as compared to primary laryngectomy, these increased risks affect only the minority of patients who fail organ preservation. The overall surgical complication rate for salvage laryngectomy in a large cohort treated with primary larynx-sparing treatment may be similar to a similar cohort treated with primary laryngectomy. Regardless, quality of life appears equivalent in patients after early or late salvage laryngectomy [18].

In the presented case, there are no indications that the larynx is unstable or that pretreatment dysphagia or aspiration is present (good lung function in preoperative assessment). Although aspiration is a risk following chemoradiation, improvement of pretreatment-detected aspiration events occur following treatment and posttreatment aspiration and dysphagia can be managed [13,29,30]. Despite the risk of pneumonia that is associated with an organ-sparing approach [29], overall survival rates are the same as patients receiving laryngectomy [1,4,24].

Laryngectomy can also result in aversion to eating in public [23], which is thought to be related to the physical consequences of surgery (such as a stoma) and interference with social activities [31,32], a potentially large impact on a salesman. In addition, laryngeal voice quality is clearly superior to alaryngeal voice quality [18]; even with cord paralysis, thyroplasty may improve voice quality posttreatment [33].

In conclusion, in this patient with high-risk, bulky, T4aN2c supraglottic laryngeal cancer, the final treatment decision should be made by the patient after being well informed of the risks and benefits of larynx-sparing treatment versus laryngectomy. If his larynx is preserved, he will have a corresponding higher quality of life posttreatment and could retain his current job in sales. As there is no difference in overall survival, we would endorse an initial attempt at larynx preservation by either induction chemotherapy followed by chemoradiation or concurrent chemoradiation. The available data support a larynx preservation rate of least 60%. Modern trials incorporating novel concurrent therapies demonstrate larynx preservation rates of 80% or better and the success rates appear to be improving. With continued advancement in larynx-sparing therapies, laryngectomy should be reserved for salvage.

COMMUNITY PRACTITIONER COMMENT

James Piephoff

This case is a reminder that as radiation oncologists we do not treat cancer, but rather people that have cancer. It is necessary to understand what factors are important to individual patients when helping them arrive at a treatment decision.

For this patient with a T4aN2cM0 supraglottic cancer, I would first discuss a total laryngectomy followed by radiation therapy with or without chemotherapy. This approach is felt to offer the best overall survival [9]. A total laryngectomy also eliminates the risk of aspiration, which in this patient could be a fatal event. The risk that aspiration presented because of his COPD would be made clear to the patient and that a total laryngectomy effectively eliminates this risk. To try to alleviate concerns about the loss of normal voice, he would be seen in speech pathology and meet with total laryngectomy patients. Hopefully, he

would realize that losing his larynx does not mean losing his ability to speak.

If he was unable to accept a total laryngectomy followed by radiation therapy with or without chemotherapy, I would offer him radiation therapy and concurrent high-dose cisplatin. The study that led to this approach being a standard for larynx preservation in advanced larynx cancer (RTOG 91-11 [3,4]) did not include patients with significant thyroid cartilage destruction. Other studies have also indicated trends of lower overall survival and higher rates of salvage laryngectomy when thyroid cartilage invasion and fixed vocal cords are present [4–7]. These are all factors the patient needs to understand. If the medical oncologist and I felt that the patient would have a difficult time tolerating concurrent high-dose cisplatin, a reasonable option would be to substitute cetuximab for cisplatin [34]. If he was not felt to be a good candidate for either cisplatin or cetuximab, or just refused both, he could be offered radiation therapy alone [8]. His history of tobacco abuse would also need to be addressed. This patient has a 35-pack-year history, but it was not clear if he was a former or current smoker. If he was a current smoker, the importance of smoking cessation would be stressed. Both decreased rates of laryngeal preservation and overall survival have been associated with continued tobacco abuse [12].

Recently, there has been renewed interest in induction chemotherapy. The initial trials establishing laryngeal preservation as an accepted treatment option used induction chemotherapy followed by radiation therapy alone [1,3,4]. The current focus with induction chemotherapy is to follow it with combined radiation therapy and chemotherapy. Off protocol, I generally do not recommend induction chemotherapy followed by radiation therapy and concurrent chemotherapy for reasons of increased toxicity without a demonstrated improvement in overall survival [35]. It is difficult enough to get a patient through radiation therapy and concurrent high-dose cisplatin without induction chemotherapy. After induction chemotherapy, many patients are not able to tolerate concurrent high-dose cisplatin, which I consider a standard for larynx preservation in advanced laryngeal cancer. I generally only consider offering induction chemotherapy followed by radiation therapy and concurrent chemotherapy for patients facing a total laryngectomy who are highly motivated to preserve their natural voice and have both a high performance status and a willingness to have a total laryngectomy if the disease does not respond to the induction chemotherapy. While the patient's performance status was unknown other than COPD with lung function "just adequate for surgery," it was made clear that he refused surgical intervention.

In summary, this is a patient with a T4aN2cM0 supraglottic cancer with features that make him a less-than-ideal laryngeal preservation candidate. If he was unable to accept a total laryngectomy followed by radiation therapy with or without chemotherapy, I would offer radiation therapy with concurrent high-dose cisplatin, but would substitute cetuximab for cisplatin if his performance status was marginal. For a patient who is unable to accept a total laryngectomy, this approach strikes a reasonable balance between the most effective treatment for the cancer and what is the best treatment for the patient as a whole.

SECTION EDITOR'S NOTE

Wade Thorstad

Bulky laryngeal cancer represents a unique treatment challenge. I agree with the sentiments of the section authors in that a detailed discussion regarding the risks, benefits, and anticipated side effects of the treatment options is warranted so the patient can make an informed decision. In the United States, laryngectomy is the preferred and most commonly employed option for this case example [20–22]. For the patient who refuses surgery, the practitioner would be well-supported treating with concurrent chemoradiotherapy as was done in the RTOG 91-11 trial [3,4]. As outlined in the earlier sections, newer approaches including induction chemotherapy followed with concurrent chemoradiotherapy, or induction chemotherapy to select responders for continued nonsurgical therapy, can be supported with smaller phase 2 and retrospective trials, and may be appropriate for selected patients [14,15]. The Canadian perspective outlined in the "Academic Comment" section eloquently argues against surgery for most patients with bulky laryngeal cancer. For those who practice in the United States, you can certainly enliven a tumor board discussion by arguing along these lines.

REFERENCES

1. Induction chemotherapy plus radiation compared with surgery plus radiation in patients with advanced laryngeal cancer. The Department of Veterans Affairs Laryngeal Cancer Study Group. *N Eng J Med.* 1991;324(24):1685–1690.

2. Terrell JE, Fisher SG, Wolf GT. Long-term quality of life after treatment of laryngeal cancer. The Veterans Affairs Laryngeal Cancer Study Group. *Arch Otolaryngol Head Neck Surg.* 1998;124(9):964–971.

3. Forastiere AA, Zhang Q, Weber RS, et al. Long-term results of RTOG 91-11: A comparison of three nonsurgical treatment strategies to preserve the larynx in patients with locally advanced larynx cancer. *J Clin Oncol.* 2013;31(7):845–852.

4. Forastiere AA, Goepfert H, maor M, et al. Concurrent chemotherapy and radiotherapy for organ preservation in advanced laryngeal cancer. *N Engl J Med.* 2003;349(22):2091–2098.

5. Bradford CR, Wolf CT, Carey TE, et al. Predictive markers for response to chemotherapy, organ preservation, and survival in patients with advanced laryngeal carcinoma. *Otolaryngol Head Neck Surg.* 1999;121(5):534–538.

6. Gourin CG, Conger BT, Sheils WC, et al. The effect of treatment on survival in patients with advanced laryngeal carcinoma. *Laryngoscope.* 2009;119(7):1312–1317.

7. Patel UA, Howell LK. Local response to chemoradiation in T4 larynx cancer with cartilage invasion. *Laryngoscope.* 2011;121(1):106–110.

8. Mendenhall WM. T3-4 squamous cell carcinoma of the larynx treated with radiation therapy alone. *Semin Radiat Oncol.* 1998;8(4):262–269.

9. American Society of Clinical Oncology, Pfister DG, Laurie SA, et al. American Society of Clinical Oncology clinical practice guideline for the use of larynx-preservation strategies in the treatment of laryngeal cancer. *J Clin Oncol.* 2006;24(22):3693–3704.

10. Beitler JJ, Muller S, Grist WJ, et al. Prognostic accuracy of computed tomography findings for patients with laryngeal cancer undergoing laryngectomy. *J Clin Oncol.* 2010;28(14):2318–2322.

11. Li B, Bobinski M, Gandour-Edwards R, et al. Overstaging of cartilage invasion by multidetector CT scan for laryngeal cancer and its potential effect on the use of organ preservation with chemoradiation. *Br J Radiol.* 2011;84(997):64–69.

12. Rodriguez CP, Adelstein DJ, Rybicki LA, et al. Clinical predictors of larynx preservation after multiagent concurrent chemoradiotherapy. *Head Neck.* 2008;30(12):1535–1542.

13. Nguyen NP, Frank C, Moltz CC, et al. Aspiration rate following chemoradiation for head and neck cancer: An underreported occurrence. *Radiother Oncol.* 2006;80(3):302–306.

14. Urba S, Wolf G, Eisbruch A, et al. Single-cycle induction chemotherapy selects patients with advanced laryngeal cancer for combined chemoradiation: A new treatment paradigm. *J Clin Oncol.* 2006;24(4):593–598.

15. Worden FP, Kumar B, Lee JS, et al. Chemoselection as a strategy for organ preservation in advanced oropharynx cancer: Response and survival positively associated with HPV16 copy number. *J Clin Oncol.* 2008;26(19):3138–3146.

16. Pointreau Y, Garaud P, Chapet S, et al. Randomized trial of induction chemotherapy with cisplatin and 5-fluorouracil with or without docetaxel for larynx preservation. *J Natl Cancer Inst.* 2009;101(7):498–506.

17. Posner MR, Hershock DM, Blajman CR, et al. Cisplatin and fluorouracil alone or with docetaxel in head and neck cancer. *N Engl J Med.* 2007;357(17):1705–1715.

18. Fung K, Lyden TH, Lee J, et al. Voice and swallowing outcomes of an organ-preservation trial for advanced laryngeal cancer. *Int J Radiat Oncol Biol Phys.* 2005;63:1395–1399.

19. O'Sullivan B, Mackillop W, Gilbert R, et al. Controversies in the management of laryngeal cancer: Results of an international survey of patterns of care. *Radiother Oncol.* 1994;31:23–32.

20. Groome PA, Mackillop WJ, Rothwell DM, et al. Management and outcome of glottic cancer: A population-based comparison between Ontario, Canada and the SEER areas of the United States. Surveillance, Epidemiology and End Results. *J Otolaryngol.* 2000;29:67–77.

21. Groome PA, O'Sullivan B, Irish JC, et al. Glottic cancer in Ontario, Canada and the SEER areas of the United States. Do different management philosophies produce different outcome profiles? *J Clin Epidemiol.* 2001;54:301–315.

22. Groome PA, O'Sullivan B, Irish JC, et al. Management and outcome differences in supraglottic cancer between Ontario, Canada, and the Surveillance, Epidemiology, and End Results areas of the United States. *J Clin Oncol.* 2003;21:496–505.

23. Browman GP, Wong G, Hodson I, et al. Influence of cigarette smoking on the efficacy of radiation therapy in head and neck cancer. *N Engl J Med.* 1993;328:159–163.

24. Soo KC, Tan EH, Wee J, et al. Surgery and adjuvant radiotherapy vs concurrent chemoradiotherapy in stage III/IV nonmetastatic squamous cell head and neck cancer: A randomised comparison. *Br J Cancer.* 2005;93:279–286.

25. Knab BR, Salama JK, Stenson KM, et al. Definitive chemoradiotherapy for T4 laryngeal squamous cell carcinoma. *Int J Radiat Oncol Biol Phys.* 2006;66(3):S14.

26. Lefebvre J, Pointreau Y, Rolland F, et al. Sequential chemoradiotherapy (SCRT) for larynx preservation (LP): Results of the randomized phase II TREMPLIN study. ASCO Meeting Abstracts. *J Clin Oncol.* 2011;29(Suppl):abstract 5501.

27. Furuta Y, Homma A, Oridate N, et al. Surgical complications of salvage total laryngectomy following concurrent chemoradiotherapy. *Int J Clin Oncol.* 2008;13:521–527.

28. Starmer HM, Ishman SL, Flint PW, et al. Complications that affect postlaryngectomy voice restoration: Primary surgery vs salvage surgery. *Arch Otolaryngol Head Neck Surg.* 2009;135:1165–1169.

29. Eisbruch A, Lyden T, Bradford CR, et al. Objective assessment of swallowing dysfunction and aspiration after radiation concurrent with chemotherapy for head-and-neck cancer. *Int J Radiat Oncol Biol Phys.* 2002;53:23–28.

30. Rosenthal DI, Lewin JS, Eisbruch A. Prevention and treatment of dysphagia and aspiration after chemoradiation for head and neck cancer. *J Clin Oncol.* 2006;24:2636–2643.

31. Mohide EA, Archibald SD, Tew M, et al. Postlaryngectomy quality-of-life dimensions identified by patients and health care professionals. *Am J Surg.* 1992;164:619–622.

32. DeSanto LW, Olsen KD, Perry WC, et al. Quality of life after surgical treatment of cancer of the larynx. *Ann Otol Rhinol Laryngol.* 1995;104:763–769.

33. Tirado Y, Lewin JS, Hutcheson KA, et al. Office-based injection laryngoplasty in the irradiated larynx. *Laryngoscope.* 2010;120:703–706.

34. Buiret G, Combe C, Favrel V, et al. A retrospective, multicenter study of the tolerance of induction chemotherapy with docetaxel, cisplatin, and 5-fluorouracil followed by radiotherapy with concomitant cetuximab in 46 cases of squamos cell carcinoma of the head nad neck. *Int J Radiat Oncol Biol Phys.* 2010 Jun;77(2):430–437.

35. Hitt R, Grau JJ, Lopez-Pousa A, et al. Final results of a randomized phase III trial comparing induction chemotherapy with cisplatin/5-FU or docetaxel/cisplatin/5-FU follow by chemoradiotherapy (CRT) versus CRT alone as first-line treatment of unresectable locally advanced head and neck cancer (LAHNC) [abstract]. *J Clin Oncol.* 2009; 27(Suppl 15):abstract 6009

Oral Tongue Cancer With Lymph Node Recurrence

CLINICAL PROBLEM

After cancer of the lip, oral tongue cancers are among the most common head and neck (H&N) malignancies. Surgical resection is often performed, and whether or not lymph node (LN) dissection is performed is based on the perceived degree of risk of involvement. Phase 2 data suggest that the LN risk is low for tumors with 4 mm or less of invasion. However, how does one manage a patient after primary surgery for an oral tongue cancer who has a subsequent neck recurrence within 1 year of surgery?

CASE EXAMPLE

A 47-year-old female presented with a 2-month history of a painful sore on her left lateral oral tongue. She was found to have a 2 × 1 cm shallow ulcerated lesion biopsy proven to be squamous cell carcinoma (SCC). CT scan of the neck showed no tongue or neck abnormalities. Ultrasonography (USG) exam showed a 3-mm deep lesion. She had a wide local excision and pathology confirmed SCC extending no deeper than 3.5 mm. Perineural invasion (PNI) was present, otherwise there were no high-risk features. Surgical margins were over 5 mm in all directions. The surgeon elected to watch her neck, and did not refer her for any adjuvant therapy. Five months later she noted a lump under her chin. A CT scan showed a 2-cm left level IB LN, and a 1.7-cm left level II LN (see Figure 6.2.1). A selective neck dissection (level IB–IV) was performed and pathology showed 2 LNs positive for metastatic SCC with extracapsular extension (ECE) in a level Ib LN and no ECE in a level II LN. A total of 28 additional LNs were negative. She is now referred for postoperative adjuvant therapy.

Management Decisions

- What is the "correct" level(s) of the neck to treat?
- What doses should be delivered to the level(s) of the neck that is treated?
- Should the bilateral or ipsilateral neck be treated?
- Should one include the oral tongue in the clinical target volume?

MAJOR OPINION

Kenneth Hu

The patient is a 47-year-old female with an early-stage oral tongue cancer who underwent wide local excision with appropriate margins. Data from several centers indicate that a tumor with superficial invasion does not warrant elective management of the neck because of the low risk of nodal disease [1–3]. The threshold depth of invasion for which neck management is indicated varies with some institutions that recommend 2 mm as a cutoff, whereas others suggest 4 to 5 mm. In this patient, a 4-mm depth of invasion was used to justify neck observation, yet the tumor recurred suggesting that a more stringent depth of 2 mm is to be favored [4]. One could argue for adjuvant radiotherapy up front in this case because of the presence of PNI [5,6], which is considered an intermediate-risk factor for recurrence. For intermediate-risk patients, RTOG 0920 is currently testing whether the addition of cetuximab concurrently with postoperative radiotherapy improves outcome over postoperative radiotherapy alone. One soft factor in which clinical judgment dictates when to consider adjuvant treatment is the presence of pain. Nonsmoking early-stage oral cavity cancers in young patients in their early 30s are thought to be more aggressive, but this is not clearly verified in the literature [7].

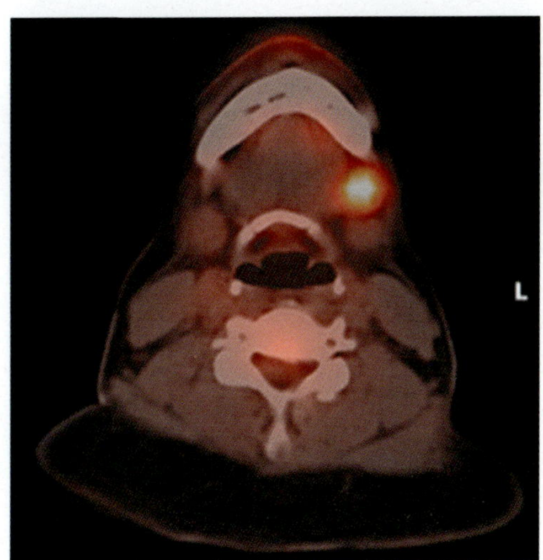

FIGURE 6.2.1 ■ PET/CT scan showing a left level IB lymph node recurrence 5 months after surgical resection of a shallow T1 SCC of the left oral tongue. The patient was treated with resection of the primary tumor and observation of the neck(s). No adjuvant therapy was delivered initially.

The prognostic implication of withholding neck management in early-stage oral cavity cancer has been tested in 2 randomized trials. The trials failed to show a survival benefit in patients randomized to receive elective neck dissection compared to observation with salvage neck dissection if nodal disease developed. In one study, the primary site was managed with primary brachytherapy, while in the other study the primary site was managed with radical resection [8,9]. In the Vandenbrouck study, a 49% incidence of nodal involvement was reported in electively treated patients while nodal disease subsequently developed in 47% in the observation group [10]. In the observation arm, the nodal disease appeared to become more aggressive with a higher incidence of ECE (25% vs. 13%) compared to the electively treated patients, and 10% of patients could not undergo therapeutic dissection. However, no survival difference could be detected between the 2 groups. Nevertheless, in this patient's situation, recurrence in the neck with multiple nodes and the presence of ECE are highly concerning and warrant aggressive adjuvant therapy.

Current management of the nodal recurrence with ECE clearly indicates the need for adjuvant radiotherapy with concurrent cisplatin chemotherapy as the standard postoperative treatment. Two landmark studies were organized independently in Europe (European Organisation

for Research and Treatment of Cancer [EORTC] 22931) and in the United States (Radiation Therapy Oncology Group [RTOG] 95-01) [11,12,37]. Both tested whether the addition of 3 cycles of high-dose cisplatin concurrent with conventionally fractionated postoperative radiation could benefit patients at high risk for recurrence. The dose of cisplatin was 100 mg/m² every 3 weeks in both the trials while the dose of radiation in the RTOG study was 60 to 66 Gy and 66 Gy in the EORTC trial. Definition of "high risk" included ECE and positive margins in both studies; however, each study had other nonoverlapping eligibility criteria including multiple nodes in RTOG 95-01 and lymphovascular invasion, PNI, stage III/IV disease, or level IV or V nodal involvement in oral cavity/oropharynx primaries in EORTC 22931. The primary endpoint in the RTOG trial was locoregional control (LRC) while progression-free survival was the primary objective in the EORTC study. Table 6.2.1 compares the patient characteristics and the outcomes of both trials. Oral cavity cancers comprised about 1/4 of patients in each study. More N2/3 patients were entered in the RTOG study (94% vs. 57%). The incidence of ECE was similar between the 2 studies (RTOG 53% vs. EORTC 57%), but more positive margins were noted in the EORTC study (29% vs. 10%). Also, the majority of patients in the EORTC study received 66 Gy while only about 1/10 of patients in the RTOG study did so. At a median follow-up of 60 months in the EORTC study and 46 months in the RTOG, the addition of chemotherapy improved the primary endpoints. Both studies showed about 9% to 13% improvement in locoregional and disease-free survival (DFS), with no difference in incidence of distant metastasis. Overall survival (OS) was statistically improved in the EORTC study with a 13% absolute improvement at 5 years and tended toward significance in the RTOG trial with a 9% absolute 4-year increase.

A pooled analysis of the 2 studies was reported by Bernier et al. [13]. For all 750 patients, the chemoradiation group had improved LRC (hazard ratio [HR] = 0.581), DFS (HR = 0.772), and OS (HR = 0.776) compared to radiation-only patients. Among the 479 patients with either ECE or positive margins, the benefit of concurrent chemoradiation was even larger for all 3 endpoints: LRC (HR = 0.524), DFS (HR = 0.695, $p = 0$), and OS (HR = 0.702, $p = 0$), respectively. However, chemoradiation showed no benefit in RTOG patients with multiple nodes in any of the 3 endpoints and tended toward a LRC advantage

TABLE 6.2.1 ■ *Comparison of Phase 3 Postoperative Chemoradiation Versus Radiation*

	RTOG 95-01	EORTC 22931
Number of patients	459	334
Patient Characteristic		
OPX/OC/LX/HPX	42%/27%/21%/10%	30%/26%/22%/20%
% T3–4	61%	66%
% N2–3	94%	57%
High-Risk Criteria		
% with ECE negative margin	49%	41%
% with positive margins without ECE	6%	13%
% with ECE and positive margins	4%	16%
% with ECE and/or positive margins	59%	70%
RT: % receiving 66 Gy	13%	91%
Greater than grade 3 acute toxicity (CT/RT vs. RT)	77% vs. 34% ($p < .0001$)	44% vs. 21% ($p = .001$)
All late toxicity (CT/RT vs. RT)	21% vs. 17% ($p = .29$)	38% vs. 41% ($p = .25$)
Median follow-up	46 months	60 months
Outcomes (CT/RT vs. RT)		
Locoregional failure	3 yr: 22% vs. 33% ($p = .01$)	5 yr: 18% vs. 31% ($p = .007$)
DFS	3 yr: 47% vs. 36% ($p = .04$)	5 yr: 47% vs. 36% ($p = .04$)
OS	3 yr: 56% vs. 47% ($p = .09$)	5 yr: 53% vs. 40% ($p = .02$)
Distant metastases	3 yr: 20% vs. 23% ($p = .46$)	5 yr: 21% vs. 24% ($p = .61$)

CT, chemotherapy; DFS, disease-free survival; ECE, extracapsular extension; HPX, hypopharynx; LX, larynx; OPX, oropharynx; OC, oral cavity; OS, overall survival; RT, radiation therapy.

($HR = 0.42$, $p = .10$) and OS benefit ($HR = 0.75$, $p = .06$) in the EORTC patients who qualified on the basis of the other criteria without ECE or positive margin. There was no detectable impact on distant metastasis. A follow-up phase 2 RTOG 0234 trial for high-risk resected tumors compared concurrent weekly Taxotere/cetuximab to weekly cisplatin with standard radiotherapy and showed similar LRC; however, a survival benefit in the Taxotere/c225 arm was demonstrated owing to a halving of distant metastasis from 26% to 13% [14]. Comparing the Taxotere/cetuximab arm to the concurrent chemoradiation group from RTOG 95-01 demonstrated a potential survival benefit, but this has yet to be confirmed in a prospective randomized trial.

Altered Fractionation Postoperative Radiation

For patients who are unable to undergo concurrent chemoradiation, the treatment package time is crucial in high-risk patients to achieve optimal LRC and survival. The value of accelerated postoperative radiation to decrease the total treatment package time (defined as time from surgery to completion of adjuvant therapy) was demonstrated in 2 studies. Ang et al. reported on a multi-institutional randomized trial [15]. Patients were stratified by risk according to the risk factors identified in the aforementioned study. Patients with no adverse pathologic factors were deemed low risk and not given postoperative radiation therapy (PORT). Patients with 1 pathologic risk factor were deemed as at intermediate risk and treated with conventional fractionated radiation to a dose of 57.6 Gy in 6.5 weeks. Those with ECE or the presence of 2 or more risk factors were deemed high risk and treated with-high dose conventional radiation to 63 Gy in 7 weeks or accelerated radiation by delayed concomitant boost to 63 Gy in 5 weeks. At a median follow-up of 59 months, LRC was excellent for low-risk patients who were observed and intermediate-risk patients (5 year actuarial LRC 90% vs. 94%, respectively). High-risk patients had a 5-year actuarial LRC and survival rate of 68% and 42%, respectively. Within this cohort, patients who underwent accelerated postoperative radiation had a nonsignificant improvement in LRC (p = .11) and survival (p = .08). The value of accelerated treatment was based on the ability to keep the treatment package time to 11 weeks or less, whether treated by conventional or accelerated radiotherapy. Therefore, if standard fractionation is to be used, treatment should start within 4 weeks of surgery to keep the overall treatment time to 11 weeks. Suwinski reported on a second trial of postoperative accelerated radiotherapy treating 7 days per week versus conventional fractionation and showed that for the subset of oral cavity/oropharynx cancer patients, those who received accelerated radiotherapy had improved local control. If high-risk patients are unable to start within 4 weeks of surgery, accelerated radiotherapy may be considered [16].

Target Coverage and Dosing

With regard to radiotherapy details, the target area would include comprehensive treatment of the ipsilateral neck level IA–V and with treatment of the retrostyloid nodes to the skull base at the jugular foramen and selective treatment of contralateral level IA–III and sparing of the retrostyloid nodes. Surgical series of radical neck dissections serve as the basis for such a treatment approach (Tables 6.2.2 and 6.2.3). Elective nodal irradiation (ENI) including level IV LNs should be considered for those with tumors involving the tip of the oral tongue because of the direct drainage to this area that bypasses the orderly contiguous progression in the anterior jugular nodes [17,18]. Involvement of the ipsilateral level V LNs in node-negative oral cavity tumors is rare, occurring in less than 1%, and does not warrant ENI. However, with increasing involvement of levels I to III or the involvement of level IV, the risk for level V involvement increases warranting ENI. There are no surgical data regarding the treatment of retropharyngeal (RP) nodes, but I would include the ipsilateral lateral RP nodes especially, as this would entail relatively minor expansion from the retrostyloid jugular nodes. Given that there was PNI, I would consider obtaining an MRI to ensure that no gross disease has developed. I would include the primary site because of the concern for in-transit lymphatic involvement. It is important to cover the primary site to the insertion sites to the floor of mouth and bone. I would consider using bolus to treat the skin ipsilaterally in the level I/II

TABLE 6.2.2 ■ *Percentage Incidence and Distribution of Pathologically Involved Nodes in a Clinical Node-Negative Neck After Elective Radical Neck Dissection*

	I	II	III	IV	V
Oropharynx n = 48	2	25	19	8	2
Oral cavity N = 192	20	17	9	3	0.5

Source: Adapted from [19].

TABLE 6.2.3 ■ *Percentage Incidence and Distribution of Pathologically Involved Nodes in a Clinical Node-Positive Neck After Therapeutic Radical Neck Dissection*

	I	II	III	IV	V
Oropharynx n = 165	14	71	42	28	9
Oral cavity N = 324	46	43	33	15	3

Source: Adapted from [17].

areas given that the scar should be included in the field and that there was ECE.

The value of dose escalation with postoperative radiation was explored in a prospective, randomized trial reported by Peters, where 302 radically resected patients were stratified as low, intermediate, or high risk for locoregional recurrence on the basis of an empirically derived scoring system that evaluates margin status, stage, and pathologic factors [20]. Patients were randomized to 4 dose levels at 52.2 Gy, 57.6 Gy, 63 Gy, and 68.4 Gy to the resection bed while 54 Gy was delivered to nonsurgically treated areas of potential subclinical disease. Analysis of 240 patients at a median followup of 45 months showed that ECE was the overriding risk factor for locoregional recurrence (30% vs. 19%, p = .04). For the 110 patients with ECE, a dose of 63 Gy was superior compared to a dose of 57.6 Gy or less (locoregional recurrence 26% vs. 48%, respectively), but there was no further benefit at 68.4 Gy (locoregional recurrence 28%) and more complications. For patients stratified to the high-risk group, there did not appear to be any significant benefit with regard to neck control rates (84% vs. 77%) when the 63 Gy dose level was compared with the 68.4 Gy dose level. Although these observations may reflect an underpowered analysis, it has been concluded that a dose of at least 63 Gy is warranted to postoperative sites at greatest risk. The study did show that the presence of 2 or more risk factors predicted a high risk for failure. Based on this trial, minimum doses of 57.6 Gy are recommended to the whole operative bed with a boost to

63 Gy to areas at high risk, especially where ECE is present. With regard to dose painting, 63 Gy in 35 fractions should be adequate to cover the high-risk areas, ipsilateral level I and II with dose painting to 60 Gy in the postoperative bed, and 54 Gy for elective treatment. Alternatively, one might consider 60 Gy in 30 fractions with sequential intensity-modulated radiation therapy (IMRT) plans and the use of cone beam CT (CBCT) image-guided treatment to reduce margins.

In summary, the use of PORT remains an integral component in the management of high-risk postoperative oral cavity patients. The presence of nodal ECE is a dominant factor that influences the risk for regional relapse. This patient suffered a neck recurrence, had a neck dissection with pathologic evidence of ECE, and thus management can be considered in the same vein as a high-risk postoperative patient. There is compelling level I evidence supporting the use of concurrent chemotherapy with PORT to reduce locoregional relapse and improve survival. Patients undergoing surgical resection, in which PORT is deemed to be likely, should be jointly evaluated prior to surgery to minimize treatment delay. Standard PORT remains with a daily fractionated schedule to a dose of 60 to 66 Gy to high-risk areas with the use of accelerated schedules in patients unable to proceed with concurrent chemoradiation.

ACADEMIC COMMENT

W. Ken Zhen

This case illustrates the difficulty and the controversies in the management of a clinically negative (N0) neck in a patient with early-stage oral tongue SCC. The argument for observation is on the basis of the fact that lymphatic metastases will develop in only 20% to 30% of patients with early oral cancer. Therefore, a selective nodal treatment either with neck dissection or irradiation would result in overtreatment for a majority of patients without a clear survival advantage. On the other hand, the proponents for elective treatment contend that elective neck treatment would be more effective for subclinical disease with less morbidity. Elective neck dissection may also provide better patient selection for more aggressive adjuvant therapy, thus better outcomes. A study reported by Lydiatt et al. comparing glossectomy with or without neck dissection for T1/T2N0 oral tongue SCC demonstrated better LRC (91% vs. 50%) and survival (55% vs. 31%) with elective neck dissection [21].

Wendt et al. reported a 44% rate of neck recurrence in patients with T1/T2N0 oral tongue SCC without elective neck irradiation. The rate of neck failure was reduced to 27% when less than a dose of 40 Gy, and to 11% when a dose of 40 Gy or higher dose of elective irradiation was given [22]. Furthermore, there is a greater concern for neck recurrence with more aggressive disease. A study by Andersen et al. demonstrated that a high incidence (77%) of patients with clinical N0 necks at initial observation had adverse prognostic findings at the time of salvage neck dissection, among which 49% of these patients had ECE [23]. The rate of ECE in Lydiatt's study was 58% in patients who were observed initially. A study comparing 5-year survival in T1/T2N0 oral tongue SCC also showed a worse survival rate, 44.8% versus 80.5% when a salvage neck dissection was performed for recurrent neck disease [24].

The presence of PNI has been associated with poorer prognosis for oral tongue SCC with a higher rate of regional failure and decreased survival. A study by Brown et al. showed 30% incidence of PNI in patients with initially N0 oral cavity SCC [5]. Among the patients with PNI, 71% eventually developed regional disease, whereas 36% of patients without PNI recurred in the neck. The 2-year disease-specific survival rates were 52% and 82% with and without the presence of PNI. Therefore, the presence of PNI should be strongly considered as an indication for elective neck dissection or irradiation. For this patient, I would have preferred elective irradiation after the initial surgery because of multiple intermediate-risk factors for occult nodal disease; namely a T2 ulcerative tumor with depth of invasion of 4 mm and the presence of PNI (I would also consider poorly differentiated histologic grade and lymphovascular invasion as intermediate-risk factors). However, elective neck dissection for this patient would also have been appropriate because of her young age and the desire to avoid multimodality treatment for an early-stage oral tongue cancer.

As to the levels of neck nodes to be irradiated, it is critical to treat both sides of the neck, which consists of postoperative radiation to the involved neck and elective irradiation for the contralateral neck. When there are multiple levels of ipsilateral nodes involved, as seen in this patient, the risk of contralateral metastasis will increase significantly. A study reported by Kurita et al. showed the incidence of contralateral nodal metastasis of 50% when multiple ipsilateral nodes were involved, as compared to 26% in those patients with single nodal disease illustrating the importance of comprehensive irradiation for nodal-positive patients [25].

I would agree with Dr. Hu's detailed description of target coverage and dosing. I, however, would not routinely obtain an MRI scan for PNI. I think the yield of MRI for microscopic and asymptomatic PNI is low. With regard to IMRT dose painting, I would not use a dose of 63 Gy in 35 fractions because this would result in a potentially inadequate fraction size (1.54 Gy fraction) when 54 Gy is used for elective treatment. I would use a dose of 63 to 64 Gy in 30 fractions to ipsilateral level I and II of the neck, 60 Gy to the rest of the involved neck, and 54 Gy to the contralateral neck field. It is important to initiate postoperative radiation as soon as possible, preferably within 4 weeks, to maximize the efficacy of the radiation. It is also important to have patients undergo a dental evaluation prior to the surgery so any unrestorable teeth can be extracted during the surgery to avoid unnecessary delay of postoperative radiation when it is indicated. When radiation therapy is used for oral tongue cancers, it is important to immobilize the tongue using a bite block, preferably a customized bite block, which not only restricts the tongue mobility during the treatment, but can also displace the upper oral cavity and upper lip out of the high dose field, thus reducing mucositis in the hard palate and upper buccal mucosa/lip.

COMMUNITY PRACTITIONER COMMENT

Kimberly Creach

Currently there is much controversy regarding the appropriate management of a clinical N0 neck after definitive surgical resection of a shallow oral tongue cancer as thoroughly discussed by both Dr. Hu and Dr. Zhen [26,27]. One can argue about the appropriateness of this patient's initial treatment; regardless, she has developed a regional recurrence and as such requires further treatment.

If one draws from data regarding the utility of adjuvant therapy in the definitive setting, this patient should benefit from chemoradiation therapy given the ECE has been identified in a dissected LN [11,12,37]. Both the EORTC and the RTOG independently conducted clinical trials that evaluated the addition of cisplatin to adjuvant radiation in patients with resected head and neck

cancer with "high-risk features." Although each study defined "high-risk features" differently, both of them included ECE. The EORTC trial found not only an improvement in LRC with the addition of chemotherapy, but also an improvement in OS [12]. The RTOG trial also demonstrated an improvement in LRC with a trend in improvement of OS in the initial publication [11]. The RTOG trial has recently been updated with nearly 10 year follow-up. For the entire cohort, there is no longer a statistically significant difference in outcome between the treatment groups; however, in an unplanned subgroup analysis, a benefit in LRC and DFS in favor of the chemotherapy arm remains for patients with ECE and or a positive surgical margin [37].

We know from landmark surgical series that at presentation, the ipsilateral neck levels IA through V were at risk for disease, with levels IB and II as highest risk with 34% and 89% of patients having involved LNs at those levels, respectively [28]. On the other hand, the contralateral neck had a much lower rate of positive LNs: no level had greater than a 10% rate of LN involvement [28]. These findings have been supported by more modern series as well [29]. However, as pointed out by Dr. Zhen, the risk of contralateral LN involvement or recurrence increases with ipsilateral LN involvement [25,30,31]. As such, I would recommend that the patient receives radiation to the bilateral neck. I would treat the ipsilateral levels IA–V and the contralateral levels IA–IV. On the contralateral side, I would not include the level II LNs superior to where the posterior belly of the digastric muscle crosses the jugular vein, as it allows for contralateral parotid sparing without an increased risk of failure in a clinically node-negative contralateral neck [32]. I would also treat the bilateral lateral RP LNs superiorly to the skull base [32]. If the LN with ECE had been located in level II, III, or IV, I would take the lateral border of the affected level's contours to the platysma to ensure coverage of the circumference of the sternocleidomastoid muscle. I do not routinely use bolus while treating head and neck cancers with IMRT, even in the setting of ECE.

With regard to the primary site, though treatment of the oral tongue can be quite toxic acutely, I would include it in the treatment volume. Although we do not have data regarding the risk of local recurrence after regional recurrence, we do know that involved LNs at presentation are associated with increased risk of recurrence in the primary site [4,33,32]. ECE has also been found to correlate with local recurrence and the presence of PNI tends toward an association with local recurrence [34]. Further, the median time to recurrence is more than 7 months (a time point this patient has not yet reached) [34].

Lastly, if the patient were to recur locally after undergoing radiation therapy to the neck only, her salvage options would be quite limited. In order to limit some of the acute toxicity, I would advocate the use of a custom-made bite block that would allow for spatial displacement of the lips, buccal mucosa, and hard palate from the tongue. The use of the bite block will decrease the dose these organs receive, thus limiting acute oral mucositis.

The dose I would utilize is 66 Gy in 2 Gy fractions to the primary site and affected neck levels IB and II, with the remainder of the treated volume receiving 54 Gy in 1.64 Gy fractions with simultaneous integrated boost technique. Groups using this dose/fractionation with simultaneous integrated boost have reported excellent LRC [34–36].

SECTION EDITOR'S NOTE

Wade Thorstad

I concur with the recommendations for concurrent chemoradiation on the basis of the patient's pathologic risk factors and data drawn from prospective randomized trials in the definitive management setting. I agree with the target volumes outlined by the authors for this case. If the neck recurrence were to occur after 24 months rather than 5 months as in the case example, I would not include the primary tumor as a target, as most local recurrences tend to occur within 2 years.

It is interesting that the 3 authors used slightly different dose/fractionation schemes. I do share Dr. Zhen's concern about a dose painting fraction size of 54 Gy in 35 fractions, but otherwise consider all of the dose/fraction schemes to be within standard practice. The current RTOG postoperative trial (0920) uses a dose of 60 Gy in 30 fractions (200 cGy/day) to the high-risk areas concurrently with 56 Gy in 30 fractions (180 cGy/day) to the low-risk areas. A dose of 66 Gy in 30 fractions (220 cGy/day) is acceptable in this trial. As treatment of the oral tongue is toxic, I prefer not to exceed 200 cGy/fraction for the high-dose region in the oral cavity. In practice, I use a dose/fraction scheme similar to that outlined by the community practitioner author, Dr. Creach.

REFERENCES

1. Spiro RH, Huvos AG, Wong GY, et al. Predictive value of tumor thickness in squamous carcinoma confined to the tongue and floor of the mouth. *Am J Surg.* 1986 Oct;152(4):345–350.

2. Byers RM, El-Naggar AK, Lee YY, et al. Can we detect or predict the presence of occult nodal metastases in patients with squamous carcinoma of the oral tongue? *Head Neck.* 1998 Mar;20(2):138–144.

3. Shim SJ, Cha J, Koom WS, et al. Clinical outcomes for T1-2N0-1 oral tongue cancer patients underwent surgery with and without postoperative radiotherapy. *Radiat Oncol.* 2010 May 27;5:43.

4. Ganly I, Patel S, Shah J. Early stage squamous cell cancer of the oral tongue-clinicopathologic features affecting outcome. *Cancer.* 2011 Jun; 118(1):101–111.

5. Brown B, Barnes L, Mazariegos J, et al. Prognostic factors in mobile tongue and floor of mouth carcinoma. *Cancer.* 1989;64:1195–1202.

6. Rahima B, Shingaki S, Nagata M, Saito C. Prognostic significance of perineural invasion in oral and oropharyngeal carcinoma. *Oral Surg Oral Med Oral Pathol Oral Radiol Endod.* 2004 Apr;97(4): 423–431.

7. Popovtzer A, Shpitzer T, Bahar G, et al. Squamous cell carcinoma of the oral tongue in young patients. *Laryngoscope.* 2004 May;114:915.

8. Spiro RH, Guillamondegui O Jr, Paulino AF. Pattern of invasion and margin assessment in patients with oral tongue cancer. *Head Neck.* 1999 Aug;21(5):408–413.

9. Fakih AR, Rao RS, Borges AM, et al. Elective versus therapeutic neck dissection in early carcinoma of the oral tongue. *Am J Surg.* 1989; 158(4):309–313.

10. Vandenbrouck C, Sancho-Garnier H, Chassagne D, et al. Elective versus therapeutic radical neck dissection in epidermoid carcinoma of the oral cavity: Results of a randomized clinical trial. *Cancer.* 1980;46(2):386–390.

11. Cooper JS, Pajak TF, Forastiere AA, et al. Postoperative concurrent radiotherapy and chemotherapy for high-risk squamous-cell carcinoma of the head and neck. *N Engl J Med.* 2004;350(19):1937–1344.

12. Bernier J, Domenge C, Ozsahin M, et al. Postoperative irradiation with or without concomitant chemotherapy for locally advanced head and neck cancer. *N Engl J Med.* 2004;350(19):1945–1952.

13. Bernier J, Cooper JS, Pajak TF, et al. Defining risk levels in locally advanced head and neck cancers: A comparative analysis of concurrent

postoperative radiation plus chemotherapy trials of the EORTC (#22931) and RTOG (#9501). *Head Neck.* 2005;27(10):843–850.

14. Kies M. et al. RTOG 0234: Phase II randomized trial of post-op chemoradiation plus C225 for high Risk SCC of head and neck. ASTRO 2009.

15. Ang KK, Trotti A, Brown BW, et al. Randomized trial addressing risk features and time factors of surgery plus radiotherapy in advanced head-and-neck cancer. *Int J Radiat Oncol Biol Phys.* 2001;51(3):571–578.

16. Suwinski R, Bankowska-Wozniak M, Majewski W, et al. Randomized clinical trial of 7-days-week postoperative radiotherapy for high-risk squamous cell carcinoma. *Radiat and Oncol.* 2008;87:155–163.

17. Shah JP. Patterns of cervical lymph node metastasis from squamous carcinomas of the upper aerodigestive tract. *Am J Surg.* 1990;160(4):405–409.

18. Byers RM, Weber RS, Andrews T, et al. Frequency and therapeutic implications of "skip metastases" in the neck from squamous carcinoma of the oral tongue. *Head Neck.* 1997;19(1):14–19.

19. Shah JP, Candela FC, Poddar AK. The patterns of cervical lymph node metastases from squamous cell carcinoma of the oral cavity. *Cancer.* 1990 Jul 1;66(1):109–113.

20. Peters LJ, Goepfert H, Ang KK, et al. Evaluation of the dose for postoperative radiation therapy of head and neck cancer: First report of a prospective randomized trial. *Int J Radiat Oncol Biol Phys.* 1993;26(1):3–11.

21. Lydiatt DD, Robbins KT, Byers RM, et al. Treatment of stage I and II oral tongue cancer. *Head Neck.* 1993;15:308–312.

22. Wendt CD, Peters LJ, Delclos L, et al. Primary radiotherapy in the treatment of stage I and II oral tongue cancers: importance of the proportion of therapy delivered with interstitial therapy. *Int J Radiat Oncol Biol Phys.* 1990;18:1287–1292.

23. Andersen PE, Cambronero E, Shaha AR, et al. The extent of neck disease after regional failure during observation of the N0 neck. *Am J Surg.* 1996;172:689–691.

24. Haddadin KJ, Soutar DS, Oliver RJ, et al. Improved survival for patients with clinically T1/T2, N0 tongue tumors undergoing a prophylactic neck dissection. *Head Neck.* 1999;21(6):517–525.

25. Kurita H, Koike T, Narikawa JN, et al. Clinical predictors for contralateral neck lymph node metastasis from unilateral squamous cell carcinoma in the oral cavity. *Oral Oncol.* 2004;40:898–903.

26. Yuen AP, Ho CM, Chow TL et al. Prospective randomized study of selective neck dissection versus observation for N0 neck of early tongue carcinoma. *Head Neck.* 2009;31(6):765–772.

27. Lim YC, Lee JS, Koo BS et al. Treatment of contralateral N0 neck in early squamous cell carcinoma of the oral tongue: Elective neck dissection versus observation. *Laryngoscope.* 2006;116(3):461–465.

28. Linberg R. Distribution of cervical lymph node metastases from squamous cell carcinoma of the upper respiratory and digestive tracts. *Cancer.* 1972;29(6):1446–1449.

29. Mukherji SK, Armao D, Joshi VM. Cervical nodal metastases in squamous cell carcinoma of the head and neck: What to expect. *Head Neck.* 2001;23(11):995–1005.

30. Gonzalez-Garcia R, Naval-Gias L, Rodriguez-Campo FJ, et al. Contralateral lymph neck node metastasis of squamous cell carcinoma of the oral cavity: A retrospective analytic study in 315 patients. *J Oral Maxillofac Surg.* 2008;66(7):1390–1398.

31. Capote-Moreno A, Naval L, Munoz-Guerra MF. Prognostic factors influencing contralateral neck lymph node metastases in oral and oropharyngeal carcinoma. *J Oral Maxillofac Surg.* 2010;68(2):268–275.

32. Eisbruch A, Marsh LH, Dawson LA, et al. Recurrences near the base of skull after IMRT of head-and-neck cancer: Implication for target delineation in high neck and for parotid gland sparing. *Int J Radiat Oncol Biol Phys.* 2004;59(1):28–42.

33. Goldstein DP, Bachar GY, Lea J, et al. Outcomes of squamous cell cancer of the oral tongue managed at the princess margaret hospital. *Head Neck.* 2012 (epub ahead of print).

34. Yao M, Dornfeld KJ, Buatti JM, et al. Intensity-modulated radiation treatment for head-and-neck squamous cell carcinoma – the University of Iowa experience. *Int J Radiat Oncol Biol Phys.* 2005;63(2):410–421.

35. Yao M, Chang K, Funk GY, et al. The failure patterns of oral cavity squamous cell carcinoma after intensity-modulated radiotherapy-the university of Iowa experience. *Int J Radiat Oncol Biol Phys.* 2007;67(5):1332–1341.

36. Chao KS, Ozyigit G, Tran BN, et al. Patterns of failure in patients receiving definitive and postoperative IMRT for head-and-neck cancer. *Int J Radiat Oncol Biol Phys.* 2003;55(2):312–321.

37. Cooper JS, Zhagn Q, Pajak TF, et al. Long-term follow-up of the RTOG 9501/Intergroup Phase III trial: Postoperative concurrent radiation therapy and chemotherapy in high-risk squamous cell carcinoma of the head and neck. *Int J Radiat Oncol Biol Phys.* 2012;84(5):1198–2205.

Management of Carcinoma Metastatic to the Neck From an Occult Primary Site

CLINICAL PROBLEM

Asymptomatic carcinoma metastatic to the neck is a common presentation of squamous cell cancer from mucosal sites of the pharynx. On initial presentation, many of these patients are therefore diagnosed as having carcinoma metastatic to the neck from an unknown primary site.

CASE EXAMPLE

A 52-year-old male with a 15-pack-year smoking history, but who quit 7 years ago, presents with painless right neck lymphadenopathy. His only previous surgery was a bilateral tonsillectomy as a child. Workup including physical examination, office nasopharyngoscopy, CT scan of the neck with contrast, and a whole-body PET/CT scan that revealed a 4.5-cm right side level II lymph node (LN) without evidence of a primary tumor (see Figure 6.3.1). The patient underwent triple endoscopy with no mucosal abnormalities detected. Directed biopsy of the nasopharynx, bilateral base of tongue, and larynx was negative.

An incisional biopsy of the LN was performed and was positive on being frozen for squamous cell carcinoma, prompting a modified radical neck dissection. Final pathology revealed that 2 of 36 LNs were positive for poorly differentiated squamous cell carcinoma with extracapsular extension (ECE). Immunohistochemistry (IHC) staining for p16 was positive, consistent with a human papilloma virus (HPV)-related tumor (see Figure 6.3.2).

Management Decisions

- What is the clinical target volume (CTV) to be treated? Neck(s) and/or mucosa?
- What are the mucosal targets?
- What is the dose to the operative bed?
- What is the dose to subclinical sites?
- If mucosal sites are treated, can one limit treatment to the tongue base in this case because of the HPV status and surgically absent tonsils?

MAJOR OPINION

Adam S. Garden and Steven J. Frank

The case described is a relatively typical presentation of both HPV-positive oropharynx cancer and carcinoma metastatic to the neck from an unknown

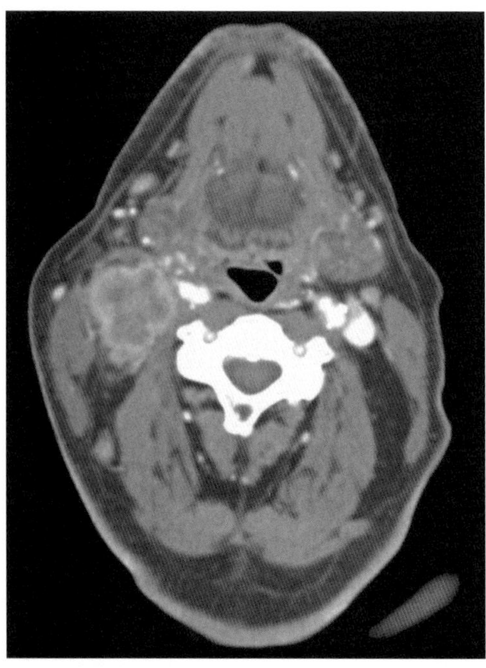

FIGURE 6.3.1 ■ CT scan with contrast demonstrates a (palpable) 4-cm LN in the right level II region without evidence for a primary site of disease.

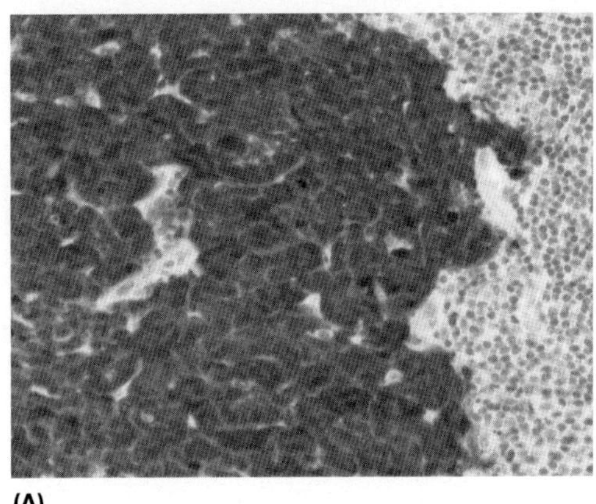
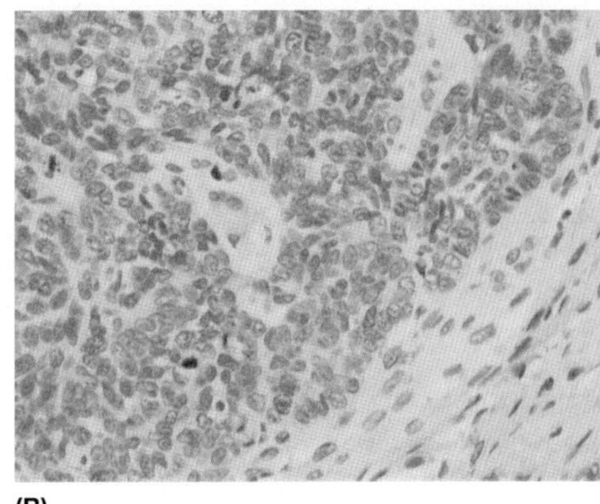

(A)

(B)

FIGURE 6.3.2 ■ (A) p16-positive tumor by immunohistochemistry showing strong nuclear and cytoplasmic staining (×400). (B) p16-negative tumor by immunohistochemistry (×400).

primary site. The patient is male, in his 50s, and presents with asymptomatic lymphadenopathy. While not a never-smoker, his smoking history is limited.

Diagnostic recommendations for metastatic carcinoma from an unknown primary site vary, but these patients should undergo a thorough evaluation including diagnostic imaging of the head and neck. Often, if the primary site remains elusive, an examination under anesthesia using directed biopsies of multiple locations within the pharynx and tonsillectomy are components of the staging process. In this case, the patient's thorough staging evaluation is consistent with National Comprehensive Cancer Network (NCCN) consensus guidelines [1], and it is suggested that if the patient had tonsils, these would be removed as part of the diagnostic workup.

Frequently, the primary site is identified in either the tonsil or the base of the tongue. This is not surprising, as the lymphoidal tissue in these locations makes visualization of disease in these sites difficult. It has been observed that HPV-positive oropharynx cancer patients often present with adenopathy as their first sign of malignancy and the majority tend to have low-volume primary disease (ie, T-stage). It is therefore probable that the primary site of disease in a patient with HPV-positive carcinoma metastatic to the neck, in whom a primary tumor cannot be identified, is still the oropharynx.

NCCN guidelines [1] agree that there is no category 1 evidence regarding a specific therapy for these patients. The guidelines recommend a wide variety of options including: neck dissection

± radiation (± concurrent chemotherapy), concurrent chemoradiation, radiation alone, or induction chemotherapy followed by radiation (± concurrent chemotherapy). The nonsurgical choices are followed by a neck dissection if there is residual disease. These 4 options range from uniform consensus for neck dissection to major disagreement for radiation alone or induction chemotherapy.

Prior to the routine use of chemotherapy for head and neck cancer, the principal controversy in patients presenting with an unknown primary was whether neck dissection or up-front radiotherapy was the better option. Reports varied, some favoring surgery, some radiation, and some, particularly from our institution [2], not supporting either modality as being clearly superior. Results of radiation were occasionally biased as these cohorts often included patients for whom surgery was not an option. At the University of Texas MD Anderson Cancer Center (UTMDACC) and other institutions, the approach of up-front surgery evolved into using radiation more frequently, in part owing to a parallel shift in philosophy toward organ preservation as a general approach for patients with pharyngeal and laryngeal cancer. Even prior to the understanding of HPV and its relationship to prognosis, there was a general philosophy that patients with T0N+ carcinoma had a disease whose natural history was similar to oropharyngeal carcinoma, and therefore these patients could effectively be treated with radiation, with neck dissection reserved for residual disease.

The addition of chemotherapy is now strongly advocated for "advanced" head and neck cancer [3] and by definition nodal disease constitutes advanced disease. Many of the randomized trials included patients with T3–T4 disease, and often trials excluded patients with T1 disease, so whether chemotherapy is necessary for patients with unknown primary (T0) disease, especially without a large nodal burden, is moot. Our use of chemotherapy has been relatively limited in the management of patients with unknown primary tumors. Despite this, our local and regional control rates are greater than 90% [4].

In the current case described, the patient did have a neck dissection. We still rely on postoperative indications for making a recommendation for radiation, and in the case of unknown primaries, our recommendations for radiation are on the basis of the surgical and pathological findings in the neck. Indications for radiation include multiple nodes, nodes greater than 3 cm, and ECE; therefore, a recommendation for radiation should be made for this patient.

Two seminal reports both strongly support concurrent chemotherapy (2 cycles of high-dose cisplatin) in patients operated on for head and neck cancer who are found to have extracapsular nodal extension [5,6,27]. While this suggests that there is category 1 evidence for adding concurrent chemotherapy, neither series included patients with unknown primary tumors. When we evaluated our unknown primary tumor patients treated (principally in the 1970s to the 1980s) with neck dissection and postoperative radiation, ECE was predictive of regional relapse [7]. Although we believe that HPV-positive disease is more radiosensitive, and the benefit of chemotherapy in this situation is less than that demonstrated in the randomized trials, use of concurrent chemotherapy should be considered on a case-by-case basis taking into consideration both the radiographic and, if available, the pathologic extent of ECE.

Once the commitment to radiation is made, the next question is "what are the target volumes?" Should treatment be limited to the involved part of the neck, or to both sides of the neck and the putative mucosal primary sites? NCCN guidelines [1] recommend either approach; ipsilateral therapy was recommended though there was major disagreement among the panel. The literature is quite varied on this subject, and the vast majority of reports predate the routine use of PET and tonsillectomies as components of the staging workup. As the diagnostic evaluation has improved, it is probable that estimates of patients ultimately developing primary site tumor if the mucosa is untreated

should be lower than what is sometimes quoted in the historical literature. In 2000, Nieder and colleagues reviewed the management of patients with cervical nodes from an unknown primary site and compared reports on ipsilateral neck versus comprehensive mucosal and bilateral neck therapy [8]. Some reports suggested that patients who were treated with ipsilateral therapy have higher rates of disease recurrence and poorer survival, while other reports describe patient outcomes with ipsilateral therapy as comparable to outcomes of those treated more comprehensively. With regard to disease control, there is no support that comprehensive therapy is inferior to ipsilateral therapy. Thus, the question becomes "is comprehensive therapy of value in light of its greater rate of acute and late toxicity?"

Nieder and colleagues had suggested a randomized trial between ipsilateral therapy and comprehensive treatment, but efforts to launch this trial in a cooperative group setting failed [8]. One reason for the failure of this trial was the advent of intensity-modulated radiation therapy (IMRT), which in theory might allow for a decrease in toxicity with comprehensive therapy. This is the approach we and others have taken, and small series seem to suggest favorable outcomes, albeit with moderate rates of acute toxicity and modest rates of late xerostomia [4].

While many groups advocate comprehensive therapy, an additional controversy is about which mucosal sites should be irradiated. In the late 1980s, we advocated irradiating the entire pharyngeal axis [9]. More recently, some have advocated eliminating radiation of the larynx and hypopharynx in the belief that these sites are at low risk for development of a primary tumor, and treating these sites adds morbidity [10]. At UTM-DACC, we consider radiation of the larynx and hypopharynx on a case-by-case basis. For example, we began to eliminate the hypopharynx and larynx from treatment in never-smokers, and in patients presenting with cystic nodes located in level 2 of the neck. Currently, we do not treat the larynx or hypopharynx in patients with HPV- or p16-positive disease. In this case, his remote history of smoking does not override his HPV status in our consideration of treatment volume, and we would not irradiate the hypopharynx and larynx.

Should the nasopharynx be treated in HPV-positive disease? We still treat the nasopharynx for two reasons. First, the retropharyngeal nodes are irradiated, so much of the nasopharynx would automatically receive the prescribed dose; second, there have been recent small series of HPV-positive disease arising in the nasopharynx [11]. It is possible that the entire Waldeyer's ring is at risk for HPV disease, though certainly the vast majority of cases are in the tonsils and tongue base. When we delineate the nasopharynx in the treatment of unknown primary disease, we contour the nasopharynx only, and tend to be much tighter on this structure than for a patient presenting with T1 disease of the nasopharynx, for whom we would contour a portion of the pterygoids, sinuses, and clivus.

In theory, the soft palate is likely at very low risk in HPV disease, so we may be able to further reduce our treatment volume at the superior-anterior-medial aspect adjacent to the junction with the hard palate; however, we have not made these changes routinely. Even in patients who have had tonsillectomies as a child, we would also treat the tonsillar fossae. Often, there is residual tonsillar tissue and if covering the base of tongue, especially in a closed mouth position, the lateral pharyngeal walls are routinely in the target volume.

When using IMRT, we have delivered our doses routinely in 30 fractions. The preoperative tumor bed receives a dose of 60 Gy, though we have often added a built-in boost to a small volume in cases of extracapsular disease, ranging from 63 to 66 Gy, recognizing that there are little data supporting doses beyond 60 Gy. The remaining operative bed receives a dose of 57 Gy. The uninvolved contralateral neck (excluding level 1) and putative mucosal sites are treated to 54 Gy. The development of in-field mucosal tumors and regional recurrences with this dose is extremely low with radiation alone; however, with ECE of disease, consideration should be made for concurrent chemotherapy. Further escalation in dose does not seem warranted, especially as the emerging data demonstrate that HPV-related disease is fairly radiosensitive.

In conclusion, for patients presenting with carcinoma metastatic to the neck from an unknown primary site, a multidisciplinary approach is necessary to optimize patients' cure rates and quality of life following treatment. Our most commonly used treatment approach is radiation; however, consideration of chemotherapy and surgical neck management may be complementary. We treat patients (unless circumstances dictate otherwise) with comprehensive irradiation to both sides of the neck and the pharyngeal axis, though we now eliminate the hypopharynx and larynx in patients with HPV-positive disease.

For this patient with T0pN2b p16-positive SCC, we would recommend postoperative radiation. While controversial, we favor treating both sides of the neck and the naso- and oropharynx. The tumor bed would receive a dose of 60 Gy, the operative bed a dose of 56 to 57 Gy, and the uninvolved, undissected sites would receive a dose of 54 Gy. At the present time, as there was ECE of the nodal disease, we would likely add concurrent cisplatin, though there is a growing body of retrospective data suggesting that the addition of chemotherapy may not add significant benefit for patients with p16-positive disease and ECE.

ACADEMIC COMMENT

Christopher L. Hallemeier and Yolanda I. Garces

For patients with biopsy-proven SCC in a cervical node with no primary site evident after appropriate workup, there are 2 different approaches to initial management. Patients can be treated with a primary surgical approach consisting of neck dissection with selective use of postoperative radiotherapy with or without chemotherapy. Alternatively, patients can be treated with a primary radiotherapy approach with or without chemotherapy, with neck dissection only performed following radiotherapy in cases of initial bulky nodal disease (N2c or N3) or residual nodal disease after radiotherapy. As there is no level I evidence to guide selection of a primary treatment modality, both approaches are considered acceptable in the 2012 NCCN Guidelines [1].

At our institution, patients who are medically able to tolerate surgery are typically managed initially with neck dissection, as in the case presented. With this approach, gross disease is removed up front and patients are accurately staged on the basis of pathologic information, allowing the subsequent management strategy to be risk-stratified. For patients found to have early nodal disease (ie, a single LN less than 3 cm) without evidence of ECE, data from our institution and others suggest that the rate of nodal recurrence is very low with no further therapy. Thus, close observation alone is an appropriate strategy [7,12]. Therefore, these patients can be spared the morbidity of radiotherapy. Patients found to have more advanced nodal disease and/or ECE are at a significantly higher risk for both regional and distant progression and thus may benefit from more intensified therapy that would include radiotherapy with or without chemotherapy [7,12].

When treating patients with unknown primary head and neck squamous cell carcinoma, we would use IMRT to "paint" specified radiation doses to different CTVs on the basis of the risk of disease. In addition, retrospective series suggest that IMRT can reduce the dose to critical normal structures, resulting in lower rates of complications compared to conventional radiotherapy techniques [4,13]. Radiotherapy would be initiated 4 to 6 weeks following the neck dissection and would be given in 30 daily fractions over 6 weeks. "CTV high risk" would receive a dose of 63 Gy (2.1 Gy per fraction), "CTV intermediate risk" would receive a dose of 60 Gy (2.0 Gy per fraction), and "CTV low risk" would receive a dose of 54 Gy (1.8 Gy per fraction). "CTV high risk" would include the location of the original gross involved node with ECE, as reconstructed from the preoperative imaging, plus a margin of 1 cm. This dose is based on data from an MD Anderson prospective trial of patients with squamous cell carcinoma of the head and neck receiving postoperative radiotherapy, which suggested that a dose of 63 Gy or higher improves disease control in patients with nodal ECE [14]. "CTV intermediate risk" would include the ipsilateral neck postoperative changes and dissected LN levels. "CTV low risk" would include the contralateral neck LN levels II–V, bilateral retropharyngeal LNs, bilateral pterygoid plates, and target mucosal sites, as outlined subsequently. In the contralateral neck, the superior extent of the CTV would be contoured at the level where the posterior belly of the digastric muscle crosses the jugular vein in order to maximize sparing of the contralateral parotid gland [15].

We agree that the mucosal site CTV should include the oropharynx (including the tonsillar beds) and the nasopharynx. We would not include the larynx and hypopharynx in the CTV given the positive p16 immunohistochemical stain, as well as data from investigators at the University of Florida that suggest that these sites can be omitted from the treatment field without compromising disease control [16]. As this patient did not have LN level IB involvement, we would not include the mucosa of the oral cavity in the CTV, given the relatively infrequent incidence of failure at this site, the ability to easily monitor for recurrence, and the acute toxicity associated with treatment to the oral cavity.

As mentioned by Dr. Garden and Dr. Frank, for patients with high-risk SCC of the head and neck, there is level I evidence that demonstrates that high-dose cisplatin (100 mg/m^2 every 3 weeks) administered concurrently with postoperative radiotherapy significantly reduces the risk of locoregional failure and increases disease-free survival, compared to postoperative radiotherapy alone [5,10]. This benefit was most prominent in patients with ECE or positive surgical margins. Although these studies did not include patients with an unknown primary, there is no reason to believe that these data would not apply to this clinical situation as well. In a single institution retrospective series in which patients with unknown primary head and neck squamous cell carcinoma were treated with resection and postoperative radiotherapy without chemotherapy, the reported rates of neck recurrence in patients with ECE ranged from 16% to 38% [7,17]. Therefore, for this relatively young and healthy patient with high-risk disease, we would strongly recommend concurrent administration of high-dose cisplatin during the radiotherapy course to maximize the chances of regional control and disease-free survival.

COMMUNITY PRACTITIONER COMMENT

Najeeb Mohideen

Patients with cervical node metastases from a head and neck squamous cell carcinoma of unknown primary (HNSCCUP) present a rare but challenging diagnostic and therapeutic dilemma. Thorough diagnostic imaging and panendoscopy with biopsies may reveal the primary in approximately 40% of patients and the majority of these detected lesions are located within the oropharynx (43% in the tonsil and 39% in the base of the tongue) [18]. The presence of HPV positivity in the cervical node metastases makes it highly likely that the primary is of oropharyngeal origin. A study from Johns Hopkins University Hospital showed that all patients whose neck dissection specimens were HPV 16-positive by in situ hybridization (ISH) had a primary in the oropharynx and none of the node metastases from the other sites were HPV-positive [19]. p16 is often advocated as a surrogate marker of HPV on the basis of findings that HPV integration with the transcription of viral oncoproteins induces overexpression of p16. On a direct comparison of p16 IHC and HPV-16 ISH, a discordancy rate of 7% was noted in 1 study. The discrepancies exclusively involved cancers that were negative for HPV-16 by ISH but p16-positive by IHC. In 1 of 3 of these discordant cases, high p16 expression existed because of the presence of a non-16 HPV type, as confirmed by HPV ISH for additional oncogenic types [20]. The remaining discordant cases may reflect the imperfections of p16 as a surrogate marker, a factor to keep in mind in this patient who also may have other causative factors like a 15-pack-year smoking history.

What Is the Volume to Be Treated?

This is an area of controversy. The radiation fields have classically covered all potential mucosal disease sites and LNs on both sides of the neck. While effective, it has also been associated with significant long-term side effects, such as xerostomia and dysphagia, prompting studies to reduce this volume in appropriately selected patients. Investigators from the Universities of Florida and Wisconsin recently reported their pooled experience at successfully eliminating the larynx and hypopharynx from their mucosal volumes (unless level III nodes are present) with a 5-year mucosal control rate of 92% with radiotherapy [10]. Although the median neck relapse rates (calculated from multiple retrospective studies) for unilateral neck irradiation versus bilateral neck irradiation were reportedly lower for bilateral neck radiation (51.5% vs. 19%), it may well be secondary to the confounding effect of patient selection and imbalances in known prognostic variables in the various retrospective studies [8]. The European Organisation for Research and Treatment of Cancer (EORTC) study 24001–22005, which randomized patients with HNSCCUP to ipsilateral radiation therapy (RT) or bilateral RT and whole mucosal RT, would have helped answer this question; however, it was closed early owing to very poor accrual. The advent of IMRT planning and the low probability of primary tumor occurrence in the laryngeal axis offer the potential to reduce morbidity from comprehensive radiation of both sides of the neck and all mucosal sites in this patient.

This patient who has a 4.5 cm level II LN metastases from an HNSCCUP may be managed by a number of options as outlined by the authors earlier and in the NCCN guidelines. The most likely option in our hospital would be neck dissection followed by concurrent chemoradiation. The presence of ECE would be the primary reason to consider chemoradiation. The pooled analysis of the patients from the EORTC and Radiation Therapy Oncology Group (RTOG) postoperative chemoradiation trials did not include patients with unknown primaries nor did it account for HPV status. However, it did show that the subset of patients who might benefit the most from the addition of chemotherapy to radiotherapy in the postsurgical setting were those with microscopic positive margins and extracapsular nodal extension [21].

What Is the Dose to the Operative Bed and Subclinical Sites?

In this patient, the radiation target volume will be as follows: The high-risk CTV is the tumor bed with a 1-cm margin; the intermediate-risk CTV is LN levels I, II, III on the ipsilateral side, ipsilateral tonsillar fossa, and the base of tongue; the low-risk CTV is levels 4 and 5 on the ipsilateral side, contralateral neck nodes (except level 1), retropharyngeal nodes and remaining mucosal surfaces of the oropharynx (including contralateral tonsillar fossa and the base of tongue), and nasopharynx. For this patient, the larynx, hypopharynx, and oral cavity will not be included, except for portions of these volumes that are included by proximity to the nodal volume. The doses are as follows: high-risk CTV is treated to 63 Gy in 30 fractions, intermediate-risk CTV to 57 Gy in 30 fractions, and low-risk CTV to 54 Gy in 30 fractions with IMRT and cisplatin-based chemotherapy.

Some patients have also been treated after initial biopsy with primary concurrent chemoradiation followed by neck dissection for residual disease. In these patients, the high-risk CTV is the gross tumor volume (the palpable and visible disease on clinical and radiological evaluation) with a 1.5 cm margin, while the intermediaterisk and low-risk CTVs are similar to that used after neck dissection. The doses are as follows: The low-risk CTV is treated to 57.75 Gy in 35 fractions, intermediate-risk CTV to 63 Gy in 35 fractions, and high-risk CTV to 70 Gy in 35 fractions. In patients who have no residual disease on clinical and radiological examination after chemoradiation, a routine neck dissection is not done. A large body of evidence supports that approach [22].

If Mucosal Sites Are Treated, Can One Limit Treatment to the Tongue Base in This Case Because of the HPV Status and Surgically Absent Tonsils?

As HPV has a propensity for the epithelium overlying the lymphoid tissue of the lower portions of Waldeyer's ring, it is plausible that the faucial tonsils and adenoids also provide a site for HPV-induced cancer of the nasopharynx. There are reports in the literature on HPV-positive head and neck cancer occurring outside the oropharynx [22–25]. A primary tumor at these other sites can be excluded by clinical exam, imaging, and panendoscopy with biopsy. The fossa of Rosenmuller in the nasopharynx is a potential site for an occult primary and needs special attention by imaging and endoscopy-directed biopsies (rather than blind biopsies). As mentioned earlier, emerging data point to HPV 16 in the cervical nodes as a useful biomarker for discerning tumor origin in the oropharynx [19]. As outcomes continue to improve, we also need to consider quality-of-life issues and reducing long-term toxicities. This calls for reevaluating the low-risk mucosal and nodal targets and dose in an attempt to reduce dose to the opposite parotid gland and constrictor muscles to limit xerostomia and swallowing difficulties. Possible strategies include limiting nasopharyngeal coverage, avoiding the laryngeal axis and oral cavity in appropriate patients, avoiding the high neck nodes on the opposite neck, limiting low-risk mucosal dose below 60 Gy, judicious rather than routine use of chemotherapy, and individualizing treatment considering all clinical, pathological, biological, and technical factors. This coupled with continued refinements in treatment planning and delivery will help optimize the therapeutic ratio for these patients.

SECTION EDITOR'S NOTE

Wade Thorstad

Treatment for patients similar to this case with unknown primary cancer metastatic to the neck is controversial, and, with respect to the ongoing epidemic of HPV-related disease, still evolving. In this case treated with up-front surgery with pathologically proven ECE in the LNs, I agree with the authors' recommendations of radiation or concurrent chemoradiation based on data extrapolated from randomized trials. In terms of target volume, the authors all recommend treatment of bilateral neck and oropharyngeal to nasopharyngeal mucosa, and all favor omission of the laryngeal axis and hypopharynx in the setting of HPV-related disease.

In contrast, at Washington University in St. Louis, we often treat these patients with a neck dissection and radiation therapy (± concurrent chemotherapy) limited to the ipsilateral neck. Recent results in a small series of patients failed to reveal significant outcome differences between ipsilateral and comprehensive treatment [26]. As noted earlier, the 2012 NCCN guidelines recommended either approach (ipsilateral vs. comprehensive treatment), albeit with significant disagreement among the panel members [1]. Unfortunately, as previously mentioned, efforts to complete a randomized trial comparing ipsilateral versus comprehensive therapy have been unsuccessful [8].

REFERENCES

1. Head and Neck Cancers (Version 2.2012, NCCN Clinical Practice Guidelines in Oncology, NCCN.org, 2012 (Accessed at http://www.nccn.org)

2. Wang RC, Goepfert H, Barber AE, et al. Unknown primary squamous cell carcinoma metastatic to the neck. *Arch Otolaryngol Head Neck Surg.* 1990;116:1388–1393.

3. Pignon JP, le Maitre A, Maillard E, et al. Meta-analysis of chemotherapy in head and neck cancer (MACH-NC): An update on 93 randomised trials and 17,346 patients. *Radiother Oncol.* 2009;92:4–14.

4. Frank SJ, Rosenthal DI, Petsuksiri J, et al. Intensity-modulated radiotherapy for cervical node squamous cell carcinoma metastases from unknown head-and-neck primary site: M. D. Anderson Cancer Center outcomes and patterns of failure. *Int J Radiat Oncol Biol Phys.* 2010;78:1005–1010.

5. Bernier J, Domenge C, Ozsahin M, et al. Postoperative irradiation with or without concomitant chemotherapy for locally advanced head and neck cancer. *N Engl J Med.* 2004;350:1945–1952.

6. Cooper JS, Pajak TF, Forastiere AA, et al. Postoperative concurrent radiotherapy and chemotherapy for high-risk squamous-cell carcinoma of the head and neck. *N Engl J Med.* 2004;350:1937–1944.

7. Colletier PJ, Garden AS, Morrison WH, et al. Postoperative radiation for squamous cell carcinoma metastatic to cervical lymph nodes from an unknown primary site: Outcomes and patterns of failure. *Head Neck.* 1998;20:674–681.

8. Nieder C, Gregoire V, Ang KK. Cervical lymph node metastases from occult squamous cell carcinoma: Cut down a tree to get an apple? *Int J Radiat Oncol Biol Phys.* 2001;50:727–733.

9. Carlson LS, Fletcher GH, Oswald MJ. Guidelines for radiotherapeutic techniques for cervical metastases from an unknown primary. *Int J Radiat Oncol Biol Phys.* 1986;12:2101–2110.

10. Wallace A, Richards GM, Harari PM, et al. Head and neck squamous cell carcinoma from an unknown primary site. *Am J Otolaryngol.* 2011;32(4):286–290.

11. Lo EJ, Bell D, Woo JS, et al. Human papillomavirus and WHO type I nasopharyngeal carcinoma. *Laryngoscope.* 2010;120:1990–1997.

12. Coster JR, Foote RL, Olsen KD, et al. Cervical nodal metastasis of squamous cell carcinoma of unknown origin: Indications for withholding radiation therapy. *Int J Radiat Oncol Biol Phys.* 1992;23:743–749.

13. Chen AM, Li BQ, Farwell DG, et al. Improved dosimetric and clinical outcomes with intensity-modulated radiotherapy for head-and-neck cancer of unknown primary origin. *Int J Radiat Oncol Biol Phys.* 2011;79:756–762.

14. Peters LJ, Goepfert H, Ang KK, et al. Evaluation of the dose for postoperative radiation therapy of head and neck cancer: First report of a prospective randomized trial. *Int J Radiat Oncol Biol Phys.* 1993;26:3–11.

15. Eisbruch A, Marsh LH, Dawson LA, et al. Recurrences near base of skull after IMRT for head-and-neck cancer: Implications for target delineation in high neck and for parotid gland sparing. *Int J Radiat Oncol Biol Phys.* 2004;59:28–42.

16. Barker CA, Morris CG, Mendenhall WM. Larynx-sparing radiotherapy for squamous cell carcinoma from an unknown head and neck primary site. *Am J Clin Oncol.* 2005;28:445–448.

17. Iganej S, Kagan R, Anderson P, et al. Metastatic squamous cell carcinoma of the neck from an unknown primary: Management options and patterns of relapse. *Head Neck.* 2002;24:236–246.

18. Mendenhall WM, Mancuso AA, Amdur RJ, et al. Squamous cell carcinoma metastatic to the neck from an unknown head and neck primary site. *Am J Otolaryngol.* 2001;22(4):261–267.

19. Begum S, Gillison ML, Ansari-Lari MA, et al. Detection of human papillomavirus in cervical lymph nodes: A highly effective strategy for localizing site of tumor origin. *Clin Cancer Res.* 2003;9:6469–6475.

20. Singhi A, Westra WH. Comparison of human papillomavirus in situ hybridization and p16 immunohistochemistry in the detection of human papillomavirus associated head and neck cancer based on a prospective clinical experience. *Cancer.* 2010 May 1;116(19):2166–2173.

21. Bernier J, Cooper JS, Pajak TF, et al. Defining risk levels in locally advanced head and neck cancers: A comparative analysis of concurrent postoperative radiation plus chemotherapy trials of the EORTC (#22931) and RTOG (#9501). *Head Neck.* 2005 Oct;27(10):843–850.

22. Ferlito A, Corry J, Silver CE, et al. Planned neck dissection for patients with complete response to chemoradiotherapy: A concept approaching obsolescence. *Head Neck.* 2010 Feb;32(2):253–261.

23. Maxwell JH, Kumar B, Feng FY, et al. HPV-positive/p16-positive/EBV-negative nasopharyngeal carcinoma in white North Americans. *Head Neck.* 2010;32(5):562–567.

24. Punwaney R, Brandwein MS, Zhang DY, et al. Human papillomavirus may be common within nasopharyngeal carcinoma of Caucasian Americans: investigation of Epstein-Barr virus and human papillomavirus in eastern and western nasopharyngeal carcinoma using ligation-dependent polymerase chain reaction. *Head Neck.* 1999;21(1):21–9.

25. Bozdayi G, Kemaloglu Y, Ekinci O, et al. Role of human papillomavirus in the clinical and histopathologic features of laryngeal and hypopharyngeal cancers. *J Otolaryngol Head Neck Surg.* 2009;38:119–125

26. Perkins SM, Spencer CR, Chernock RD, et al. Radiotherapeutic management of cervical lymph node metastases from an unknown primary site. *Arch Otolaryngol Head Neck Surg.* 2012;138:656–661.

27. Cooper JS, Zhagn Q, Pajak TF, et al. Long-term follow-up of the RTOG 9501/Intergroup Phase III trial: Postoperative concurrent radiation therapy and chemotherapy in high-risk squamous cell carcinoma of the head and neck. *Int J Radiat Oncol Biol Phys.* 2012:84(5);1198–1205.

■ THORAX ■

Section Editor: Gregory Videtic

Limited-Stage Small Cell Lung Cancer in High-Risk Patients

CLINICAL PROBLEM

For patients with limited-stage small cell lung cancer (L-SCLC) with clinical or tumor characteristics that would have made them ineligible for phase 3 trials (eg, impaired performance status, impaired pulmonary function, large tumors precluding "safe" delivery of radiotherapy), the optimal timing, dose, and fractionation of radiotherapy, and its sequencing with chemotherapy remain areas of controversy.

CASE EXAMPLE

A 62-year-old female, former smoker, presented to an emergency department with left subscapular pain radiating to the medial aspect of the left arm in the ulnar distribution. A cardiac event was ruled out but a chest x-ray revealed an 8 × 4 cm spiculated lesion in the left upper lung apex extending into the mediastinum. A subsequent chest CT revealed a 7.8 × 6 cm infiltrating soft tissue mass in the anterior mediastinum with middle mediastinal and left hilar extension and encasement of the mediastinal structures with postobstructive pneumonitis. Her physical exam was remarkable for a BMI of 41.5. Her chest exam was unremarkable. Serum chemistries and complete blood count (CBC) were normal. Serum lactate dehydrogenase (LDH) was mildy eleveated at 234 (normal value is 220 or lesser).

Bronchoscopy revealed a mass in the left bronchial tree and transbronchial needle aspiration biopsy of the left upper lobe mass was consistent with small cell undifferentiated carcinoma. Pulmonary function testing was not done. She underwent staging: An MRI brain scan was negative for metastases. A PET/CT showed a large, intensely hypermetabolic mediastinal mass with extension into the left upper lobe and left hilum encasing the left upper lobe bronchus with left upper lobe collapse, consistent with the primary diagnosis of small cell carcinoma and no evidence for distant hypermetabolic metastatic disease (Figure 7.1.1).

The medical oncologist who saw her initially started chemotherapy the day after his consultation with her because of her symptoms and the size and extent of the disease.

Management Decisions

- What are your comments on the decision of the medical oncologist to start chemotherapy immediately?
- What is the impact of very large tumors on therapy, timing, and sequencing of RT?
- How is the treatment volume defined for the radiotherapy if initiated after cycle(s) of chemotherapy?
- What is the impact of volume and location of disease on RT and risk of radiation pneumonitis and other toxicities such as plexopathy?
- What is the role of pulmonary function testing (PFT) in decision making?
- Where does prophylactic cranial irradiation (PCI) timing fit in the management plan?

MAJOR OPINION

Paul D. Aridgides and Jeffrey A. Bogart

This is a challenging and common presentation for patients with L-SCLC. The most relevant factors in determining a treatment plan relate to the extent of disease and the patient's ability to withstand aggressive therapy. In this patient's favor is the fact that limited stage disease has been confirmed by FDG-PET imaging, whereas the majority of available data reflect outcomes for patients found to have limited disease on the basis of traditional

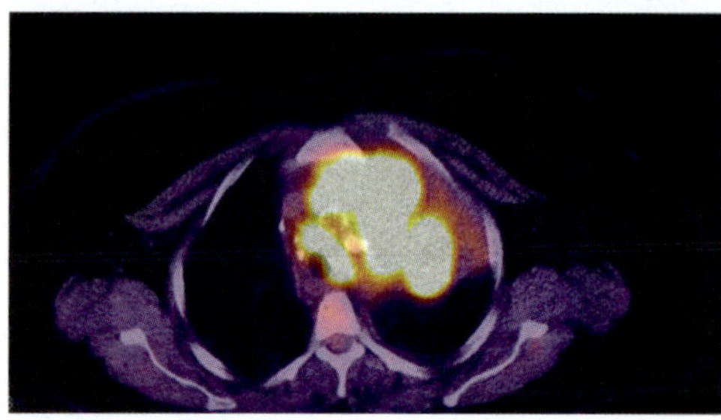

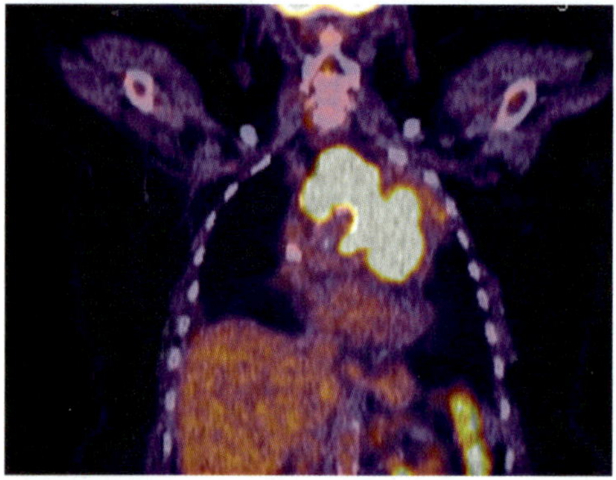

FIGURE 7.1.1 ■ Representative axial and coronal images from the fused FDG-PET/CT scan of a 62 year old patient with small cell lung cancer demonstrating intense hypermetabolic uptake in the left upper lobe into the mediastinum.

imaging (eg, CT imaging, bone scintigraphy, and plain chest x-ray). An overview of published series suggests that approximately 10% of patients will be upstaged to extensive disease on the basis of findings on FDG-PET imaging [1]. Another favorable sign is that the patient appears to have a relatively good performance status (interestingly, most phase 3 studies for L-SCLC have included Eastern Cooperative Oncology Group performance status [ECOG PS] 2 patients), which would not preclude the delivery of concurrent combined modality therapy, and she has not lost weight. Moreover, the patient quit smoking many years ago, a positive sign both in terms of prognosis as well as tolerating therapy without interruptions. On the other hand, the locally aggressive and bulky nature of the tumor is concerning given both the large tumor volume and the neurologic and respiratory compromise noted in the evaluation. In this patient, the T and N status appear difficult to discern given the direct extension of the tumor into the mediastinum. So, it is not clear if there are separate mediastinal lymph nodes involved with

tumors, although given the nature of small-cell lung cancer this is very likely.

One question to address is whether the patient should undergo any additional evaluation prior to initiation of therapy. The only obvious exam that has been overlooked at this time is the PFTs. Although PFTs may give some indication of the patient's ability to withstand thoracic radiotherapy, I think they are of little value in directing therapy in a patient who otherwise looks well and has obvious pulmonary compromise by tumor, and I would not delay treatment in order to obtain PFTs. That said, I would plan to obtain "baseline" PFTs, including diffusing capacity of carbon monoxide, once the primary tumor has responded to therapy and is no longer obstructing the left upper lobe bronchus (hopefully this will lead to re-expansion of the left upper lobe). Even if PFTs are poor, the fact that L-SCLC is a serious disease with a 20% to 25% 5-year survival [2] following aggressive combined modality therapy should be taken into account. So I would rarely deny someone concurrent therapy purely on the basis of PFTs as long as they understand and accept the risks of therapy. Concurrent chemoradiotherapy is associated with improved survival compared with sequential therapy [3], and I would hypothesize that the impact of combined therapy may be even greater in such a patient with bulky disease.

The first major decision to be made in consultation with the medical oncologist is the timing of thoracic radiotherapy—whether the patient should be treated initially with systemic chemotherapy alone (delaying the initiation of thoracic radiotherapy) or with concurrent chemotherapy and thoracic radiotherapy. The relevant question is whether initiating concurrent therapy earlier would improve the disease response and/or result in improved long-term survival. While we generally believe that adding radiotherapy will result in a more rapid resolution of local signs and symptoms, there are little data that attest to this belief in patients with small cell lung cancer. At presentation, the patient has virtually no respiratory symptoms and her pain is under excellent control with modest doses of narcotics. I would be comfortable in this situation to start with chemotherapy alone as the likelihood of getting an objective tumor response with improvement in pain control is very good. For example, Cancer and Leukemia Group B (CALGB) studies suggest that greater than 75% of patients will achieve at least a radiographic partial response following 2 cycles of induction chemotherapy [4]. That said, I would monitor the patient closely and consider starting radiotherapy urgently in the unlikely situation that there was not prompt resolution of symptoms. I would not ask the medical oncologist to delay starting chemotherapy in order to have adequate time to appropriately simulate and plan radiotherapy for the patient.

The issue of thoracic radiotherapy timing and impact on survival continues to be controversial. While Intergroup Study 0096 (INT 0096) started thoracic radiotherapy with the first cycle of chemotherapy, there are little data to support "cycle 1" radiotherapy as a standard of care. The seminal study that demonstrated improved survival for early thoracic radiotherapy, conducted by the National Cancer Institute of Canada Clinical Trials Group, compared cycle 2 radiotherapy with cycle 6 radiotherapy [5]. While survival was significantly improved with cycle 2 radiotherapy, study results must be tempered by the limitations of staging (CT imaging was not required) and treatment planning (spinal cord blocks that shielded gross disease were routinely used) at the time the trial was conducted. Interestingly, the study design was repeated by the London Lung Cancer Group (LLCG) and earlier radiotherapy did not result in better survival in that study [6]. One major criticism of the LLCG study was the reduced intensity of chemotherapy delivered in the early radiotherapy arm. Overall, several reviews of radiotherapy timing suggest that earlier radiotherapy may be associated with improved survival, particularly when intensive thoracic radiotherapy is given [7–9]. For the patient under consideration, I would consider initiating thoracic radiotherapy with either the second or third cycle of chemotherapy to allow for some reduction in tumor burden. Several prospective cooperative group studies have started radiotherapy with either the third chemotherapy cycle without obvious detriment. In the current randomized phase 3 trial in the United States (CALGB 30610/RTOG 0538), starting radiotherapy with either the first or second cycle of chemotherapy is permitted, while the European phase 3 study assessing radiotherapy dose and schedule (CONVERT) mandates cycle 2 radiotherapy.

The issue of radiotherapy dose and fractionation is at present being studied in the above mentioned US and European trials. That said, I strongly encourage the use of a dose of 1.5 Gy twice-daily to 45 Gy in patients that do not go on trial. In fact, the phase 3 trial that showed superiority of twice-daily radiotherapy over once-daily radiotherapy

(INT 0096) is one of the few studies ever to show that fractionation, particularly in conjunction with chemotherapy, impacts overall survival [1]. An increase in 5-year survival from 16% to 26% should be taken seriously in deciding whether to commit somebody to a once-daily regimen. The main argument against using twice-daily radiotherapy is that a relatively modest dose of once-daily radiotherapy was used in the standard arm in the phase 3 study. While recent trials have shown that doses as high as 70 Gy are feasible with once-daily fractionation, there is still no convincing evidence that high-dose once-daily radiotherapy equals or exceeds the 45 Gy twice-daily regimen [4]. Perhaps there is a lesson to be learned from the recently reported results of Radiation Therapy Oncology Group (RTOG) 0617, which demonstrated that a higher dose of conventionally fractionated radiotherapy (74 Gy) was not more effective than a standard dose of conventionally fractionated radiotherapy (60 Gy) [10]. The third regimen tested in CALGB 30610/RTOG 0538 was a concomitant boost regimen piloted by the RTOG. Although the initial experience with this regimen appeared promising, reported outcomes on the RTOG phase 2 trial have been somewhat disappointing and I would not use it outside of a clinical trial setting [11,12]. The main concern with the twice-daily regimen is severe esophagitis and this should be managed supportively (pain medication, nutrition consultation, intravenous hydration, etc.) with vigilance during the treatment course.

Treatment volume correlates with the choice of dose and fractionation. While there is a growing body of evidence on dose/volume relationships for patients who are treated with once-daily radiotherapy for locally advanced non-small cell lung cancer, there are little data for patients with L-SCLC. In part, this is because very few prospective trials have mandated the use (and submission) of conformal planning techniques. So, a threshold lung V20 (percentage of lung volume receiving 20 Gy) has not been defined for patients who are treated with twice-daily fractionation, nor is it clear whether this metric correlates well with pulmonary toxicity. A recent analysis of CALGB trials that used high dose (eg, 70 Gy) once-daily radiotherapy actually suggested a higher lung V20 threshold (compared with data for non-small cell lung cancer) with few severe pulmonary toxic events [13]. That said, every effort should be made to minimize the volume of normal tissue irradiated. CT simulation should be routinely performed with consideration of 4-D simulation to measure tumor motion with respiration. We routinely fuse FDG-PET imaging studies with the planning CT to facilitate treatment planning. When the 45 Gy twice-daily regimen is used, meeting accepted dose constraints may be less challenging for some structures, such as the brachial plexus, when compared to high-dose once-daily radiotherapy. I would not hesitate to include a part of the brachial plexus throughout the entire treatment course for apical tumors (or involved ipsilateral supraclavicular adenopathy), but I would generally try to limit the brachial plexus dose to less than 66 Gy when high-dose daily fractionation is used. On the other hand, paying meticulous attention to spinal cord tolerance is critical and the maximum spinal cord dose is typically limited to 36 Gy when 1.5 Gy twice-daily fractionation is given. The integration of conformal techniques may allow continuation of a single plan throughout the treatment course, as opposed to completely shielding the spinal cord during the afternoon session of the final 2 weeks of therapy (as was mandated in INT 0096).

One issue that has been studied in some detail is whether it is appropriate to use the postchemotherapy target volume after induction chemotherapy when radiotherapy is delayed. The results of a seminal randomized phase 3 trial from the Southwest Oncology Group (SWOG) demonstrated less myelosuppression and equal survival for patients treated to a "postchemotherapy" volume [14], and recent prospective randomized data from China, which used a more modern concurrent chemoradiotherapy approach, confirm this result [15]. Moreover, very few marginal relapses have been reported from studies where the postchemotherapy volume is used for radiotherapy planning. So I would certainly take advantage of the reduced tumor burden following induction chemotherapy. However, as per the current CALGB 30610/RTOG 0538 study, I would include all initially involved nodal regions as part of the gross tumor volume (GTV) even if there were a complete response in these nodal regions after induction chemotherapy. Other considerations relevant to target volume are whether to electively treat clinically uninvolved regional lymph nodes and appropriate expansions for target volumes. The available literature suggests that isolated mediastinal relapse is uncommon when FDG-PET/CT is utilized to determine target volumes for radiotherapy, although mediastinal lymph nodes were typically included in the treatment volume in past phase 3 trials. Integrating

available advanced technology can be critical in limiting target volumes, and I routinely use image guidance, preferably with a cone-beam CT, on a daily basis. This allows for limited expansion of target volumes, particularly into lung parenchyma, and also allows for assessment of tumor response during radiotherapy. In the current patient, I would consider "adaptive" therapy and repeat simulation during therapy depending on rapidity of response. This would likely be of greatest value the earlier radiotherapy was initiated. While there are no prospective data regarding adaptive therapy in small cell lung cancer, theoretical considerations in using a shrinking field technique to protect lung parenchyma are similar to the rationale for using postchemotherapy volumes. CALGB 30610 does allow for resimulation once during therapy on each of the experimental arms.

After completion of 4 cycles of chemotherapy and thoracic radiotherapy, this patient would be considered for PCI pending restaging evaluation including a chest and abdomen CT and a brain MRI. Some investigators have suggested that earlier administration of PCI may be beneficial, but safely integrating PCI between chemotherapy cycles is a difficult challenge in my experience. Although the meta-analysis of randomized trials was restricted to patients with a "complete response" to initial treatment [16,17], most protocols would allow PCI for patients with a good partial response to therapy as well. The standard dose of PCI appears to be 2500 cGy in 10 fractions based on recent randomized data from the United States and Europe, as the administration of 3600 cGy (in once- or twice-daily fractionations) resulted in a similar incidence of brain metastases (at 2 years) but apparent increased mortality [18]. Analysis of the RTOG 0212 trial found older age and higher dose to be associated with increased risk of chronic neurotoxicity [19]. Older age is not a factor in the patient under consideration, but comorbid medical illness including ischemic heart disease, hypertension, longstanding diabetes, and atherosclerotic disease may be considered when discussing the option of PCI with the patient.

Whether there is a role for early assessment of response by functional (FDG-PET) imaging has not been well studied, but a small prospective trial suggested that FDG-PET response to induction chemotherapy (prior to thoracic radiotherapy) may predict survival in L-SCLC [20]. This issue would appear to merit further prospective study as perhaps early response to induction therapy could help guide the intensity of thoracic radiotherapy and the choice of further systemic therapy. FDG-PET/CT imaging may also be of value in following patients after completion of all therapy. This may be particularly true in patients with residual masses (more likely in patients with bulky disease as in the present case), as prospective trials show that many patients who scored as having a partial response by CT criteria never actually experience local tumor relapse.

ACADEMIC COMMENT

Thomas J. Dilling

Dr. Bogart has provided a superb outline of the medical literature regarding the treatment of L-SCLC. In response to his review are my perspectives as an academic radiation oncologist.

I completely agree with Dr. Bogart that up front PFTs are not necessary. These patients are typically heavy smokers with significant chronic obstructive pulmonary disease (COPD). The typically large size of these tumors often causes a respiratory compromise as well. However, the tumors also shrink significantly (and quickly) with aggressive therapy. Consequently, subjective pulmonary function typically improves after treatment is initiated. One can question, then, whether up-front PFTs are relevant. I certainly would not delay therapy in order to perform the PFTs.

I strongly believe that concurrent chemoradiotherapy should be employed in almost every case. Out of approximately 50 to 60 cases of L-SCLC we have treated at our institution in the past 5 years, we have only treated 3 or 4 sequentially. The remainder has been treated to a dose of 45 Gy in 150 cGy fractions BID (twice daily), per the Intergroup regimen [2]. It is important to bear in mind that this is the only large, completed, phase 3, multi-institutional trial of concurrent chemoradiotherapy in L-SCLC in the United States. With aggressive management of the patient during therapy, it is possible to complete this aggressive treatment successfully.

It remains to be seen whether a once-daily fractionation schema is equivalent or superior. It has been shown that a dose of 70 Gy in 35 fractions can be readily accomplished without undue toxicity [21]. But it has not been proven equivalent to a dose of 45 Gy BID in a randomized trial. This is not to say that 45 Gy BID is ideal—the local control is only 36% in the Intergroup trial [2]. The

currently enrolling CALGB 30610/RTOG 0538 is testing a concomitant boost regimen against 45 Gy BID and 70 Gy QD (once daily). This trial will yield valuable insight.

These tumors typically have a rapid doubling time. Consequently, our typical practice is to initiate the first cycle of chemotherapy as quickly as possible. Most commonly, we simulate the patient at that time and then begin radiation treatment 2 or more weeks later, on day 1 of cycle 2. This allows for adequate planning time for the radiotherapy. If the patient is asymptomatic (as in this case), one could consider simulating the patient and then starting chemotherapy and radiation together during the first cycle of chemotherapy, if this does not delay treatment significantly. In the case provided, it should not prove difficult to develop a treatment plan that is within standard dosimetric constraints. If this were not so, one can consider giving 1 to 2 cycles of chemotherapy and then initiating radiation during cycle 2 of chemotherapy. The chemotherapy should result in significant cytoreduction.

Academic thoracic radiation oncologists predominantly perform selective nodal irradiation for SCLC. It is quite reasonable to define the GTV using the PET/CT scan [22,23]. In these cases, one must take extra care in the analysis of supraclavicular lymph nodes, because of the risk of isolated failure in those nodes [23]. Furthermore, defining the disease only with a CT scan is likely inadequate to assess for the presence of disease owing to increased risk of failure in lymph nodes outside the treatment volume [24]. I use PET/CT scan to determine the GTV, occasionally adding PET-negative but enlarged nodes that are evident on the CT scan, on the basis of independent clinical judgment. I also treat supraclavicular nodes if I see even a faint enhancement whatsoever on the PET/CT scan.

When simulating/treating a patient after chemotherapy, it is important to utilize the initial staging PET/CT to determine the treatment volumes. Even if a node "melts away" before radiotherapy, that nodal station should be irradiated if it was previously enlarged and PET-positive. The postchemotherapy volumes may be utilized, reducing the overall treatment field size, but no areas of prior involvement may be omitted from the selective irradiation fields [25]. Again, I would take special care to analyze the original PET/CT scan for possible disease in the supraclavicular fossae.

It is important to aggressively manage these patients throughout therapy. At our institution, they have weekly meetings with a dietician. I stress to the patients on the urgency of not losing weight while on treatment. They are counseled extensively regarding the use of nutritional supplements to increase their caloric intake. I treat radiation esophagitis aggressively, with liberal use of short-acting and long-acting narcotics as necessary. I also have a very low threshold to treat patients for presumptive esophageal thrush (minimum of 15 days of fluconazole).

At my institution, patients are restaged approximately 1 month after the completion of the fourth cycle of chemotherapy (typically 10–13 weeks after completing radiotherapy). We repeat the brain MRI (CT with contrast if MRI is not possible) and CT of the thorax. If there is evidence of near or complete response and the brain is negative for metastatic disease, we offer PCI. Certainly there are concerns about possible neurological sequelae, but the increase in overall survival is clear [17]. I treat patients to a dose of 2500 cGy in 10 fractions of 250 cGy each. In an attempt to minimize hot spots in the treatment plan, I CT-simulate these patients and treat them with a field-in-field plan (typically 3–4 control points) to better homogenize the dose delivered and thereby potentially reduce treatment toxicity.

COMMUNITY PRACTITIONER COMMENT

Stephen T. Lutz

The clinical scenario described and reviewed presents commonly in the community setting. The proper choice for treatment includes an evaluation of factors involving: the patient (ie, age, performance status, weight loss, pulmonary function, comorbid disease), the cancer (ie, stage, bulky presentation, nodal status), and both the capability and willingness of the patient and her caretakers to seek out aggressive therapy. Although we have made great strides in the length of survival of patients with L-SCLC, this woman's overall survival based on current standards of care remains modest. Nonetheless, treatment with curative intent remains appropriate for selected patients, because it also offers the best hope of locally controlling the disease.

It is difficult to accurately predict her baseline pulmonary functioning given the obstruction of her left upper lobe bronchus. Still, PFT prior to irradiation might provide information regarding her pulmonary reserve and the degree to which she might be at risk for long-term shortness of breath or oxygen dependence, depending on what volume of the normal lung receives radiotherapy. If she has very little reserve, then I might be more inclined to begin treatment to the postchemotherapy volume present after either the second or third cycle of chemotherapy rather than with the first. Also, in that situation I might be slightly more judicious about the amount of non-PET-positive mediastinal lymph node stations I would include in my clinical treatment volume. In general, I would not offer sequential chemoradiotherapy unless her performance status declines dramatically owing to the toxicity of her first or second cycle of chemotherapy. I would, however, offer emergent radiotherapy if she shows symptoms or radiographic findings consistent with suboptimal response or progression of disease with the initial chemotherapy.

While I recognize the statistically significant improvement in survival for patients who receive twice-daily radiotherapy versus daily treatment, my experience in the community hospital setting is that patients often tend to choose once-daily therapy because of convenience issues or because of fear of increased acute toxicity. So, while I offer twice-daily treatments and explain the rationale for that dosing schema, I do so in a way that does not cause the patient to feel that if they chose daily treatment they have made an "incorrect" decision.

If she were to accept twice-daily radiation, I would prescribe a dose of 45 Gy while sparing the spinal cord after 36 Gy and decreasing the treated volume once or twice during treatment as repeat CT simulations would suggest feasible. My preferred single-fraction regimen for this patient would be to achieve a total dose of between 60 and 66 Gy, depending on the dosimetric constraints of the spinal cord, normal lung, and brachial plexus. My recommendation would be for PCI to a dose of 25 Gy in 10 fractions for complete or near-complete response to the entire chemotherapy dose. While the evidence does suggest that PCI should be initiated as early as the end of the fourth cycle of chemotherapy, most patients have treatment-related fatigue that causes them to defer PCI until after all of their chemotherapy is done.

Finally, given the reality that this patient has what will likely prove to be a fatal illness, I find it critical that she be offered a consultation with the palliative care service at the time of her initial diagnosis. This meeting provides several valuable enhancements to care, including an emotional acknowledgment of the most likely outcome of this disease, the opportunity for the palliative care team to help manage disease- and treatment-related effects, and a means by which to seamlessly transition the patient to the hospice service should the disease fail to respond or eventually come to recur. Furthermore, even though the data were gathered in patients with non-SCLC, there is literature which suggests that patients with advanced lung cancer survive longer when receiving active palliative care along with curative treatment [26].

SECTION EDITOR'S NOTE

Gregory Videtic

I agree overall with the approach described by the various authors. I would generally have planned on starting radiotherapy with cycle 2 of chemotherapy and ensure that baseline PFTs (always including diffusion capacity) would have been carried out prior to starting radiotherapy. In my practice, I frequently use the hypofractionated regimen described in the National Cancer Institute of Canada phase 3 trial in SCLC [5], as it was a cycle 2 start and was accelerated, with outcomes similar to the Turrisi et al. trial [2].

REFERENCES

1. Thomson D, Hulse P, Lorigan P, Faivre-Finn C. The role of positron emission tomography in management of small cell lung cancer. *Lung Cancer.* 2011;73:121–126.
2. Turrisi, AT III, Kim K, Blum R, et al. Twice-daily compared with once-daily thoracic radiotherapy in limited small-cell lung cancer treated concurrently with cisplatin and etoposide. *N Engl J Med.* 1999;340:265–271.
3. Takada M, Fukuoka M, Kawahara M, et al. Phase III study of concurrent versus sequential thoracic radiotherapy in combination with cisplatin and etoposide for limited-stage small-cell lung cancer: Results of the Japan Clinical Oncology Group Study 9104. *J Clin Oncol.* 2002 Jul 15;20:3054–3060.
4. Bogart JA, Herndon JE 2nd, Lyss AP, et al. 70 Gy thoracic radiotherapy is feasible concurrent with chemotherapy for limited-stage small-cell lung cancer: Analysis of Cancer and Leukemia Group B study 39808. *Int J Radiat Oncol Biol Phys.* 2004 1;59:460–468.
5. Murray N, Coy P, Pater JL, Hodson I, et al. Importance of timing for thoracic irradiation in the combined modality treatment of limited-stage small-cell lung cancer. The National Cancer Institute of Canada Clinical Trials Group. *J Clin Oncol.* 1993;11:336–344.
6. Spiro SG, James LE, Rudd RM, et al. Early compared with late radiotherapy in combined modality treatment for limited disease small-cell lung cancer: A London Lung Cancer Group multicenter randomized clinical trial and meta-analysis. *J Clin Oncol.* 2006 Aug 20;24:3823–3830.
7. Pijls-Johannesma MC, De Ruysscher D, Lambin P, et al. Early versus late chest radiotherapy for limited stage small cell lung cancer. *Cochrane Database Syst Rev.* 2005;(1):CD004700.
8. Fried DB, Morris DE, Poole C, et al. Systematic review evaluating the timing of thoracic radiation therapy in combined modality therapy for limited stage small-cell lung cancer. *J Clin Oncol.* 2004;22:4837–4845.
9. De Ruysscher D, Pijls-Johannesma M, Vansteenkiste J, et al. Systematic review and meta-analysis of randomised, controlled trials of the timing of chest radiotherapy in patients with limited-stage, small-cell lung cancer. *Ann Oncol.* 2006;17:543–552.
10. RTOG Broadcast, June 17, 2011. Accessed online at: http://ww6.rtog.org/LinkClick.aspx?fileticket=tN4D8xvlHW4%3D&tabid=290
11. Komaki R, Swann RS, Ettinger DS, et al. Phase I study of thoracic radiation dose escalation with concurrent chemotherapy for patients with limited small-cell lung cancer: Report of Radiation Therapy Oncology Group (RTOG) protocol 97-12. *Int J Radiat Oncol Biol Phys.* 2005 Jun 1;62:342–350.
12. Komaki R, Paulus R, Ettinger DS, et al. A phase II study of accelerated high-dose thoracic radiation therapy (AHTRT) with concurrent chemotherapy for limited small cell lung cancer: RTOG 0239. *J Clin Oncol.* 2009;27:15s.
13. Salama JK, Hodgson L, Pang H, et al. Predictors of pulmonary toxicity in limited-stage (LS) small cell lung cancer (SCLC) patients treated with concurrent chemotherapy (CTX) and high-dose (70 Gy) daily radiotherapy (RT): A pooled analysis of three CALGB studies. *J Clin Oncol.* 2011;29:(suppl; abstr 7078).
14. Kies MS, Mira JG, Crowley JJ, et al. Multimodal therapy for limited small-cell lung cancer: A randomized study of induction combination chemotherapy with or without thoracic radiation in complete responders; and with wide-field versus reduced-field radiation in partial responders: A Southwest Oncology Group Study. *J Clin Oncol.* 1987;5:592–600.

15. Hu X, Bao Y, Zhang L, et al. Omitting elective nodal irradiation and irradiating postinduction versus preinduction chemotherapy tumor extent for limited-stage small cell lung cancer interim analysis of a prospective randomized noninferiority trial. *Cancer.* 2012 Jan 1;118(1):278–287.

16. Arriagada R, Le Chevalier T, Borie F. Prophylactic cranial irradiation for patients with small-cell lung cancer in complete remission. *J Natl Cancer Inst.* 1995; 87:183–190.

17. Auperin A, Arriagada R, Pignon JP. Prophylactic cranial irradiation for patients with small-cell lung cancer in complete remission. Prophylactic Cranial Irradiation Overview Collaborative Group. *N Engl J Med.* 1999;341:476–484.

18. Le Pechoux C, Dunant A, Senan S, et al. Standard-dose versus higher-dose prophylactic cranial irradiation (PCI) in patients with limited-stage small-cell lung cancer in complete remission after chemotherapy and thoracic radiotherapy (PCI 99-01, EORTC 22003-08004, RTOG 0212, and IFCT 99-01): A randomised clinical trial. *Lancet Oncol.* 2009;10:467–474.

19. Wolfson AH, Bae K, Komaki R, et al. Primary analysis of a phase II randomized trial radiation therapy oncology group (RTOG) 0212: Impact of different total dose schedules of prophylactic cranial irradiation on chronic neurotoxicity and quality of life for patients with limited-stage small-cell lung cancer. *Int J Radiat Oncol Biol Phys.* 2011;81:77–84.

20. Yamamoto Y, Kameyama R, Murota M, et al. Early assessment of therapeutic response using FDG PET in small cell lung cancer. *Mol Imaging Biol.* 2009;11:467–472.

21. Choi NC, Herndon JE 2nd, Rosenman J, et al. Phase I study to determine the maximum-tolerated dose of radiation in standard daily and hyperfractionated-accelerated twice-daily radiation schedules with concurrent chemotherapy for limited-stage small-cell lung cancer. *J Clin Oncol.* 1998;16:3528–3536.

22. Shirvani SM, Komaki R, Heymach JV, et al. Positron emission tomography/computed tomography-guided intensity-modulated radiotherapy for limited-stage small-cell lung cancer. *Int J Radiat Oncol Biol Phys.* 2012 Jan 1;82(1):e91–e97.

23. vanLoon J, De Ruysscher D, Wanders R, et al. Selective nodal irradiation on basis of (18)FDG-PET scans in limited-disease small-cell lung cancer: A prospective study. *Int J Radiat Oncol Biol Phys.* 2010;77:329–336.

24. DeRuysscher D, Bremer R-H, Koppe F, et al. Omission of elective node irradiation on basis of CT-scans in patients with limited disease small cell lung cancer: A phase II trial. *Radiother Oncol.* 2006;80:307–312.

25. Liengswangwong V, Bonner JA, Shaw E, et al. Limited-stage small-cell lung cancer: Patterns of interathoracic recurrence and the implications for thoracic radiotherapy. *J Clin Oncol.* 1994;12:496–502.

26. Ternel J, Greer J, Muzinkansky A, et al. Early palliative care for patients with metastatic non-small-cell lung cancer. *N Engl J Med.* 2010;363:733–742.

■ **CASE 2** ■

Recurrent Non-Small Cell Lung Cancer After Resection of Early-Stage Disease

CLINICAL PROBLEM

The management of regional nodal recurrence after definitive management of an early-stage non-small cell lung cancer (NSCLC) is unclear and controversial. The role of radiotherapy (RT) in that setting, whether alone or in combination with chemotherapy, and the appropriate sequencing if used in a combined modality program, is unknown.

CASE EXAMPLE

A 72-year-old male with history of pT1aN0M0, stage I adenocarcinoma, following a right upper lobectomy in 2006, presents with a new isolated right-sided mediastinal recurrence, and is being referred for a RT opinion. The pathology from the initial operation had revealed lymph nodes R4, 7, L4, 9, and R11 negative for neoplasm and a right lung specimen with a mucinous bronchoalveolar adenocarcinoma with an acinar component, lymphovascular invasion, and negative margins. Adjuvant therapy was not administered. A surveillance chest CT of 7/2009 revealed interval development of mediastinal lymphadenopathy, with the largest node (LN) seen at the right tracheobronchial angle, and measuring 2.1×2.6 cm. On ultrasound-guided biopsy of the right paratracheal node, adenocarcinoma was found. Restaging with PET was done and only showed a 2.7×1.7 cm right paratracheal LN with increased fludeoxyglucose (FDG) uptake with maximum standardized uptake value (SUV) = 3.7. In addition, there is an FDG avid right hilar LN with maximum SUV = 3.6. Brain MRI shows a negative result. Pulmonary testing showed a forced vital capacity (FVC) 3.46 L or 73% predicted and forced expiratory volume (FEV1) of 2.43 L or 68% predicted. His performance status is good and his exam unremarkable.

Management Decisions

- What is the optimal management for regionally recurrent lung cancer and what patient, tumor, and treatment variables impact the decision?
- What is the expected goal of treatment?
- What are the roles of surgery, chemotherapy, and RT in the management of such a presentation?
- What is the rationale for RT? If employed, how are the volumes defined, and what is the recommended dose/fractionation schedule?

MAJOR OPINION

Ronald C. McGarry

NSCLC treatment can often be controversial, even in an apparently early disease. Aside from the management decisions regarding the primary mass, significant management decisions are often dependent on mediastinal nodal involvement. Regional nodal failure can be difficult to predict and, depending on the patient, present with some difficult treatment decisions.

The gold standard for preoperative staging of the mediastinum is a mediastinoscopy. However, in an attempt to determine the need for mediastinoscopy after PET and CT imaging, a recent meta-analysis evaluated the association between the size of mediastinal LNs and the probability of malignancy [1]. In patients with a negative PET scan and LNs of 10 to 15 mm size on CT scanning, the probability for N2 disease was only 5%. Indeed, in patients with T1 lung cancer and good performance status, the finding of PET-negative nodes of lesser than 10-mm size on CT scanning would favor surgical resection without preoperative invasive nodal sampling owing to the high negative predictive value of a PET scan [1].

The resected tumor showed lymphovascular invasion and negative margins. While lymphovascular invasion might make one concerned about the risk of nodal spread, the pathological report showed sampling of 3 perihilar (level 10), level 4R, 4L (right and left tracheobronchial), and 9L (left pulmonary ligament) nodes. All were found to be negative for tumor metastasis. Eastern Cooperative Oncology Group (ECOG) performed a randomized prospective trial that compared the impact of RT alone versus chemoradiation on patients with systematic sampling (SS) of LNs versus complete MLND. SS was defined as at least one LN removed from level 4, 7, and 10 during a right thoracotomy and levels 5, 6, and 7 during a left thoracotomy. By definition, complete MLND required complete removal of all LNs from those levels. There appeared to be no major advantage of MLND versus SS, as long as the appropriate nodal regions were sampled. Current National Comprehensive Cancer Network (NCCN) guidelines suggest that N1 and N2 nodal mapping and resection are standard with minimum sampling of 3 N2 nodal stations or complete nodal resection [2]. From the pathological report, the patient under investigation received a barely adequate LN sampling, with the majority of nodes from the contralateral mediastinum. While contralateral LN metastases are not uncommon, most nodal failures in this setting would likely be ipsilateral, which would suggest that better surgical staging in this case would also include level 7 (subcarinal) nodes. Left-sided lung cancers have a higher incidence of contralateral mediastinal nodal metastasis than those arising on the right [3].

The lungs have a rich lymphatic supply consisting of a pleural and parenchymal network. The pleural lymphatics course over the parietal and visceral pleural surfaces and drain into the medial aspect of the lung near the hilum. Hilar nodes drain into the mediastinum but the mediastinal pathways are variable depending on the lobe of the lung in which the tumor arises. Lesions of the right upper lobe commonly drain into the right paratracheal and anterior mediastinal nodes. Right middle and lower lobe tumors commonly drain into the subcarinal nodes, and then toward the right paratracheal and anterior mediastinal nodes. Left upper lobe tumors drain to the subaortic and para-arotic nodes, while left lower lobe tumors drain to subcarinal and subaortic nodes [3]. Skip metastases to N2 nodes clearly occur in the absence of hilar positivity with a rate of about 15% to 22%. It is therefore incumbent on the surgeon to accurately stage the nodal regions at risk [4]. Before

PET scanning, it was clear that the potential for a 20% inaccuracy rate in staging was not acceptable and mediastinal exploration was mandatory. It appears that PET/CT has significant utility in the detection of LN metastases. In an early trial, the American College of Surgeons Oncology Group (ACSOG) [5] found that PET was significantly better than CT for detection of nodal disease during lung cancer staging and could potentially avoid unnecessary thoracotomy in 1 of 5 patients.

Histopathological subtyping of NSCLC is relevant at present in treatment decisions because of a differential activity of specific therapeutic agents particularly in some adenocarcinomas. As the tumor was thyroid transcription factor 1 (TTF-1) immunoreactive, a diagnosis of a lung-derived primary was confirmed. TTF-1 has commonly been associated with a diagnosis of lung cancers, particularly adenocarcinomas [6]. In a review of 103 FNA samples, TTF1 positivity was highly correlated with adenocarcinoma [7]. Diffuse coexpression of TTF-1 and p63 was observed in one-half of the adenocarcinomas with signet ring cancer cells (Ad-SRCCs) present with a significant number of these tumors (40% of cases in a small study) harboring anaplastic lymphoma kinase (ALK) translocations. This may have significance in future studies for chemotherapy responsiveness, particularly for the case under discussion in the event of new metastasis or further local failure [8].

Given the overall scenario presented above, the decision for routine follow-up was reasonable with no obvious need for chemotherapy and/or radiation. The expected 5-year survival for stage Ia NSCLCs that are resected by lobectomy is 60% to 70% [9]. CT scans of the chest are commonly done every 4 to 6 months for surveillance because the risk of developing a second lung cancer can be as high as 2% to 3% per year [10]. Surveillance CT scan at almost 2 years following initial diagnosis showed interval development of mediastinal adenopathy at the right tracheobronchial angle. The CT report does not fully describe the observed adenopathy, but only that the "largest" node is present at the right tracheobronchial angle (level 4R). It would be important to clarify with the radiologist which other levels of nodal disease were enlarged. PET/CT revealed uptake in the malignant range (cutoff often taken to be in the SUV 3.0–4.0 range) for LNs in the right paratracheal and hilar regions. There were also several new non-FDG avid ground-glass opacities (GGOs) in the right lower lobe. Also noted were several non-FDG avid nodules in the left lung, presumably all were new. The significance of these findings is uncertain.

Endobronchial ultrasound (EBUS) was done with a biopsy of the enlarged right paratracheal node, which was positive for adenocarcinoma. Interestingly, this area was sampled at the time of the original lobectomy. In the initial resected tumor, a component of bronchoalveolar carcinoma (BAC) was noted. This component of the biopsy represents a subtype usually considered a subtype of adenocarcinoma and is characterized by its ability to spread via airway dissemination. On CT imaging of the lung, BAC may present with a ground glass (GGO) appearance and is commonly not FDG avid. In general, because their differential diagnosis includes inflammatory processes, GGOs are more often of uncertain significance and are usually followed with serial imaging; however, depending on clinical suspicion, excisional biopsy ("wedge resection") could be considered for diagnosis.

In an analysis of patterns of failure, Kelsey et al. [3] reviewed 61 patients who underwent resection of NSCL at Duke University. Patterns of failure in the mediastinum were relatively predictable and for those patients who underwent resection of a right upper lobe (RUL) lesion, the most common site of nodal recurrence was in the 4R nodal level that corresponds to the tracheobronchial angle consistent with what we have noted in our case report. The other most common sites of recurrence expected in a RUL lesion were the bronchial stump and the level 7 nodes (subcarinal). There were other less common isolated recurrences throughout the mediastinum. Median interval to time of recurrence was 12 months.

Suggested Treatment

In summary, the case involves a 72-year-old male with biopsy-proven recurrent NSCLC in a mediastinal LN about 2 years after lobectomey and LN dissection. He has good pulmonary reserve with an FEV1 of 68% predicted. He has relatively few comorbidities. In my opinion, he is an appropriate candidate for definitive therapy to potentially achieve cure. As per the NCCN guidelines, in the setting of locoregionally recurrent disease in a patient with good performance status, chemotherapy combined with radiation would be the treatment of choice. There are many chemotherapy regimens that could be used for advanced or metastatic disease, however, newer agent/platinum combinations seem to have reached a plateau in overall response rates (25–35%), time to progression (4–6 months), median survival (8–10 months), 1-year survival (30–40%) and 2-year survival rates (10–15% in physically fit patients) [2]. In this particular case of a chemotherapy-naïve patient with limited mediastinal nodal recurrence, I would expect median survival to be more similar to a patient with stage IIIa NSCLC, in the 20-month range.

Overall, it appears he would be able to tolerate combined chemoradiation. Cisplatinum can be combined with a number of other agents, most commonly etoposide or gemcitabine, with reasonable effectiveness. Having never had chemotherapy and in the setting of a relatively healthy patient, the most common chemotherapy and standard of care for this patient would be cisplatinum/etoposide concurrent with a dose of 60 Gy of radiation to the mediastinum respecting all the usual limits to dose-limiting organs, eg, spinal cord. Chemotherapy should be given for 4 to 6 cycles [2]. One could consider the addition of a targeted agent for maintenance if the appropriate epidermal growth factor receptor (EGFR) mutation is present and EML4-ALK testing is done [2].

Radiation ports would be focused on the mediastinum and right hilum as his disease is primarily nodal although a significant number of failures can occur in the bronchial stump and subcarinal regions. The issue of size of the field treated is problematic. At present, most radiation oncologists would treat areas containing gross disease and areas at highest risk in their clinical target volume. In this setting, ie, metachronous nodal failure following resection of the stage I primary lung cancer, there is no obviously correct treatment port; however, several studies have shown no improvements in outcome in elective nodal irradiation versus involved fields only [11,12]. Fields commonly used to treat the mediastinum include initial parallel opposed antero-posterior fields to approximately 40 Gy then off cord to the final prescribed dose. Intensity modulation may be used but it is incumbent on the radiation oncologist to limit the dose to the lung, especially the lower isodose curves where intensity modulation encompasses larger volumes of the lung.

Radiation prescription dose would be selected much like chemoradiation in any stage III NSCLC. The NCCN guidelines [2] suggest doses between 60 and 70 Gy. There is no randomized data that show that doses above 60 Gy confer a significant improvement in survival. One must keep in mind that part of the rationale for treating concurrent with chemotherapy is the putative radiation sensitization of drugs like cisplatinum. Moreover, a dose to the mediastinum can be limited by the esophagus and spinal cord. By controlling the amount of lung treated to limit the V20 to the lowest possible dose attainable, the risk of pneumonitis can be significantly decreased. Expected toxicities from treating this patient would likely include esophagitis, skin erythema in the treated port, fatigue, and other more uncommon risks.

Overall, in the setting of a chemoradiotherapy-naïve patient with a reasonable performance status who has isolated nodal recurrence, the treatment of choice should be much like any other "curative" therapy in lung cancer, ie, conventionally fractionated RT to 60 Gy, using optimal current planning techniques delivered concurrently with platinum-based systemic therapy. The patient nonetheless remains at significant risk for distant metastatic disease and clearly one of the goals of future trials in lung cancer must remain to improve our systemic therapy.

ACADEMIC COMMENT

Gregory Videtic

Dr. McGarry has provided a thoughtful overview of the appropriate assessment and management of the patient who presents with a mediastinal recurrence after previous surgery for a pathologic stage I NSCLC. I agree with his approach for care in this case where there are no high-level evidence-based standards and appreciate his focus on the RT parameters in managing the patient. My brief comments in response to his discussion are made to further highlight the complex issues involving recurrent lung cancer.

Prevention of Recurrence After Resection of Early Stage Lung Cancer

In patients with early-stage NSCLC, even when complete surgical resection is offered as the primary and appropriate treatment, there remains a substantial risk of recurrence, as evidenced from the 5-year survival rates for stage I disease ranging from 50% to 70% [13]. This observation has prompted ongoing efforts to find effective adjuvant therapies to reduce the risk of recurrence and improve survival or, at least, patients' quality of life.

Adjuvant RT

There is currently no established role for adjuvant RT after standard surgical resection of early-stage disease. In 1998, the Post-operative Radiation Therapy (PORT) study, a large meta-analysis involving data from 9 randomized trials of adjuvant RT in stages I–III NSCLC, revealed a 24% reduction in local recurrence but an absolute increase in mortality of 7% at 2 years when using adjuvant radiation. On subset analysis the mortality was restricted to patients with stage I or II NSCLC [14]. In contrast, however, a relatively recent randomized single-institution trial specifically addressed the role of adjuvant RT in resected stage I NSCLC and found a decrease in local recurrence from 23% to 2% in the patients receiving adjuvant RT to the bronchial stump and hilum, but without an associated survival detriment [15]. This study has not been replicated.

Adjuvant Chemotherapy

In general, there are no prospective randomized data to support the routine use of adjuvant platinum-based chemotherapy for patients with resected stage I NSCLC. None of the contemporary randomized trials [16–20] of adjuvant cisplatin-based chemotherapy versus observation in resected stage I–III NSCLC has found an improvement in survival for the subset of patients with stage I disease, and in a recent meta-analysis of adjuvant chemotherapy [21] again no benefit was seen to its addition for resected stage I patients. Results for Cancer and Leukemia Group B (CALGB) 9633, a randomized study of resected stage IB NSCLC patients to 4 cycles of adjuvant carboplatin and paclitaxel or observation, suggested no survival benefit to the addition of chemotherapy [22], although an unplanned subset analysis suggested that patients with tumors sized 4 cm or larger may obtain a small survival benefit with adjuvant carboplatin and paclitaxel [23]. In Japan, the Japan Lung Cancer Research Group on Postsurgical Adjuvant Chemotherapy (JLCRG) study suggested a survival benefit to the adjuvant addition of Tegafur-uracil (UFT) to resected stage IB patients, and possibly stage IA when the tumor was larger than 2 cm. [24]. Of note is that this drug is not available outside that country.

Detection of Recurrence

A review of the published literature reveals that there is a lot of variability in how patterns of failure are defined. First, rates of local failure are often underreported in many prospective trials, and when done, there is a substantial variation in the rates that are reported; eg, rates for stage I disease have been reported to range from 6% to 45% [25]. Second, the definition of local failure varies widely among publications. For example, in the prospective randomized Adjuvant Navelbine International Trialist Association (ANITA) trial of chemotherapy versus observation for patients with stage IB to IIIA NSCLC, the crude rate of local failure was 12% in the arm randomized to receive chemotherapy [20]. However, only ipsilateral mediastinal recurrences were scored as local failures. In other words, a contralateral mediastinal recurrence was not considered a local recurrence. Some authors suggest that the most appropriate definition of local (ie, local/regional) failure is disease recurrence at the surgical resection margin, ipsilateral hilum, and mediastinum [24]. In that regard, the differentiation between "local" and "locoregional" is not consistent and exclusive nodal (regional) failures are rarely analyzed in most studies as a separate entity. Third, local recurrences are often not consistently reported in lung cancer trials. Many studies only report first sites of failure, and for lung cancer where distant metastases predominate, thorough evaluations for other sites of failure at the time of (distant) disease recurrence are often not carried out consistently or exhaustively. Some studies notably will only report local failures in the absence of a distant failure [24].

Management of Local Recurrence

How best to manage local (locoregional) recurrence after resection of early-stage NSCLC will be dictated both by the patient and the disease factors and only selected patients may benefit from an aggressive (curative) approach to its management equivalent to the resection used for management of the primary tumor [26]. Outcomes from treatment

will therefore be a reflection of initial selection factors. Thus, there are reports on re-resection, RT alone, chemotherapy alone, and combined modality therapies administered in the setting of relapsed cancer, as there are no standardized approaches to this disease presentation. Approximately 1% to 2% of intrathoracic recurrences of lung cancer have been reported to be managed by reoperation with curative intent; however, results from this approach have been generally modest, with survival rates at 2 years of around 20% [27]. There are series that documented the efficacy of salvage RT alone in the setting of recurrent lung cancer, with median survivals ranging from 11 to 19 months [28]. Despite these attempts at local salvage, one-half of recurrent patients will go on to fail with distant disease [16]. This has prompted the increased use of systemic therapy for local recurrences. As noted by Dr. McGarry, the use of RT with chemotherapy likely would thus represent the most common current management approach in the setting of true regional nodal recurrence.

COMMUNITY PRACTITIONER COMMENT

Andrew Vassil

As summarized by Dr. McGarry, this is a case of a 72-year-old man with a regional recurrence of stage I RUL adenocarcinoma approximately 2 years after lobectomy. At presentation, he had a mixed type adenocarcinoma with mucinous bronchioalveolar cell and acinar components. There has been a movement to reclassify patients to identify those with excellent disease-specific survival, eliminate the terms *bronchioalveolar carcinoma* and *mixed subtype adenocarcinoma*, and introduce *adenocarcinoma in situ* and *minimally invasive adenocarcinoma* [29]. This may aid in identifying those who may or may not benefit from adjuvant therapies.

Regionally recurrent NSCLC represents a significant management challenge. Thorough evaluation, including history and physical exam, biopsy to confirm recurrence versus new primary, review of prior pathology and treatment history, complete restaging (including brain imaging), and pulmonary assessment are necessary. Discussions with fellow providers are necessary to develop treatment and follow-up plan.

It is important to establish a dialog with the patient, family, and caregivers to understand the prognostic implications of a regional recurrence, goals of care, and treatment options. Review for participation in a clinical trial should also be considered.

Regarding the re-staging evaluation and prior mediastinal LN sampling, Dr. McGarry highlights the importance of understanding pathways of lymphatic spread, and assessing the extent of disease at presentation and recurrence. I agree with Dr. McGarry's recommendation that mediastinal LN sampling is unlikely to alter the treatment field design or recommendation for concurrent chemotherapy and radiation therapy. This incidence of subclinical nodal spread is not defined for patients with regional recurrence, thus it is unknown if elective nodal treatment should be applied in patients with regional nodal failure such as in this case.

Salvage radiation therapy is feasible for patients with regional recurrence and should be considered for this patient. A report of 29 patients treated with radiation therapy, with or without concurrent chemotherapy, for locally and regionally recurrent NSCLC resulted in a median survival of 17 months. Younger age and longer disease-free interval between surgery and local recurrence tended toward predicting for improved survival [28]. Recurrences confined to the bronchial stump may represent a more favorable subgroup of patients with recurrent NSCLC for salvage radiation therapy [30].

The paradigm of management of stage IIIA NSCLC could be applied given the presence of ipsilateral mediastinal disease in this physically fit 72-year-old patient. I would not recommend surgical resection because a right-sided pneumonectomy would likely be necessary given the hilar location of the recurrence. Prospective data are not available in the salvage setting, thus radiation doses and volumes applied for regional recurrence are extrapolated from clinical trials for stage III NSCLC and retrospective studies of salvage radiation therapy. Prospective data have suggested improved survival with dose-escalated radiation therapy [31]; however, preliminary results from a phase 3 dose-escalation study (Radiation Therapy Oncology Group [RTOG] 0617) did not show a benefit to treatment of 70 Gy compared to 60 Gy. Both studies did not include elective nodal radiation treatment.

As Dr. McGarry indicated, invasive mediastinal staging is unlikely to influence the radiation treatment fields. Given the propensity for involvement of bronchial stump and mediastinal level 7 involvement, as described by Kelsey et al. [3] and discussed by Dr. McGarry, I would include these and the areas positive on PET in the design of my treatment fields. This appears to be a relatively small treatment volume, and given the published results supporting escalated dose, I would aim to deliver a dose of 70 Gy to the areas of PET-positive disease. I would ensure coverage of level 7 and the bronchial stump to at least a dose adequate for elimination of microscopic disease (45–50 Gy). CT-based 3-D planning would be used, and if available, 4-D simulation. Planning must respect constraints on spinal cord, lung, esophageal, and heart doses. Given the preliminary findings of RTOG 0617, if the goals for the dose to normal tissues cannot be met, then one might consider reducing the dose, but not below 60 Gy to involved regions. The experience of salvage radiation therapy published by Kelsey et al. reported a median dose of 66 Gy [28].

In summary, this patient appears to be a physically fit 72-year-old man with regionally recurrent NSCLC for which the treatment paradigm of stage IIIA NSCLC could be applied. Application of therapy for regionally recurrent NSCLC may be altered as management of stage IIIA NSCLC evolves. I would recommend combination therapy with radiation and cisplatin-based chemotherapy. It is important to recognize that physically fit elderly patients can be successfully treated with concurrent chemoradiation, but may be at higher risk of toxicity [32,33]. Prospective data highlight the importance of patient-reported quality of life scores as an important prognostic factor in patients with locally advanced NSCLC, and this may be considered with formulating management plans [34].

SECTION EDITOR'S NOTE

Gregory Videtic

Given the patient's history and presentation, I would offer definitive concurrent chemoradiation to maximize local control and potentially impact on survival. With respect to dose and treatment approach, I would give a dose of 60 Gy in keeping with the most current phase 3 trials in lung cancer. With respect to volume, I would treat the ipsilateral hilum, subcarinal area, and ipsilateral draining mediastinum to 45 to 50 Gy and boost the true recurrent disease to full dose.

REFERENCES

1. de Langen AJ, Raijmakers P, Riphagen I, et al. The size of mediastinal lymph nodes and its relation with metastatic involvement: A meta-analysis. *Eur J Cardiothorac Surg*. 2006; 29:26–29.

2. National Comprehensive Cancer Network Guidelines, Version 2. 2012. National Comprehensive Cancer Network Inc. 2012.

3. Kelsey CR, Light KL, Marks LG. Patterns of failure after resection of non-small-cell lung cancer: Implications for postoperative radiation therapy volumes. *Int J Radiat Biol Phys*. 2006;65:1097–1105.

4. Bonner JA, Garces YI, Gould PM. Frequency of noncontiguous lymph node involvement in patients with resectable nonsmall cell lung carcinoma. *Cancer*. 1999;86:1159–1164.

5. Reed CE, Harpole DH, Posthener KE. Results of the American College of Surgeons Oncology Group Z0050 trial. *J Thor Cardiovasc Surg*. 2003;126:1943–1951

6. Rekhtman N, Ang DC, Sima CS, et al. Immunohistochemical algorithm for differentiation of lung adenocarcinoma and squamous cell carcinoma based on large series of whole-tissue sections with validation in small specimens. *Mod Pathol*. 2011;24:1348–1359.

7. Righi L, Graziano P, Fornari A, et al. Immunohistochemical subtyping of nonsmall cell lung cancer not otherwise specified in fine-needle aspiration cytology: A retrospective study of 103 cases with surgical correlation. *Cancer*. 2011;117:3416–3423.

8. Yoshida A, Tsuta K, Watanabe S, et al. Frequent ALK rearrangement and TTF-1/p63 co-expression in lung adenocarcinoma with signet-ring cell component. *Lung Cancer*. 2011;72:309–315.

9. Mountain CF. A new international staging system for lung cancer. *Chest*. 1986;89:225–232.

10. Martini N, Bains MS, Burt ME, et al. Incidence of local recurrence and second primary tumors in resected stage I lung cancer. *J Thorac Cardiovasc Surg*. 1995;109:120–129.

11. Rosenzweig KE, Sura J, Jackson A, et al. Involved field radiation therapy for inoperable non small-cell lung cancer. *J Clin Oncol*. 2007;25:5557–5561.

12. Fernandes AT, Shen J, Finlay J, et al. Elective nodal irradiation vs. involved field irradiation for locally advanced non-small cell lung cancer: A comparative analysis of toxicities and clinical outcome. *Radother Oncol*. 2010;95:178–193.

13. Mountain CF. The international system for staging lung cancer. *Semin Surg Oncol*. 2000;18(2):106–115.

14. Postoperative radiotherapy in non-small-cell lung cancer: Systematic review and meta-analysis of individual patient data from nine randomised controlled trials. PORT Meta-analysis Trialists Group. *Lancet*. 1998;352(9124):257–263.

15. Trodella L, Granone P, Valente S, et al. Adjuvant radiotherapy in non-small cell lung cancer with pathological stage I: Definitive results of a phase III randomized trial. *Radiother Oncol*. 2002;62:11–19.

16. Arriagada R, Bergman B, Dunant A, et al. Cisplatin-based adjuvant chemotherapy in patients with completely resected non-small-cell lung cancer. *N Engl J Med*. 2004;350:351–360.

17. Scagliotti GV, Fossati R, Torri V, et al. Randomized study of adjuvant chemotherapy for completely resected stage I, II, or IIIA non-small-cell Lung cancer. *J Natl Cancer Inst*. 2003;95:1453–1461.

18. Waller D, Peake MD, Stephens RJ, et al. Chemotherapy for patients with non-small cell lung cancer: The surgical setting of the Big Lung Trial. *Eur J Cardiothorac Surg*. 2004;26:173–182.

19. Winton T, Livingston R, Johnson D, et al. Vinorelbine plus cisplatin vs. observation in resected non-small-cell lung cancer. *N Engl J Med*. 2005;352:2589–2597.

20. Douillard JY, Rosell R, De Lena M, et al. Adjuvant vinorelbine plus cisplatin versus observation in patients with completely resected stage IB-IIIA non-small-cell lung cancer (Adjuvant Navelbine International Trialist Association [ANITA]): A randomised controlled trial. *Lancet Oncol*. 2006;7:719–727.

21. Pignon JP, Tribodet H, Scagliotti GV, et al. Lung adjuvant cisplatin evaluation: A pooled analysis by the LACE Collaborative Group. *J Clin Oncol*. 2008;26:3552–3559.

22. Strauss GM, Herndon JE, Maddaus MA, et al. Adjuvant paclitaxel plus carboplatin compared with observation in stage IB non-small-cell lung cancer: CALGB 9633 with the Cancer and Leukemia Group B, Radiation Therapy Oncology Group, and North Central Cancer Treatment Group Study Groups. *J Clin Oncol*. 2008;26:5043–5051.

23. Wakelee H, Dubey S, Gandara D. Optimal adjuvant therapy for non-small cell lung cancer–how to handle stage I disease. *Oncologist*. 2007;12:331–337.

24. Kato H, Ichinose Y, Ohta M, et al. A randomized trial of adjuvant chemotherapy with uracil-tegafur for adenocarcinoma of the lung. *N Engl J Med*. 2004;350:1713–1721.

25. Kelsey CR, Marks LB, Hollis D, et al. Local recurrence after surgery for early stage lung cancer. *Cancer.* 2009,115:5218–5227.

26. Curran WJ Jr, Herbert SH, Stafford PM, et al. Should patients with post-resection locoregional recurrence of lung cancer receive aggressive therapy? *Int J Radiat Oncol Biol Phys.* 1992;24:25–30.

27. Zimmermann FB, Molls M, Jeremic B. Treatment of recurrent disease in lung cancer. *Semin Surg Oncol.* 2003;21:122–127.

28. Kelsey CR, Clough RW, Marks LB, et al. Local recurrence following initial resection of NSCLC: Salvage is possible with radiation therapy. *Cancer J.* 2006;12:283–288.

29. Travis WD, Brambilla E, Noguchi M, et al. International association for the study of lung cancer/American thoracic society/European respiratory society international multidisciplinary classification of lung adenocarcinoma. *J Thorac Oncol.* 2011;6:244–285.

30. Jeremic B, Bamberg M. External beam radiation therapy for bronchial stump recurrence of non-small-cell lung cancer after complete resection. *Radiother Oncol.* 2002;64:251–257.

31. Kong FM, Ten Haken RK, Schipper MJ, et al. High-dose radiation improved local tumor control and overall survival in patients with inoperable/unresectable non-small-cell lung cancer: Long-term results of a radiation dose escalation study. *Int J Radiat Oncol Biol Phys.* 2005;63:324–333.

32. Jalal SI, Riggs HD, Melnyk A, et al. Updated survival and outcomes for older adults with inoperable stage III non-small-cell lung cancer treated with cisplatin, etoposide, and concurrent chest radiation with or without consolidation docetaxel: Analysis of a phase III trial from the Hoosier Oncology Group (HOG) and US Oncology. *Ann Oncol.* 2012;23:1730–1738.

33. Schild SE, Mandrekar SJ, Jatoi A, et al. The value of combined-modality therapy in elderly patients with stage III nonsmall cell lung cancer. *Cancer.* 2007;110:363–368.

34. Movsas B, Moughan J, Sarna L, et al. Quality of life supersedes the classic prognosticators for long-term survival in locally advanced non-small-cell lung cancer: An analysis of RTOG 9801. *J Clin Oncol.* 2009;27:5816–5822.

The Role of Adjuvant Radiotherapy in Stage III Lung Cancer

CLINICAL PROBLEM

The role of radiotherapy (RT) in the setting of resected locally advanced non-small cell lung cancer (NSCLC) remains controversial because a survival benefit is unclear. Furthermore, its role for patients who have functional or other impairments before or after surgery makes decision making on its use more challenging. It remains unclear, therefore, what the role, optimal timing, and dose of adjuvant RT in resected stage III lung cancer is if given, and its sequencing with respect to chemotherapy.

CASE EXAMPLE

A 54-year-old man presented to his primary care physician (PCP) with a progressive cough. A CT of the chest revealed a 5 × 3.5 cm neoplasm within the posterior segment of the right upper lobe adjacent to the posterior superior aspect of the right hilum. There was an enlarged lymph node at the anterior superior aspect of the right hilum. An enlarged subcarinal lymph node was also appreciated along with multiple smaller lymph nodes. Biopsy by bronchoscopy revealed poorly differentiated non-small cell carcinoma. A PET scan revealed a focally intense fluorodeoxyglucose (FDG) uptake (maximum standardized uptake value [SUV] 15.3) associated with the 4-cm right suprahilar pulmonary mass that demonstrates irregular margins on the CT images and subcarinal adenopathy (maximum SUV 8.77), suspicious for metastatic involvement. His preoperative forced expiratory volume (FEV1) was 2.44 L or 65% of predicted and his diffusion capacity of the lung for carbon monoxide (DLCO) was 71% of predicted. A mediastinoscopy, however, was negative for involved lymph nodes. The patient underwent surgical resection. The pathology specimen revealed close (at 2 mm) but negative margins, a 3.8 × 3.5 × 3.0 cm invasive squamous cell

carcinoma with 1 positive out of 9 resected lobar nodes, and metastatic disease replacing the subcarinal node. His postoperative course was complicated by a pleural effusion for which he was admitted to hospital and had a chest tube placed and talc pleurodesis. His pulmonary testing shows an FEV1 of 2.17 L (59% of predicted) and a DLCO of 59% of predicted.

Management Decisions

- What is the role of adjuvant RT in this patient?
- How does his clinical status and change in clinical and objective respiratory function influence decision making?
- If RT is recommended, what dose/fractionation schedule is recommended and how is the volume defined?
- Does the estimated risk of pneumonitis influence the radiation delivery parameters?
- How is it sequenced with chemotherapy, and implications for outcomes?
- What is the role of serial assessment of pulmonary function?

MAJOR OPINION

Steven E. Schild

Until 1998, postoperative radiation therapy (PORT) after resection of NSCLC was often recommended for patients with positive margins or whose condition involved hilar or mediastinal lymph nodes. This was based on retrospective analyses that found that PORT was associated with improved survival in these patient groups. However, the PORT Meta-analysis Trialists Group published a study in that year that challenged this relatively frequent recommendation [1]. This study included data on 2128 patients from

9 randomized trials that compared PORT to no-PORT. With a median follow-up of 3.9 years, there were 707 deaths out of 1056 (67%) patients with PORT compared to 661 of 1072 (62%) with surgery alone. The authors found a significant adverse effect of PORT on survival (hazard ratio [HR] = 1.21, p = .001). This 21% relative increase in the risk of death is equivalent to an absolute detriment of 7% at 2 years reducing survival from 55% to 48%. Subgroup analyses suggest that this adverse effect was greatest for stage I/II, N0–N1 disease, whereas for those with stage III, N2 disease, there was no evidence of an adverse effect. More specifically, the results for stage III and N2 patients were slightly in favor of PORT (HR .97 and .96, respectively), and the confidence intervals are wide, indicating no clear evidence of a difference between treatments for these groups of patients. The authors concluded that PORT is detrimental to patients with early-stage completely resected NSCLC and should not be used. They concluded that the role of PORT for N2 disease was not clear and may warrant further research.

This PORT analysis has been criticized because it was based on studies using obsolete RT techniques that were likely hazardous to patients. Following this report, there were attempts to clarify the value of PORT using data from other sources. Lally et al. evaluated the outcome of PORT for stage II or III NSCLC using the Surveillance Epidemiology and End Results (SEER) database in 2006 [2]. Included were 7465 patients with stages II–III NSCLC who underwent a lobectomy or pneumonectomy. The median follow up was 3.5 years. On multivariate analysis, older age, T3–T4 tumor stage, N2 disease, male sex, fewer sampled lymph nodes, and greater number of involved nodes had a negative impact on survival. The use of PORT did not have a significant impact on survival. However, for patients with N0 (HR = 1.176; p = .0435) and N1 (HR = 1.097; p = .0196) disease, PORT was associated with a significant decrease in survival. For patients with N2 disease (HR = .855; p = .0077), PORT was associated with a significant increase in survival. These authors concluded that PORT was associated with an increase in survival in patients with N2 disease but not with N0/N1 disease.

In 2008, Douillard et al. performed a secondary analysis of the Adjuvant Navelbine International Trialist's Association (ANITA) trial evaluating the effect of PORT in this study [3]. The ANITA trial was performed primarily to evaluate the effect of adjuvant chemotherapy. This randomized trial compared adjuvant cisplatin and vinorelbine chemotherapy versus observation in resected stages IB–IIIA NSCLC. The median survival (MS) was 65.7 months in the chemotherapy group and 43.7 months in the observation group (p = .017) [4]. PORT was recommended for pN+ disease but was neither randomized nor mandatory. Overall, PORT was given to 33.3% in the observation arm and 21.6% in the chemotherapy arm. In univariate analysis, PORT had a deleterious effect on the overall population survival. Patients with pN1 disease had an improved survival from PORT in the observation arm (MS 25.9 vs. 50.2 months), whereas PORT had a detrimental effect in the chemotherapy group (MS 93.6 months and 46.6 months). In contrast, survival improved in patients with pN2 disease who received PORT, both in the chemotherapy (MS 23.8 vs. 47.4 months) and observation arms (median 12.7 vs. 22.7 months). This retrospective evaluation suggests a positive effect of PORT in pN2 disease and a negative effect on pN1 disease when patients received adjuvant chemotherapy. Douillard concluded that the results support further evaluation of PORT in prospectively randomized studies in completely resected pN2 NSCLC.

These provocative findings led to a proposal for a phase 3 trial to clarify the value of PORT for patients with resected stage III NSCLC. This trial was called the Adjuvant Mediastinal Observation or Radiotherapy Evaluation (AMORE) and was supported by the American College of Surgeons Oncology Group (ACOSOG) and the Radiation Therapy and Oncology Group (RTOG). Patients with resected N2 NSCLC were to receive adjuvant chemotherapy and then be randomized to either a dose of 54 Gy in 30 fractions of adjuvant RT to the mediastinum or no PORT. However, this study was not approved by the reviewers.

Meanwhile several European cancer centers have collaborated to perform the Lung Adjuvant Radiotherapy Trial (Lung ART), which compares 3-D conformal PORT (54 Gy) versus no PORT for completely resected N2 patients, irrespective of chemotherapy. This study requires the inclusion of 700 patients to show a 10% difference in 3-year disease-free survival. The secondary end points include survival, patterns of relapse, local failure, secondary cancers, and toxicity. As of June 1, 2011, 104 patients were accrued of the planned 700.

The findings from the above noted studies can now be briefly summarized. The PORT Meta-analysis Trialists Group study found that PORT decreased survival for N0–N1 but not N2 resected NSCLC. The analysis from the SEER database found that PORT decreased survival for N0–N1 but increased survival for N2-resected NSCLC. The ANITA trial review revealed that PORT increased survival for all resected N2 NSCLC patients but decreased survival for N1 disease when patients received adjuvant chemotherapy, and increased survival within the no-chemotherapy arm. The results supported further evaluation of PORT in prospectively randomized studies in completely resected pN2 NSCLC. There is one randomized prospective trial (Lung ART) open in Europe to assess the value of PORT in resected N2 NSCLC patients.

Thus we are left with no clear-cut, level 1 evidence to guide us regarding PORT. Unfortunately, this is quite frequent in oncology and in these situations one must rely on the best data available. For resected N2 NSCLC, PORT with more modern techniques appears to improve the chances of survival. This is likely to be true owing to modern planning and delivery, which is likely safer and more efficacious. Generally, it is a good practice to obtain baseline complete pulmonary function studies prior to beginning RT. The preoperative CT or CT/PET provides very useful information for RT planning purposes. During the simulation (which is most often performed on a CT simulator), it is useful to determine whether both diaphragms move properly. Although phrenic nerve injury from tumor or resection is uncommon, it results in paradoxical movement of the affected diaphragm and respiratory problems for the patient. In addition, this patient is on antibiotics and it would be wise to wait until any potential infection is adequately treated or before beginning more cancer therapy. The pleural effusion would make it important to review cytology of the fluid. In addition, pleurodesis is going to make future imaging quite complex. PET scans can be quite difficult to interpret after this procedure. Return visits with a pulmonary medicine specialist to ensure that the patient's lung function is optimized medically is also helpful.

In addition, these patients benefit from the administration of adjuvant chemotherapy, which is most frequently delivered prior to RT in our institution [5]. Although concurrent therapy is best for unresected patients, there are enough uncertainties that we often deliver these treatments sequentially. For completely resected disease, it appears

reasonable to deliver a total dose of 54 Gy in 30 fractions to the volume formally containing the gross tumor in the nodal regions and the bronchial margin or stump. Krupitskaya and Loo recommended that the target volume should include, at a minimum, the bronchial stump, ipsilateral hilum, and involved nodal stations, and cover the adjacent mediastinal nodal stations [6]. This was the dose fractionation regimen (54 Gy/30 fractions) to be used in the AMORE trial. However, the patient in this example has positive margins or microscopic residual disease. In this case, it would be reasonable to increase the total dose to 60 Gy in 30 fractions as well as consider concurrent administration of chemotherapy. There is precious little data that reveal a substantial improvement in survival for the use of a greater dose. Generally, I recommend serial pulmonary function tests when there is a subjective increase in symptoms following therapy. The risk of pneumonitis can be decreased by keeping the volume of lung treated to a minimum through appropriate review of the treatment plan and the dose–volume histogram (DVH) to predict for potential lung toxicity. This can also be done through attention to technique (beam arrangement) and limiting therapy to areas of previous gross disease and close or positive margins. The preoperative imaging (especially CT/PET) is very helpful to optimize treatment planning especially when these data can be coregistered within the treatment planning system. Generally, parameters such as mean lung dose less than 20 Gy, V5 less than 65% (volume of lung receiving a dose of 5 Gy or more) and V20 less than 35% (volume of lung receiving a dose of 20 Gy or more) are monitored and attempts are made to keep these values as low as achievable, as toxicity may increase substantially when these values are exceeded [7–9].

ACADEMIC COMMENT

Kenneth Olivier

Dr. Schild has provided an excellent overview of the question of adjuvant therapy in a patient with completely resected stage IIIa NSCLC. The following are my thoughts on how to address the question of whether adjuvant RT should be recommended.

I would first review the findings that led to the diagnosis of stage III lung cancer. Notably, the CT was read as having a suspicious subcarinal lymph node. A subsequent PET scan confirmed the findings on CT, including the suspicious sub-carinal lymph node. The treating physicians proceeded to confirm the radiographic findings with a mediastinoscopy. While in 2007 that would have been the gold standard for mediastinal staging, the traditional cervical mediastinoscopy is not the ideal procedure to sample the subcarinal lymph node station (station 7). The use of endosonography (transesophageal and transbronchial ultrasound combined with fine needle sampling) allows sampling of almost every lymph node station and is significantly better at staging the mediastinum when combined with mediastinoscopy than mediastinoscopy alone [10]. The mediastinoscopy was negative and the treating physicians made the reasonable decision to proceed with lobectomy, the correct surgical procedure for appropriate management of NSCLC in patients [11].

Then I would carefully review the pathology report. In it, I see that the subcarinal node N2 was "completely replaced" by metastatic squamous cell carcinoma. Aside from "completely replaced," there is no description of extranodal extension in the subcarinal node. This is reassuring, as extranodal extension may portend a worse prognosis independent of the addition of PORT [12]. Interestingly, the pathology note also questions the bronchial stump margin, but the final summary of the pathology report states that the resection was deemed to be complete with negative margins (R0). The next important consideration is the histology itself. This patient has squamous cell carcinoma, which is worth noting for two reasons. Firstly, the patient nicely fits into the randomized trial conducted by the Lung Cancer Study Group (LCSG) looking at PORT in squamous cell carcinoma of the lung [13], which is discussed subsequently. Secondly, the patient does *not* have adenocarcinoma, so some of the newer targeted therapies (bevacizumab, pemetrexed) are contraindicated, whereas others (gefitinib and the other EGFR inhibitors) are of diminished utility should he experience recurrence (for a comprehensive summary of this topic see Langer et al. [14]). Although it is difficult to salvage a recurrence of NSCLC regardless of histology, knowing the patient will have a narrowed list of options increases my enthusiasm for more aggressive up front therapy.

Next I would carefully review the operative note. Was the resection of the primary complicated in any way? Did the station 7 lymph node look obviously malignant? Was it fixed to the surrounding tissues? I typically call the surgeon involved in the case and ask if he had any concerns about the margins or degree of resection that might not appear in the pathology note. Hearing a surgeon express concern about the resection would strongly influence me to recommend PORT.

Of note is that the postoperative course for this patient was complicated by a pleural effusion that required talc pleurodesis. We can assume that the pleural effusion was negative for malignant cells, but I would have that fact confirmed. The pleural effusion alone would not change my recommendations for postoperative treatment. Pleural effusions are present in up to 60% of patients after cardiac surgery [15].

Now we are ready to ask the main question. What should our patient do next? My opinion is that the next logical step for the patient is adjuvant chemotherapy. Numerous recent phase 3 clinical trials have independently demonstrated an improvement in overall survival at 5 years with the addition of postoperative chemotherapy [4,16–18]. Specifically, the data support a survival benefit for cisplatin-based chemotherapy so it makes the most sense to recommend drug combinations containing this agent. With respect to delivery, chemotherapy should be sequenced first. I would generally not recommend that this patient receives chemotherapy concurrent with RT, as that combination in the adjuvant setting has been tested in a phase 3 randomized trial and found to be more toxic with no significant improvement in overall survival [19]. The concurrent use of chemotherapy and RT would be of potential benefit only in patients with residual disease after surgery (R1, R2 resections) and that is an interpolated application of the unresected stage III NSCLC data [20].

Do the data support the use of radiation for this patient? As detailed by Dr. Schild, the PORT meta-analysis [1] published in 1998 showed worsened survival for patients treated with PORT but specifically, for early stage and N0/N1 the negative effect of PORT was more profound, whereas for N2 and stage III patients the best that could be said is that there was no significant difference between surgery and observation. When thinking about the PORT meta-analysis, the main question is why survival would be significantly worse with the addition of PORT. What toxicity of the treatment was shortening the life span of treated patients? The most likely culprit is pneumonitis and pulmonary toxicity attributable to the use of hypofractionated regimens and outdated delivery techniques. The editorial that accompanied the publication included a telling comparison of intercurrent death and biological effective dose (BED) [21] where the two variables appeared to be strongly correlated.

A study included in the PORT meta-analysis but worth considering separately is the LSCG 773 [13] trial as was mentioned earlier. It has a specific bearing on our discussion here for a couple of reasons. First, this study avoided some of the pitfalls of other studies included in the meta-analysis by using the more traditional fractionation of 50 Gy in 1.8 to 2 Gy fractions. Second, the study was exclusively of squamous cell carcinomas, which parallels nicely with our patient. LSCG 773 was a negative study in that no survival advantage was seen for the use of RT (regardless of nodal stage), but it did show a dramatic improvement in local control with the addition of PORT. In the observation group, 41% of failures were local failures as compared with only 3% of failures in the RT group. The overall rate of recurrence was also less in the patients with positive N2 nodes who received RT compared with observation ($p = .031$).

While this study has a special bearing on our case, we have to keep in mind that our patient is not being treated with observation versus RT. Our patient will have received 4 cycles of cisplatin-based chemotherapy prior to the discussion of RT. From the randomized data presented earlier we can conclude that the benefit of RT is primarily related to a reduction in local failure. The benefit of chemotherapy is the improvement in overall survival, but likely there is some effect on local failure as well. Of the major adjuvant chemotherapy trials, the ANITA trial [4] reported the patterns of failure such that estimates of the effect of chemotherapy on local failure could be assessed. Local failure was 12% in the chemotherapy arm versus 18% in the observation arm ($p = .025$). Muddying the waters is the fact that PORT was variably used in this trial, but PORT was more frequently used in observation patients than in chemotherapy patients (33% vs. 22%, $p = .0002$). So, cautiously stated, chemotherapy using vinorelbine and cisplatin reduces local failure by at least 6% as compared with observation.

As noted by Dr. Schild, the ANITA investigators also published a retrospective analysis of the PORT data used in their trial [22]. It is important to remember that these data are still retrospective despite their origination in a phase 3 clinical trial. Nonetheless, for patients with N2 nodes, PORT

improved survival whether they were randomized to chemotherapy (MS 47 months vs. 24 months) or observation (MS 23 months vs. 12 months). There are other data that support a possible survival benefit of PORT in patients with N2 disease at the time of surgery. These include a SEER database study [11] of 7000 patients who received PORT for adjuvant treatment of node-positive lung cancer. PORT prolonged survival for patients with N2 involvement ($p = .007$). Lastly, we have a phase 3 randomized trial of PORT in patients with N2 disease that is currently accruing patients in Europe. The Lung ART trial is accruing slowly, but the results may answer the question of whether PORT improves survival in this group of patients.

Returning to our patient, what can we accurately say? PORT reliably decreases local failure and that alone is probably worth considering in this patient. If he opts for observation, he may have an 18% risk of local failure (ANITA [22]) and PORT would decrease that to lesser than 5% (LCSG [13]). The modern retrospective data are strongly suggestive that updated techniques may improve survival in N2 patients but the phase 3 data are lacking at this point. When the perennial question is asked "What would you do if it were you?," I would recommend that he receives PORT. We now need to decide on (a) dose and (b) volumes.

My choice for dose would be 50 Gy in 25 fractions. That was the dose used in the LCSG trial discussed earlier and resulted in outstanding local control. I might consider 50.4 Gy in 28 fractions (1.8 Gy/day), but our patient is 56 years old and I would be considering his need to return to work and routine life. I would like a start date that is at least 2 weeks after the completion of chemotherapy (the recommendation of the ANITA trial) but 4 weeks would also be okay to allow a more thorough recovery from chemotherapy.

Perhaps the more important discussion is what volumes we should treat to a dose of 50 Gy. As we discussed earlier, the toxicity that has given PORT a bad name is likely pulmonary and is strongly related to both dose (which we have decided) and volumes treated. The ANITA trial made no recommendations regarding field arrangement so we have no direction from that data. The LCSG trial required full mediastinal RT in addition to treating the bronchial stump. Do we need to treat large elective mediastinal volumes knowing it will increase the risk of pulmonary toxicity?

In patients with unresectable stage III NSCLC, the use of large field RT has been radically curtailed. Whereas we would have treated a field very similar to the LCSG PORT trial in the 1990s, we are mostly treating "involved field" RT, which places only nodal stations positive on PET, by biopsy, or greater than 1 cm within the clinical target volume (CTV). The reason for that shift was the accumulated data that very few patients experience treatment failure in nodal stations that were not included in the CTV of the involved field. There is ample evidence from prospective clinical trials that use involved field RT [23,24] that the isolated untreated elective nodal failure rate is lesser than 6%. The primary reason the isolated elective nodal is not common is the presence of significant local and distant failure. As we are not getting local control in the regions we directly target, there is little benefit in adding nodal stations that are not obviously involved.

Although it is tempting to want to shrink the fields for PORT in unresectable NSCLC, we should do so cautiously. Our patient has had an excellent local therapy already (surgery) and the addition of PORT will make local failure unlikely. We want to create a CTV that includes the areas at highest risk for local recurrence, and ignores areas at lower risk, remembering we have chemotherapy to help us with local/regional failure as well. Patterns of failure data are always a great place to start when trying to define a CTV. Investigators at Duke University reviewed the patterns of failure of 61 patients who experienced local failure after an R0 resection for early-stage NSCLC [25]. Overall, the most common site of regional failure was the bronchial stump, making it a priority CTV target in all patients treated with PORT. The authors also nicely lay out patterns of failure for all the different lobes of the lung allowing for individualized CTVs based on location of the primary lung cancer. For patients with right upper lobe lung cancers, the most common sites of failure were station 4R, the bronchial stump, and station 7. Contouring those sites would be the backbone for an individualized PORT CTV for our patient. Very little has been published on the use of smaller fields in the setting of PORT. There is 1 clinical trial using smaller-than-traditional RT fields for PORT. An Italian randomized trial of PORT in stage I NSCLC used 50.4 Gy in 1.8 Gy fractions and treated only the bronchial stump and ipsilateral hilum for patients after R0 resection [26]. Local failure in the RT arm was only 2.2% versus 23% for the patients who were randomized to observation. Toxicity was limited to 12% grade 1 pulmonary toxicity for PORT patients. No grade 2+ toxicity was seen. Although the entry criteria for that trial were different than our patient, the principle of covering only high-risk sites is applicable. It would also be reasonable to treat larger, more traditional fields for PORT as long as the dose was reasonable (45–60 Gy) and the bronchial stump was included.

Finally we should discuss the image guidance approach for our patient. A daily cone-beam CT initially aligned to the bony anatomy and refined to cover the bronchial stump would be the optimal approach [27]. This approach decreases the required planning target volume (PTV) expansion substantially and PTV expansions of 5 to 7 mm from the CTV can be appropriate and applied in this scenario. An alternative would be to perform daily kilovolt orthogonal x-rays to align bony anatomy. While simpler than cone-beam CT, there is no method to ensure that the bronchial stump is included in the PTV. Traditional, weekly imaging is also reasonable but requires larger expansions for PTV.

So, in summary, after a long and thorough discussion, I recommend adjuvant chemotherapy for the clear and strong survival benefit associated with its use. I would also recommend the consideration of PORT, firstly for improved local control, and secondly for some possible benefit in overall survival. I recommend a conservative dose of 50 Gy, a limited CTV focusing on high-risk sites, and the use of daily image guidance to decrease the required expansions from CTV to PTV.

COMMUNITY PRACTITIONER COMMENT

Thomas Carlson

Dr. Schild has nicely outlined the controversy surrounding patients with N2 disease and overall I agree with how he has summarized the literature and reviewed the approach to managing such cases. For the questions he posed, my responses are as follows.

What Is the Role of Adjuvant RT in This Patient?

This patient has stage IIIA, N2 disease. As outlined in Dr. Schild's review, he fits in the category of patients who would benefit from adjuvant therapy. As a community radiation oncologist, I tend to rely on guidelines and protocols as much as possible to provide insight into treatment recommendations. The National Comprehensive Cancer Network (NCCN) Clinical Practice Guidelines in Oncology [28] recommend that this patient receives adjuvant chemotherapy and radiation.

How Does His Clinical Status and Change in Clinical and Objective Respiratory Function Influence Decision Making?

The complications he experienced during the postoperative course and his objective respiratory function changes have a high probability of being associated with the surgery itself. If the patient's performance status is adequate and the plan developed to deliver the radiation falls within dosimetric guidelines, I would continue to recommend adjuvant treatment.

It would be my preference that the pleural fluid was evaluated prior to pleurodesis, as a positive finding would make the decision to treat much more controversial.

Pleurodesis can make subsequent scanning very difficult. In these situations, fusion of the preoperative CT and PET to the postoperative treatment planning data set is performed to maximize the ability to localize the anatomy and visualize the anatomic changes caused by the procedure.

If RT Is Recommended, What Dose/Fractionation Schedule Is Recommended and How Is the Volume Defined?

Assuming that the patient's performance status is acceptable, I would recommend PORT. From a dose perspective, I agree that 50 to 54 Gy is appropriate for a negative margin and 60 Gy appropriate for a positive margin. One remaining question is whether or not this patient actually has a positive margin. Discussions with the surgeon and pathologist should be undertaken to assess apparent close or positive margins as they may not represent the true margin. In this situation, the medial surface of the right mainstem detached tissue may have been cleared when the separate subcarinal lymph node dissection was performed. If the surgeon confirmed that this area was cleared with the dissection, then I would recommend the lower dose (54 Gy).

The volume should be based on the patterns of failure. In this RUL case, the most common sites of isolated failure are the bronchial stump and station 4R and 7 [25].

The Lung ART protocol provides reasonable guidelines for contouring and in this case, with a positive 7 node and a right-sided tumor, the CTV should include station 4R and have a maximal upper limit at the top of the aortic arch and a maximal lower limit at 5 cm below the carina [29].

Does the Estimated Risk of Pneumonitis Influence the Radiation Delivery Parameters?

Improved technology has increased our ability to deliver more aggressive treatment while maintaining compliance to the mean dose, V5, and V20 dosimetric constraints. As long as the treatment plan is capable of meeting these constraints (V20 is 35% or less; V5 is 65% or less) I would not compromise on the coverage. However, if it became difficult to meet these constraints, I would reevaluate the motion characteristics of the CTV and change my volume superiorly and inferiorly on the basis of this motion evaluation in an effort to meet these constraints.

How Is Radiation Sequenced With Chemotherapy, and Is There an Implication on Outcome?

With negative margins the NCCN guidelines recommend sequential therapy, with positive margins treatment should be concurrent. Whether or not chemotherapy increases the risk of pneumonitis when given with concurrent radiation or prior to radiation is also a controversial topic. If on discussion with the thoracic surgeon it is felt that he has positive margins, I would recommend concurrent chemotherapy, otherwise it will be sequential.

What Is the Role of Serial Assessment of Pulmonary Function?

I do not generally do serial testing of pulmonary functions as I am unaware of any data that suggest that this will modify outcomes after I complete my therapy. In the event of the patient complaining of respiratory symptoms after adjuvant RT, I will include these tests in my workup of the patient. The results of these tests may help in determining the origin of the patient's symptoms and also influence my management. As an aside, I empirically recommend patients either to use an inspiratory spirometer regularly or to perform deep breathing exercises as a form of respiratory physical therapy after having undergone surgery and adjuvant RT.

SECTION EDITOR'S NOTE

Gregory Videtic

In the setting of resected stage III NSCLC, it has been my practice to routinely offer adjuvant RT as part of care because it has a demonstrated impact on achieving optimal local control. With respect to sequencing with chemotherapy, I typically administer RT after chemotherapy, except in the setting of positive margins after surgery, where I believe that expeditious local management is important. RT dosing will depend on marigns, so that 50 Gy is used for margin-negative and 60 Gy is used for margin-positive cases, all at 2Gy/fraction. Patient performance and postoperative pulmonary status are critical in determining the recommendation for adjuvant therapy. For severely impaired patients after surgery, eg, Karnofsky performance status (KPS) less than 70, newly O_2-dependent, or with objectively impaired pulmonary function (DLCO less than 45%), I would recommend pulmonary rehabilitation as part of care and may opt to put on hold RT administration for fear of heightened lung injury.

REFERENCES

1. Postoperative radiotherapy in non-small-cell lung cancer: Systematic review and meta-analysis of individual patient data from nine randomised controlled trials. PORT Meta-analysis Trialists Group. *Lancet.* 1998;352:257–263.
2. Lally BE, Zelterman D, Colasanto JM, et al. Postoperative radiotherapy for stage II or III non-small-cell lung cancer using the surveillance, epidemiology, and end results database. *J Clin Oncol.* 2006;24:2998–3006.
3. Douillard JY, Rosell R, De Lena M, et al. Impact of postoperative radiation therapy on survival in patients with complete resection and stage I, II, or IIIA non-small-cell lung cancer treated with adjuvant chemotherapy: The adjuvant Navelbine International Trialist Association (ANITA)

Randomized Trial. *Int J Radiat Oncol Biol Phys.* 2008;72:695–701.
4. Douillard JY, Rosell R, De Lena M, et al. Adjuvant vinorelbine plus cisplatin versus observation in patients with completely resected stage IB-IIIA non-small-cell lung cancer (Adjuvant Navelbine International Trialist Association [ANITA]): A randomised controlled trial. *Lancet Oncol.* 2006;7:719–727.
5. Lad T. The comparison of CAP chemotherapy and radiotherapy to radiotherapy alone for resected lung cancer with positive margin or involved highest sampled paratracheal node (stage IIIA). LCSG 791. *Chest.* 1994;106:302S–306S.
6. Krupitskaya Y, Loo BW, Jr. Post-operative radiation therapy (PORT) in completely resected non-small-cell lung cancer. *Curr Treat Options Oncol.* 2008;9:343–356.
7. Emami B, Lyman J, Brown A, et al. Tolerance of normal tissue to therapeutic irradiation. *Int J Radiat Oncol Biol Phys.* 1991;21:109–122.
8. Graham MV, Purdy JA, Emami B, et al. Clinical dose-volume histogram analysis for pneumonitis after 3D treatment for non-small cell lung cancer (NSCLC). *Int J Radiat Oncol Biol Phys.* 1999;45:323–329.
9. Kwa SL, Lebesque JV, Theuws JC, et al. Radiation pneumonitis as a function of mean lung dose: An analysis of pooled data of 540 patients. *Int J Radiat Oncol Biol Phys.* 1998;42:1–9.
10. Annema JT, van Meerbeeck JP, Rintoul RC, et al. Mediastinoscopy vs endosonography for mediastinal nodal staging of lung cancer. *JAMA.* 2010 Nov 24;304:2245–2252.
11. Kraev A, Rassias D, Vetto J, et al. Wedge resection vs lobectomy*. *Chest.* 2007;131:136–140.
12. Moretti L, Yu DS, Chen H, et al. Prognostic factors for resected non-small cell lung cancer with pN2 status: Implications for use of postoperative radiotherapy. *Oncologist.* 2009;14:1106–1115.
13. Effects of postoperative mediastinal radiation on completely resected stage II and stage III epidermoid cancer of the lung. *N Engl J Med.* 1986;315:1377–1381.
14. Langer CJ, Besse B, Gualberto A, et al. The evolving role of histology in the management of advanced non-small-cell lung cancer. *J Clin Oncol.* 2010;28:5311–5320.
15. Light RW, Rogers JT, Moyers JP, et al. Prevalence and clinical course of pleural effusions at 30 days after coronary artery and cardiac surgery. *Am J Respir Crit Care Med.* 2002;166:1567–1571.
16. Chemotherapy in non-small cell lung cancer: A meta-analysis using updated data on individual

patients from 52 randomised clinical trials. *BMJ*. 1995;311:899–909.

17. Winton T, Livingston R, Johnson D, et al., Vinorelbine plus cisplatin vs. observation in resected non-small-cell lung cancer. *N Engl J Med*. 2005;352:2589–2597.

18. Arriagada R, Dunant A, Pignon JP, et al. Long-term results of the International Adjuvant Lung Cancer Trial evaluating adjuvant cisplatin-based chemotherapy in resected lung cancer. *J Clin Oncol*. 2010;28:35–42.

19. Keller SM, Adak S, Wagner H, et al. A randomized trial of postoperative adjuvant therapy in patients with completely resected atage II or IIIa non-small-cell lung cancer. *N Engl J Med*. 2000;343:1217–1222.

20. Curran WJ, Paulus R, Langer CJ, et al. Sequential vs concurrent chemoradiation for stage III non-small cell lung cancer: Randomized phase III trial RTOG 9410. *J Natl Cancer Inst*. 2011;103:1452–1460.

21. Munro AJ. What now for postoperative radiotherapy for lung cancer? *Lancet*. 1998;352:250–251.

22. Douillard JY, Rosell R, De Lena M, et al. Impact of postoperative radiation therapy on survival in patients with complete resection and stage I, II, or IIIA non-small-cell lung cancer treated with adjuvant chemotherapy: The adjuvant Navelbine International Trialist Association (ANITA) Randomized Trial. *Int J Radiat Oncol Biol Phys*. 2008;72:695–701.

23. Yuan S, Sun X, Li M, et al. A randomized study of involved-field irradiation versus elective nodal irradiation in combination with concurrent chemotherapy for inoperable stage III nonsmall cell lung cancer. *Am J Clin Oncol*. 2007;30:239–244.

24. Bradley JD, Graham M, Suzanne S, et al. Phase I results of RTOG L-0117; a phase I/II dose intensification study using 3DCRT and concurrent chemotherapy for patients with inoperable NSCLC. *J Clin Oncol*. 2005;23(16 Suppl): abstract 7063.

25. Kelsey CR, Light KL, Marks LB. Patterns of failure after resection of non–small-cell lung cancer: Implications for postoperative radiation therapy volumes. *Int J Radiat Oncol Biol Phys*. 2006;65:1097–1105.

26. Trodella L, Granone P, Valente S, et al. Adjuvant radiotherapy in non-small cell lung cancer with pathological stage I: Definitive results of a phase III randomized trial. *Radiother Oncol*. 2002;62:11–19.

27. Yeung AR, Li J, Shi W, et al. Optimal image-guidance scenario with cone-beam computed tomography in conventionally fractionated radiotherapy for lung tumors. *Am J Clin Oncol*. 2010;33:276–280.

28. Non-Small Cell Lung Cancer Version 2.2012, NCCN Clinical Practice Guidelines in Oncology. 10/04/11 © National Comprehensive Cancer Network, Inc. 2011.

29. Spoelstra FOB, Senan S, LePechoux C, et al. Variations in target volume definition for postoperative radiotherapy in stage III non-small-cell lung cancer: Analysis of an international contouring study. *Int J Radiat Oncol Biol Phys*. 2010;76:1106–1113.

■ CASE 1 ■

Anaplastic Oligodendroglioma

"HOT-OFF-THE-PRESS" UPDATE

This case was formulated and discussed by the authors prior to the recently published manuscripts that represent mature data from the Radiation Therapy Oncology Group (RTOG) – Intergroup and European Organisation for Research and Treatment of Cancer (EORTC) trials addressing codeleted anaplastic oligodendroglioma (AO) patients relative to survival advantage with chemoradiotherapy; therefore, the discussion and conclusions do not reflect these data [1].

CLINICAL PROBLEM

The "correct" treatment for patients with AO is a matter of considerable debate and controversy. Although some aspects have been studied in randomized trials, many aspects of treatment remain highly variable. This dilemma has been accentuated by the recognition that patients with these tumors have survival rates considerably superior to those of patients with glioblastoma (GBM) following a variety of different treatment combinations, especially if they harbor certain favorable molecular characteristics. The decision-making process for these patients, especially in terms of combination therapy and sequence of therapies, remains controversial.

CASE EXAMPLE

A 30-year-old right-handed woman presented to the emergency department with an episode of a partial simple seizure affecting the right hand. Evaluation included an MRI of the brain that showed a T1 hypointense area in the left frontal lobe with heterogeneous signal on T2-weighted images. No significant enhancing areas were seen within the abnormality. Biopsy showed an AO with 1p/19q codeletion. Resection confirmed a pure AO, and postoperative imaging showed no obvious residual tumor, with minimal residual T2 signal abnormality.

Management Decisions

- What postoperative therapy is required in this patient, and are there data to support the choices?
- What chemotherapy regimen (if any) should be given to the patient?
- What options are available to the patient at the time of a recurrence?

MAJOR OPINION

Haider A. Shirazi and Minesh P. Mehta

High-grade gliomas are categorized into World Health Organization (WHO) grade 3 tumors that include anaplastic astrocytomas, AOs, and anaplastic oligoastrocytomas, or WHO grade 4 tumors (GBMs) [2]. Pure anaplastic tumors and mixed oligodendrogliomas are relatively rare primary brain tumors with a better outcome than other malignant gliomas [3]. A recent population-based registry study showed an increasing incidence of oligodendroglial tumors and a corresponding decrease in astrocytic tumors, underscoring the importance of accurate histologic diagnosis of grade 3 gliomas, especially because oligodendrogliomas have comparatively favorable outcomes [4]. Reported median overall survival (OS) for pure AO is about 4.5 years, with an inferior outcome for mixed AOs likely secondary to an increased astrocytic component and less frequent 1p/19q codeletion [5]. Molecular studies from the 1990s showed the prognostic importance of allelic loss of 1p and 19q as indicators of chemo- and radiosensitivity and improved survival [6–10]. The role of 1p/19q codeletion in predicting response to a particular type of chemotherapy is unclear, and at present its most important significance may be in allowing more accurate characterization of oligodendroglial tumors [11].

Maximal safe resection with adequate margins is the first step in the management of AOs. Appropriate postoperative therapy remains controversial. In a survey of 99 neurooncologists regarding 1p/19q intact AOs, 34% recommended concurrent temozolomide and radiation followed by temozolomide and 20% recommended radiation alone. In contrast, for 1p/19q codeleted AOs, 42% recommended chemotherapy alone, typically temozolomide [12]. Although the most commonly recommended regimen was concurrent temozolomide and radiation with adjuvant temozolomide, the use of this regimen in the absence of adequate data on AO may be premature.

Two randomized trials have analyzed the benefits of adding chemotherapy to postoperative radiation in AOs. RTOG 94-02 was a phase 3 randomized trial that compared 4 cycles of neoadjuvant procarbazine, CCNU, and vincristine (PCV) chemotherapy followed by radiation versus radiation alone [13]. Tissue analysis for 1p/19q deletion was available for 70% of patients, and the study had a central review of neuropathology. Two hundred ninety-one patients were accrued, of whom 70% had pure AO. Median progression-free survival (PFS) for the combined regimen was 2.5 years compared to 1.9 years with radiation alone ($p = .018$), while no significant difference in median OS was noted (4.9 years with chemotherapy and 4.7 years without). Patients with 1p/19q codeletion had median OS of over 7 years versus 2.8 years without codeletion. Of patients who progressed on radiation alone, 80% ultimately received chemotherapy, usually PCV.

EORTC examined the role of adding chemotherapy to surgery and radiation by randomizing 368 patients to 6 cycles of postradiation procarbazine, CCNU, and vincristine versus radiation alone [14]. Tissue for 1p/19q deletion was available for 85% of patients, the study had a central review of neuropathology, and 72% of patients were found to have pure AO. This study also showed an improvement in median PFS with the addition of chemotherapy (23 months versus

13.2 months with radiation alone [$p = .0018$]), with no improvement in OS. Patients with 1p/19q codeletion in this study had a 74% survival rate after 60 months. At the time of progression, 82% of patients in the radiation-alone arm were given chemotherapy, mostly PCV. A toxicity analysis in the EORTC study showed increased rates of acute toxicity in the combined modality arm, but no long-term differences were noted between the 2 study arms [15].

Therefore, both randomized trials failed to show a categorical survival advantage (the primary end point of both trials) from the addition of chemotherapy (PCV) to a backbone radiotherapy (RT) regimen; both showed improved PFS, and the impact was greatest in the patients who had codeletion. This lack of survival advantage could possibly be associated with the effect of salvage PCV chemotherapy in patients who were progressing after RT, and if indeed this is the case, the unstated implication would be that the sequence of therapies may not be relevant. This question was partially addressed in a randomized German trial of 318 patients with anaplastic gliomas (including only 39 with centrally reviewed AO) who were randomized to up-front RT or chemotherapy (with a randomization to temozolomide or PCV). At progression, patients on the RT arm received chemotherapy, whereas patients who were progressing on one of the chemotherapy regimens were treated with the alternative chemotherapy, and only at second progression were these patients treated with RT. OS comparing the up-front randomization to RT or chemotherapy was statistically not different, further suggesting the possible use of multiple sequential therapies with the sequence itself possibly not having a significant impact. However, given that only 39 of 368 patients actually had a centrally validated diagnosis of AO, such an assumption could well be spurious [16].

The predictive and prognostic value of methylguanine-DNA methyltransferase (*MGMT*) promoter methylation continues to be investigated, driven in part by results from a phase 3 trial of temozolomide in GBM and the prognostic importance of *MGMT* methylation status observed in patients from this study [17,18]. Mollemann et al. observed *MGMT* promoter methylation in 80% of 1p/19q codeleted tumors [19]. Brandes et al. studied the response to temozolomide in 67 patients with recurrent primary AO or anaplastic oligoastrocytoma [19]. Although a significant correlation was observed between 1p/19q codeletion and *MGMT* methylation, no correlation between *MGMT* methylation and OS was noted. The authors concluded that temozolomide was an active agent in anaplastic oligodendroglial tumors with an overall response rate of almost 50%. A different retrospective study noted that in 28 patients with progressive low-grade oligodendrogliomas and low *MGMT*, protein expression correlated to codeletion of 1p/19q and overall response to temozolomide in pure and mixed AO [20].

Several recent phase 2 trials that included pure and mixed AO have shown that temozolomide in conjunction with radiation yields a similar response rate to PCV, but possibly with less toxicity, and have also shown the prognostic importance of 1p/19q codeletion with non-PCV regimens; however, other retrospective studies do not necessarily arrive at the same conclusion. Mikkelsen et al. studied 48 AO patients who received a combination of neoadjuvant and concurrent temozolomide with radiation [21]. Patients with codeleted 1p/19q received temozolomide alone, while those without codeleted 1p/19q received temozolomide followed by concurrent temozolomide and RT followed by further adjuvant temozolomide. Patients without codeleted tumors had an inferior PFS of 13.5 months compared to 28.7 months in codeleted patients. RTOG 01-31 was a phase 2 trial of neoadjuvant and concurrent temozolomide with radiation in AO patients [22]. Forty-two patients were enrolled with an objective preRT response rate of 32% (18% vs. 39% in favor of codeleted patients). Analysis of toxicity data when compared to results from RTOG 94-02 and the EORTC study suggested that temozolomide may be better tolerated than PCV.

Chemotherapy alone as initial therapy has been investigated in pure and mixed AO, particularly in those patients with 1p/19q codeletion. Abrey et al. reported the results of a prospective phase 2 trial of high-dose PCV-based chemotherapy with stem cell rescue in AO and found a median PFS of 78 months, with relapse observed in 46% of patients [23]. A study by Paleologos et al. analyzed 36 patients with AO who received either standard or intensive PCV. They observed a response rate of 70%, although 30% of patients required radiation during treatment owing to progression or relapse, and the authors therefore do not recommend PCV alone in this patient cohort [24]. Small studies of temozolomide alone have yielded somewhat better

results, with 1 study that analyzed 20 patients with AO who received a median of 14 cycles. The response rate was 75% with median time to progression of 24 months, with a majority of patients exhibiting improved neurologic function with chemotherapy [25].

Studies of biologic agents are also ongoing. One study by Desjardins et al. showed that after relapse or progression, imatinib provided a 12-month PFS of 29% with modest hematologic toxicity [26]. A phase 2 EORTC study showed a 6-month PFS of only 9% for pure and mixed AO [27]. In a study by Vredenburgh et al., bevacizumab and irinotecan was administered to 23 patients, including 9 grade 3 gliomas, that demonstrated relapse or progression after initial treatment [28]. PFS at 6 months was 38% with a 6-month OS of 72%. For the grade 3 gliomas, median OS was 30 weeks.

A new phase 3 Intergroup study, N0577, is enrolling patients with newly diagnosed AO with 1p/19q codeletion. Patients are randomized to radiation alone, radiation and concurrent plus adjuvant temozolomide, or temozolomide alone for 12 cycles.

Final Recommendations

Following maximal safe tumor resection in our 30-year-old patient with pure AO, we would treat the patient per the RTOG 01-31 phase 2 study. We recommend initial temozolomide alone, and if the patient does not have a complete response after 6 cycles of temozolomide, she should continue on to concurrent temozolomide and 59.4 Gy dose of radiation.

ACADEMIC COMMENT

Andrew B. Lassman

There is no universally agreed upon standard of care for newly diagnosed anaplastic AO. RT alone, RT with concurrent and/or adjuvant chemotherapy, and chemotherapy alone are all acceptable options [12]. For decades, following initial work performed by the Brain Tumor Study Group (BTSG) over 40 years ago, all high-grade gliomas were "lumped" together and treated with RT and that was shown to produce superior survival to either supportive care or chemotherapy with nitrosourea monotherapy [29,30]. Chemotherapy appeared to provide a modest improvement in long-term survival, flattening the "tail" of the survival curve, but caused substantial toxicity without prolonging the median survival [31]. However, most patients in those initial trials had GBMs, and by the late 1980s it emerged that oligodendrogliomas were a more chemosensitive entity [32]. This led to renewed interest in the use of chemotherapy, and 2 phase 3 trials evaluated the effect on survival from the addition of PCV chemotherapy either before or after RT [13,14]. These studies were a "negative" for survival as discussed previously.

However, these studies did not approach the disease as one would today because treatment did not depend on 1p/19q deletion status, as this prognostic factor was not discovered until after both trials were activated [6]. Survival among patients with 1p/19q codeleted tumors is sufficiently long placing patients at risk from delayed neurocognitive toxicity from initial therapy, especially RT, analogous to patients with low-grade gliomas [33]. Therefore, up to 42% of neurooncologists surveyed in 2005 advocated neoadjuvant chemotherapy alone for 1p/19q codeleted tumors [12]. A retrospective study demonstrated that since 2005, chemotherapy alone was administered in 57% of such cases [34]. At present, the Codeleted Tumors (CODEL) study is addressing this issue prospectively. In addition, a phase 3 study demonstrated that adding temozolomide (which is generally considered less toxic than PCV) to RT for newly diagnosed GBM, paradoxically a less chemosensitive tumor than oligodendroglioma, prolongs survival [18]. This led many physicians to advocate combined temozolomide and RT for all high-grade gliomas of any histologic subtype, and some for all gliomas [35]. This may be reasonable, but no level 1 evidence yet exists to support it.

Moreover, temozolomide has entirely replaced PCV presumably because it is less toxic and easier to prescribe. For example, in a retrospective data set of 1013 patients treated for oligoa strocytoma who were not enrolled in phase 3 trials, when chemotherapy was administered alone from 1995 to 1999, 86% received PCV and 0% received temozolomide. Since 2005, 98% received temozolomide and 2% received PCV (Lassman et al., submitted). However, no prospective randomized trial has ever been conducted that adequately compared PCV to temozolomide. Randomized trials were either conducted for recurrent astrocytomas [35], or were underpowered. For example, the German NOA-04 study randomized 318 patients with WHO grade 3 gliomas and suggested that temozolomide was

noninferior to PCV, but only 17 patients treated using primary chemotherapy had pure anaplastic oligoastrocytoma on central review [16]. Other data suggest that responses of low-grade oligodendrogliomas to temozolomide are less durable than to PCV [36]. Finally, complete responses of anaplastic oligoastrocytoma to neoadjuvant temozolomide in RTOG 0131 were rare, while responses to PCV were common [22]. A retrospective study demonstrated that patients with 1p/19q codeleted anaplastic oligoastrocytoma or mixed oligoastrocytomas had a substantially longer PFS following PCV than temozolomide (7.6 vs. 3.3 years, $n = 21$ vs. 68, $p = .019$) [34]. Although temozolomide is widely used, it remains unproven whether it is truly equal to or better than PCV, and no properly designed study will likely ever occur. Finally, the "relative value" of longer potential disease control versus greater potential toxicity has not been adequately studied. In my practice, all patients offered PCV have instead insisted on receiving temozolomide, mainly because of toxicity and quality of life concerns.

In this case, deferring RT at diagnosis appears reasonable because of the 1p/19q codeletion, pure anaplastic oligoastrocytoma histology and the young age of the patient, all favorable prognostic factors suggesting that late neurocognitive toxicity from RT represents a real concern. However, I would also seek additional molecular analysis such as *MGMT* promoter methylation and isocitrate dehydrogenase (*IDH*) mutation. These emerging prognostic factors may have a greater effect on survival than 1p/19q deletion and may underscore the unexpectedly short survival among a subset of patients with 1p/19q codeleted tumors [16,34,37,38]. If all 3 molecular analyses demonstrated favorable results (1p/19q codeleted, *MGMT* promoter methylated, *IDH* mutated), then I would more comfortably defer RT. In addition, rather than discontinuing temozolomide in favor of RT after lack of response to 6 cycles of neoadjuvant chemotherapy, I likely would have temozolomide continued, if tolerated, for 12 to 18 cycles and then followed closely with serial imaging every 2 to 3 months, reserving RT for clear recurrence. Had the patient responded to initial treatment, and to avoid RT altogether, an ongoing multicenter phase 2 clinical trial is exploring autologous stem cell transplant [39]. However, outside of a clinical trial, it would be difficult to advocate such an approach with its potential life threatening toxicities.

COMMUNITY PRACTITIONER COMMENT

Deepak Khuntia

As mentioned earlier, AO is a relatively uncommon primary central nervous system (CNS) tumor, the management of which is controversial. When further examining the case presented here, there is little controversy in the primary management. The patient is young and symptomatic and, as a result, maximal safe resection should be pursued. As a community physician I often look to national guidelines to help support treatment decisions. As per the most recent NCCN update, maximal safe resection should be pursued. However, after surgery, adjuvant recommendations are far from straightforward.

In our community-based practice, it would not be unusual for this patient to undergo temozolomide alone. The main reason for withholding RT in this subset is related to the lack of data supporting a survival advantage with up-front treatment with radiation and also the fear of neurotoxicity from radiation for a 30-year-old woman. In the NAO-04 German effort, 318 patients underwent a 2:1:1 randomization to receive up-front radiation versus PCV or temozolomide, respectively [16]. Radiation was used in the salvage setting in the second and third arms. AO represented 33 patients in the up-front radiation arm (139 patients in total) and 27 patients in the PCV or temozolomide arms (135 patients in total). Time-to-failure, PFS, and OS were not different between the up-front radiation arm and the 2 chemotherapy arms. Further, patients who underwent RT at recurrence had fewer adverse events as opposed to those patients who had chemotherapy at recurrence (45% vs. 75%). Finally, of the 138 patients who actually completed first-line chemotherapy, only 71 patients ultimately completed radiation therapy at recurrence, essentially avoiding the toxicity of radiation in nearly 1/2 of the patients. The true incidence of significant neurocognitive decline is not well defined, but it may be reasonable to conclude that the patients mostly likely to develop radiation-related dementia are those that will have extended survival. The patient in this case is 30 years old, has a 1p/19q deletion, has undergone a gross total resection, and is likely to realize a high 5-year survivorship. Finally, in regard to the choice of chemotherapeutic agents, NAO-04 showed no difference in efficacy in PCV versus temozolomide, but there was a higher rate of toxicity in the former. Given this information, delayed radiation with first-line temozolomide for adjuvant treatment is a very reasonable option for this patient.

SECTION EDITOR'S NOTE

Minesh P. Mehta

In a 30-year-old patient with an AO that has been found to be 1p/19q deleted several treatment options are available. I concur with the recommendations from the authors to initiate temozolomide in this setting in an attempt to delay or omit RT for a younger patient who may have a long-term survival and thus would be more apt to develop late toxicity associated with radiation. In the setting of progression I would recommend radiation therapy with concurrent temozolomide.

REFERENCES

1. Cairncross G, et al. Phase III trial of chemoradiotherapy for anaplastic oligodendroglioma: Long-term results of RTOG 9402. *J Clin Oncol.* 2013;31:337–343.
2. Black PM, Loeffler JS. *Cancer of the Nervous System.* 2nd ed. Philadelphia: Lippincott Williams & Wilkins; 2005.
3. *Statistical Report: Primary Brain Tumors in the United States, 1998–2002.* Central Brain Tumor Registry of the United States; 2005.
4. Hoffman S, Propp JM, McCarthy BJ. Temporal trends in incidence of primary brain tumors in the United States, 1985-1999. *Neuro Oncol.* 2006;8(1):27–37.
5. Shaw EG, Scheithauer BW, O'Fallon JR. Supratentorial gliomas: A comparative study by grade and histologic type. *J Neurooncol.* 1997;31(3):273–278.
6. Cairncross JG, Ueki K, Zlatescu MC, et al. Specific genetic predictors of chemotherapeutic response and survival in patients with anaplastic oligodendrogliomas. *J Natl Cancer Inst.* 1998;90(19):1473–1479.
7. Smith JS, Perry A, Borell TJ, et al. Alterations of chromosome arms 1p and 19q as predictors of survival in oligodendrogliomas, astrocytomas, and mixed oligoastrocytomas. *J Clin Oncol.* 2000;18(3):636–645.
8. Bauman GS, Ino Y, Ueki K, et al. Allelic loss of chromosome 1p and radiotherapy plus chemotherapy in patients with oligodendrogliomas. *Int J Radiat Oncol Biol Phys.* 2000;48(3):825–830.

9. Ino Y, Betensky RA, Zlatescu MC, et al. Molecular subtypes of anaplastic oligodendroglioma: Implications for patient management at diagnosis. *Clin Cancer Res.* 2001;7(4):839–845.

10. Hoang-Xuan K, He J, Huguet S, et al. Molecular heterogeneity of oligodendrogliomas suggests alternative pathways in tumor progression. *Neurology.* 2001;57(7):1278–1281.

11. Dunbar EM. The role of chemotherapy for pure and mixed anaplastic oligodendroglial tumors. *Curr Treat Options Oncol.* 2009;10(3-4):216–230.

12. Abrey LE, Louis DN, Paleologos N, et al. Survey of treatment recommendations for anaplastic oligodendroglioma. *Neuro Oncol.* 2007;9(3):314–318.

13. Intergroup Radiation Therapy Oncology Group Trial 9402, Cairncross G, Berkey B, et al. Phase III trial of chemotherapy plus radiotherapy compared with radiotherapy alone for pure and mixed anaplastic oligodendroglioma: Intergroup Radiation Therapy Oncology Group Trial 9402. *J Clin Oncol.* 2006;24(18):2707–2714.

14. van den Bent MJ, Carpentier AF, Brandes AA, et al. Adjuvant procarbazine, lomustine, and vincristine improves progression-free survival but not overall survival in newly diagnosed anaplastic oligodendrogliomas and oligoastrocytomas: A randomized European Organisation for Research and Treatment of Cancer phase III trial. *J Clin Oncol.* 2006;24(18):2715–2722.

15. Taphoorn MJ, van den Bent MJ, Mauer M, et al. Health-related quality of life in patients treated for anaplastic oligodendroglioma with adjuvant chemotherapy: Results of a European Organisation for Research and Treatment of Cancer randomized clinical trial. *J Clin Oncol.* 2007;25(36):5723–5730.

16. Wick W, Hartmann C, Engel C, et al. NOA-04 randomized phase III trial of sequential radiochemotherapy of anaplastic glioma with procarbazine, lomustine, and vincristine or temozolomide. *J Clin Oncol.* 2009;27(35):5874–5880.

17. Hegi ME, Diserens AC, Gorlia T, et al. MGMT gene silencing and benefit from temozolomide in glioblastoma. *N Engl J Med.* 2005;352(10):997–1003.

18. Stupp R, Mason WP, van den Bent MJ, et al. Radiotherapy plus concomitant and adjuvant temozolomide for glioblastoma. *N Engl J Med.* 2005;352(10):987–996.

19. Möllemann M, Wolter M, Felsberg J, et al. Frequent promoter hypermethylation and low expression of the MGMT gene in oligodendroglial tumors. *Int J Cancer.* 2005;113(3):379–385.

20. Levin N, Lavon I, Zelikovitsh B, et al. Progressive low-grade oligodendrogliomas: Response to temozolomide and correlation between genetic profile and O6-methylguanine DNA methyltransferase protein expression. *Cancer.* 2006;106(8):1759–1765.

21. Mikkelsen T, Doyle T, Anderson J, et al. Temozolomide single-agent chemotherapy for newly diagnosed anaplastic oligodendroglioma. *J Neurooncol.* 2009;92(1):57–63.

22. Vogelbaum MA, Berkey B, Peereboom D, et al. Phase II trial of preirradiation and concurrent temozolomide in patients with newly diagnosed anaplastic oligodendrogliomas and mixed anaplastic oligoastrocytomas: RTOG BR0131. *Neuro Oncol.* 2009;11(2):167–175.

23. Abrey LE, Childs BH, Paleologos N, et al., High-dose chemotherapy with stem cell rescue as initial therapy for anaplastic oligodendroglioma: Long-term follow-up. *Neuro Oncol.* 2006;8(2):183–188.

24. Paleologos NA, Macdonald DR, Vick NA, Cairncross JG. Neoadjuvant procarbazine, CCNU, and vincristine for anaplastic and aggressive oligodendroglioma. *Neurology.* 1999;53(5):1141–1143.

25. Taliansky-Aronov A, Bokstein A, Lavon I, Siegal T. Temozolomide treatment for newly diagnosed anaplastic oligodendrogliomas: A clinical efficacy trial. *J Neurooncol.* 2006;79(2):153–157.

26. Desjardins A, Quinn JA, Vredenburgh JJ, et al. Phase II study of imatinib mesylate and hydroxyurea for recurrent grade III malignant gliomas. *J Neurooncol.* 2007;83(1):53–60.

27. Raymond E, Brandes AA, Dittrich C, et al. Phase II study of imatinib in patients with recurrent gliomas of various histologies: A European Organisation for Research and Treatment of Cancer Brain Tumor Group Study. *J Clin Oncol.* 2008;26(28):4659–4665.

28. Vredenburgh JJ, Desjardins A, Herndon JE 2nd, et al. Phase II trial of bevacizumab and irinotecan in recurrent malignant glioma. *Clin Cancer Res.* 2007;13(4):1253–1259.

29. Walker MD, Alexander E Jr, Hunt WE, et al. Evaluation of BCNU and/or radiotherapy in the treatment of anaplastic gliomas. A cooperative clinical trial. *J Neurosurg.* 1978;49(3):333–343.

30. Walker MD, Green SB, Byar DP, et al. Randomized comparisons of radiotherapy and nitrosoureas for the treatment of malignant glioma after surgery. *N Engl J Med.* 1980;303(23):1323–1329.

31. Mason W, Louis DN, Cairncross JG. Chemosensitive gliomas in adults: which ones and why? *J Clin Oncol.* 1997;15(12):3423–3426.

32. Cairncross JG, Macdonald DR. Successful chemotherapy for recurrent malignant oligodendroglioma. *Ann Neurol.* 1988;23(4):360–364.

33. Douw L, Klein M, Fagel SS, et al. Cognitive and radiological effects of radiotherapy in patients with low-grade glioma: Long-term follow-up. *Lancet Neurol.* 2009;8(9):810–818.

34. Lassman AB, Iwamoto FM, Cloughesy TF, et al. International retrospective study of over 1000 adults with anaplastic oligodendroglial tumors. *Neuro Oncol.* 2011 Jun;13(6):649–659.

35. Brada M, Stenning S, Gabe R, et al. Temozolomide versus procarbazine, lomustine, and vincristine in recurrent high-grade glioma. *J Clin Oncol.* 2010;28(30):4601–4608.

36. Weller M. Chemotherapy for low-grade gliomas: When? How? How long? *Neuro Oncol.* 2010; 12(10):1013.

37. van den Bent MJ, Dubbink HJ, Sanson M, et al. MGMT promoter methylation is prognostic but not predictive for outcome to adjuvant PCV chemotherapy in anaplastic oligodendroglial tumors: A report from EORTC Brain Tumor Group Study 26951. *J Clin Oncol.* 2009;27(35):5881–5886.

38. van den Bent MJ, Dubbink HJ, Marie Y, et al. IDH1 and IDH2 mutations are prognostic but not predictive for outcome in anaplastic oligodendroglial tumors: A report of the European Organization for Research and Treatment of Cancer Brain Tumor Group. *Clin Cancer Res.* 2010;16(5):1597–1604.

39. Mohile NA, et al., High-dose chemotherapy with autologous stem cell rescue (ASCR) for newly diagnosed anaplastic oligodendroglial tumors: preliminary report of an oligodendroglioma study group trial [abstract TA-37]. *Neuro Oncol.* 2006;8(4):447.

■ CASE 2 ■

Elderly Patient With Newly Diagnosed Glioblastoma

CLINICAL PROBLEM

The "correct" treatment for an "elderly" patient with glioblastoma (GBM) is a matter of considerable debate and controversy and although some aspects of this clinical situation have been studied in randomized trials, many other aspects remain highly controversial and subject to significant interphysician variability. This dilemma is commonly seen in routine "community clinical practice" where the majority of these patients seek care given their advanced age, sometimes poor Karnofsky performance status (KPS), and reduced mobility, all of which lead to less-frequent referral to a multidisciplinary care program.

CASE EXAMPLE

A 77-year-old woman who resides in a large metropolitan city with limited intracity transportation, parking issues, and significant traffic challenges presented to the emergency department with a generalized tonic-clonic seizure. She underwent a brain MRI with contrast that demonstrated a T1 minimally enhancing mass in the left middle frontal gyrus, measuring approximately 3.3 × 2.5 × 2.4 cm in greatest transverse, anteroposterior, and craniocaudal dimensions. There was minimal mass effect and no significant midline shift. A 3-mm focus of enhancement was seen in the left cingulate gyrus. Following her seizure, the patient remained intubated for 4 days and was placed on anticonvulsant therapy. After extubation, she had mild right-hand weakness and generalized clumsiness, but no other focal neurologic deficits.

The patient then underwent an awake left frontal craniotomy with cortical mapping and Stealth-directed gross total resection. Pathology demonstrated a highly cellular infiltrating glioma with moderately pleomorphic astrocytic cells.

Areas of pseudopalisading necrosis and some microvascular proliferation were identified, consistent with a World Health Organization (WHO) grade 4 GBM. Following surgery, the patient had a KPS of 70 after having been weaned off all steroids, and she was free of further seizures on 500 mg BID (twice daily) levetiracetam. She returned to her own single-story home and was capable of performing most activities of daily living. She has 3 daughters who live nearby and provide considerable assistance with transportation, shopping, and other household chores. One of the patient's daughters is related to an academic oncologist in a different state who focuses his practice on central nervous system (CNS) neoplasms. The key clinical therapeutic questions include the appropriate selection of treatment options between hospice, radiotherapy (RT) alone, chemotherapy alone, combination chemoradiotherapy (CRT), duration of RT, and the choice of center for her treatment.

Management Decisions

- How aggressive should the management be of this elderly patient with newly diagnosed GBM?
- What radiation dose and fractionation would portend the highest benefit with the lowest risk of decreasing the patient's quality of life?
- Should chemotherapy be added to the regimen and is there a need for adjuvant therapy?

MAJOR OPINION

Minesh P. Mehta and Haider A. Shirazi

GBM is the most common CNS neoplasm in adults that constitutes about 80% of all cases of glioma and the majority of cases of high-grade glioma [1–3].

198

Patients from 65 to 84 years of age have the highest incidence of GBM. With increasing life expectancy, an increase in the number of cases of this aggressive disease with the associated poor prognosis is anticipated [4–7]. Several studies have shown poorer survival for older patients, as well as reduced treatment tolerance and response, and some reports indicate that tumors in older patients may have somewhat different molecular features [8–10]. Age is the most significant prognostic factor in GBM (with patients older than 50 years of age doing considerably worse), followed by KPS, histology, and mental status. The median survival of elderly patients is typically measured in terms of several months, with few long-term survivors. One study suggested that older patients undergo less aggressive therapies, which may account for their shorter survival [11–13]. A study of 133 patients aged 65 and older with newly diagnosed GBM found that older patients who underwent resection did not have increased perioperative complications compared to those who underwent needle biopsy only; further, those who underwent resection had a median survival of 5.7 months compared to 4 months for needle biopsy alone [14].

Although long-term survivors of GBM are the exception rather than the norm, with 5-year survival rates of less than 5%, recent improvements in treatment have resulted in improved survival. Updated results of the European Organisation for Research and Treatment of Cancer (EORTC)/ National Cancer Institute of Canada (NCIC) trial of biopsy or resection, followed by RT plus temozolomide (TMZ) versus RT alone, showed a 5-year survival rate of 9.8% in the combined modality group compared to 1.9% without TMZ, and the combined chemoradiation regimen has now become the standard of care in patients with GBM [15]. Unfortunately, outcomes in patients who are over 70 years of age cannot be deduced directly from the Stupp trial, which did not enroll older patients, and the benefits of chemoradiation in older patients with GBM remain controversial [16]. A trend benefit analysis of patients from the EORTC/NCIC trial found decreasing benefit of the combined modality regimen with increasing age, with a modest hazard ratio (HR) of .80 for patients aged 65 to 71 (p = .340) [17]. The obvious conclusion from this trial is that we have level 1 evidence that supports the role of CRT in prolonging survival in GBM, compared to RT alone, but this trial shows decreasing benefit with increasing age and does not address the issue of benefit in patients older than 70 years.

In a study published in 2007 by Keime-Guibert et al., 85 patients of age 70 years and older with newly diagnosed anaplastic astrocytoma or GBM were randomized to RT and supportive care or supportive care alone [18]. Patients had a KPS of 70 or higher, and the RT was given in 1.8 Gy fractions to a dose of 50 Gy to the involved part of the brain. The trial was stopped early when interim analysis showed a median survival of 29.1 weeks in the RT group versus 16.9 weeks in the supportive care–alone group, with a HR for death in the RT group of 0.47. No significant differences in quality of life and cognition were noted between the 2 groups. The obvious conclusion from this trial, therefore, is that we have level 1 evidence supporting the use of RT to prolong survival in elderly patients with GBM compared to supportive care alone, but this trial does not address the relative benefit of RT versus chemotherapy or combined modality therapy.

Other lines of evidence also support this conclusion. A population-based analysis of elderly patients with GBM found a significant improvement in cause-specific survival for patients treated with RT compared to those who were not, with a HR for radiation of 0.43 [19]. This study also found that age at diagnosis was prognostic in elderly populations. Kita et al. also noted age to be prognostic and suggested that the difference may be due to more radioresistant disease in elderly patients [20]. Optimal treatment of GBM in elderly patients, defined as gross total or subtotal resection with postoperative radiation, was found in 1 retrospective study to improve survival over suboptimal treatment from 2.4 to 7.4 months, independent of performance status [21]. Suboptimal treatment was defined as biopsy, biopsy with radiation, surgery alone, or surgery with palliative radiation.

In the elderly, where transportation could be a significant limitation, short-course RT could prove to be attractive, especially in a disease where the long-term concerns regarding hypofractionated RT are somewhat tempered by the limited survival. In a randomized study from 2004, Roa et al. found no difference between conventionally fractionated (60 Gy in 30 fractions) versus short-course radiation (40 Gy in 15 fractions), with median survival of 5.1 months for standard radiation and 5.6 months for short-course radiation [22]. Patients were 60 years or older with a median KPS of 70. Steroid requirements were significantly lower in the short-course group, and the authors concluded that short-course radiation was a reasonable option for patients with newly diagnosed GBM, especially the elderly. Other prospective studies have had similar results that demonstrate that survival for patients who receive abbreviated courses of radiation is similar to conventionally treated historic controls [23]. Bauman et al. studied 29 patients with GBM who were aged 65 years or older who were treated with a dose of 30 Gy in 10 fractions and found that 60% of patients alive at 1 month had stable or improved quality of life and performance status [24]. Eleven patients with KPS greater than 50 had a median survival of 5 months. Ford et al. found that GBM patients who had a poor prognosis, more than 1/2 of them over 60 years of age and were treated with a dose of 36 Gy in 12 fractions, had a median survival of 16 weeks [25].

None of these studies have addressed the role of chemotherapy alone or CRT in the elderly, and this has been the subject of several other trials and reports [26–29]. Brandes et al., in a prospective study published in 2003, reported outcomes in 79 elderly patients with GBM who were over 65 years of age, who were treated with surgery followed by radiation alone ($n = 24$), radiation plus adjuvant procarbazine, lomustine, and vincristine (PCV) chemotherapy ($n = 32$), or radiation plus adjuvant TMZ ($n = 22$), in a nonrandomized sequential manner. Statistically significant improved overall survival (OS) was found between the first and third groups only, with combined modality therapy with TMZ resulting in an OS of 14.9 months, compared to 11.2 months with radiation alone; the difference in time between the first patient who enrolled in the RT cohort and the last patient entered on to the TMZ/RT cohort was 7 ½ years, and with several recent trials showing an improvement in median survival with time (owing to incompletely explained variables), the conclusion that TMZ/RT is superior to RT alone in the elderly has to be tempered somewhat. However, their TMZ/RT cohort had a median age of 68 years (range 65–75, median KPS 77), an age bracket within which our patient falls and the median survival of 14.9 months in the absence of major toxicities is a useful finding that we can use to aid us in our decision making. Further, Minniti et al. treated 30 patients over 70 years of age with concomitant TMZ and radiation followed by 6 cycles of adjuvant therapy resulting in a median survival of 10.6 months and median progression-free survival (PFS) of 7 months [27]. Therefore, this would constitute level 2 evidence that in good

performance status elderly patients with GBM, postoperative CRT (TMZ) is well tolerated and appears to produce survival results not vastly different than those in younger patients, and putatively is superior to RT alone. Subsequently, Brandes et al. treated 58 additional GBM patients who were over 65 years of age with concomitant and adjuvant TMZ and radiation, resulting in a median survival of 13.7 months and median PFS of 9.5 months [28]. *MGMT* promoter methylation status was also evaluated in this study, and *MGMT* methylation was both prognostic and predictive in this elderly population. The authors noted significant neurologic and neurocognitive sequelae in these patients and concluded that although chemoradiation improved survival, its benefits may be outweighed by neurologic toxicity from addition of chemotherapy to radiation [29].

Combs et al. studied 43 elderly (age above 65 years) GBM patients who were treated with concomitant TMZ (81% received 50 mg/m^2, 19% received 75 mg/m^2) and RT that resulted in a median OS of 11 months. Importantly, in this study, small as it is, they showed that the elderly patients undergoing gross total resection followed by CRT achieved a median survival of 18 months, again, a very respectable result in this patient population, and this was achieved with few toxicities, especially because adjuvant TMZ was withheld in all but 5 patients. Gerstein et al. retrospectively assessed outcomes in 51 patients aged 65 and over with GBM treated to a dose of 60 Gy of radiation in 30 fractions and concomitant TMZ at 75 mg/m^2 [30]. Median OS was 11.5 months, and PFS was 5.5 months. Therefore, this would constitute level 2 or 3 evidence that in good performance status elderly patients with GBM, postoperative concomitant CRT without adjuvant TMZ is well tolerated and appears to produce survival results about the same as those in younger patients, and putatively is comparable to the results of using concomitant and adjuvant TMZ.

The role of TMZ alone has recently been investigated in some trials. Chinot et al. reported an open-label, single-center, phase 2 trial to evaluate the efficacy and safety of TMZ as first-line chemotherapy and exclusive treatment in elderly patients with newly diagnosed GBM [31]. Chemotherapy-naïve patients (age over 70 years) were treated with TMZ at a dose of 150 to 200 mg/m^2 per day for 5 consecutive days of a 28-day cycle until they developed disease progression. No RT was administered. Thirty-two patients (median age 75 years; median KPS score 70) experienced a median OS of 6.4 months and a median PFS of 5.0 months. Adverse events primarily were mild, with National Cancer Institute Common Terminology Criteria for Adverse Events (NCI CTCAE) grade 3–4 thrombocytopenia and neutropenia reported to occur in 6% and 9% of patients, respectively. Laigle-Donadey et al. analyzed 39 elderly newly diagnosed GBM patients who were treated with TMZ alone [32]. Median OS was 36 weeks and median PFS was 20 weeks. Survival of patients treated with TMZ who did not have second-line chemotherapy at progression was 27.4 weeks, comparable to the survival of 29 weeks in the RT arm of the Keimer-Guibert study, but significantly inferior to all of the combined CRT data in the elderly. The Nordic trial randomized elderly patients with newly diagnosed GBM to radiation alone or TMZ alone. An initial report at the American Society of Clinical Oncology (ASCO) 2010 compared two different RT schedules—either standard RT (60 Gy in 2 Gy fractions over 6 weeks) or hypofractionated RT (34 Gy in 3.4 Gy fractions over 2 weeks) or single-agent TMZ alone, without RT (6 cycles at 200 mg/m^2 day 1–5 every 28 days) [33]. A total of 342 patients were included, of which 291 were randomized among the 3 treatment options, and an additional 51 patients were separately randomized among hypofractionated RT and TMZ. Median age was 70 years (range 60–88), and 72% had undergone tumor resection, the remaining 28% had a biopsy only. Eastern Cooperative Oncology Group (ECOG) performance status was 0 to 1 for 75% of patients. Survival data were available for 334 patients (98%), with 11 (3%) remaining alive. There was no significant difference in survival among the 3 treatment arms, with median survival being 8 months for TMZ, 7.5 months for hypofractionated RT, and 6 months for 6 weeks of RT (p = .14). Subgroup analyses and determination of molecular markers is ongoing. The authors concluded that elderly patients with GBM have short survival. Time-consuming therapy that does not offer longer survival should therefore be avoided. Their study showed no advantage of standard 6 weeks RT compared to hypofractionated RT over 2 weeks or 6 cycles of TMZ chemotherapy only, but did not address the question of concomitant CRT. These results suggest that standard RT alone should no longer be offered to the elderly patient population with GBM.

Both the Radiation Therapy Oncology Group (RTOG) 05-25, a recently completed randomized trial of 2 different maintenance chemotherapy schedules, as well as RTOG 08-25 (also recently completed), which randomized patients to radiation and TMZ with or without bevacizumab, did not exclude elderly patients and may provide additional insight into the role of aggressive treatment in elderly patients. The EORTC/NCIC are conducting a phase 3 trial (NCT00482677) of short-course radiation with and without TMZ in elderly GBM patients aged 65 and over and results will also be informative regarding appropriate therapeutic choices in the elderly with GBM.

Since the compilation of this chapter, at press time new data have emerged that were *not* included in the decision making presented here. Both of these manuscripts are discussed here, but none of the complete data from these manuscripts were included in the recommendations provided.

Wick et al., in May 2012, reported the results of the NOA-08 German phase 3 randomized trial of TMZ versus RT in *The Lancet*. They compared the efficacy and safety of dose-dense TMZ alone versus RT alone in elderly patients with anaplastic astrocytoma or GBM, with "elderly" being defined as 65 years of age or older, and a minimum KPS of 60. Four hundred twelve patients were randomized to 100 mg/m^2 TMZ, given on days 1 to 7 of 1 week on/1 week off cycles, or RT of 60 Gy, in 30 fractions of 1.8 to 2.0 Gy. Three hundred seventy-three patients (195 in the TMZ group and 178 in the RT group) received at least 1 dose of treatment and were included in efficacy analyses. Median OS was 8.6 months (95% CI 7.3–10.2) in the TMZ group versus 9.6 months (8.2–10.8) in the RT group (HR 1.09, 95% CI 0.84–1.42, p [noninferiority] = .033), implying "noninferiority" of TMZ alone in comparison to RT alone in elderly patients with GBM, but this does not address the issue of concomitant CRT.

Post hoc, in a non-prespecified cohort, *MGMT* promoter methylation status was evaluated in 209 patients (56% of the cohort analyzed for survival, and 50% of the cohort actually enrolled). *MGMT* promoter methylation was observed in 73 (35%) of the patients tested. *MGMT* promoter methylation was associated with longer OS (11.9 months [95% CI 9.0 to not reached] vs 8.2 months [7.0–10.0]; HR 0.62, 95% CI 0.42–0.91, p – .014). Event-free survival (EFS) was longer in patients with *MGMT* promoter methylation who received TMZ alone than in those who underwent RT alone (8.4 months [95% CI 5.5–11.7] vs. 4.6 [4.2–5.0]), whereas the opposite was true for patients with no methylation of the *MGMT* promoter (3.3 months [3.0–3.5] vs. 4.6 months [3.7–6.3]).

The major conclusions that can be drawn from this most recent trial are that TMZ alone is noninferior to RT alone in the treatment of elderly patients with malignant astrocytoma, but this still does not address the role of concomitant CRT. Further, although available only in a subset of patients and therefore subject to some potential bias, *MGMT* promoter methylation seems to be a useful biomarker for outcomes by treatment and could aid decision making; it appears that in the unmethylated patients, TMZ alone is inferior to RT alone, and perhaps one could argue that such patients should be treated either with RT alone or combination CRT [34].

In August 2012, the manuscript from the aforementioned Nordic randomized trial became available as an e-publication ahead of print in *Lancet Oncology*. Elderly patients (60 years or older) with GBM were randomized to 1 of 3 arms, TMZ alone (200 mg/m^2 on days 1–5 of every 28 days for up to 6 cycles), hypofractionated RT (34 Gy administered in 3.4 Gy fractions over 2 weeks), or standard RT (60 Gy administered in 2.0 Gy fractions over 6 weeks). Of the 342 patients enrolled, 291 were randomized (TMZ $n = 93$, hypofractionated RT $n = 98$, standard RT $n = 100$) but 51 were randomized across only 2 groups (TMZ $n = 26$, hypofractionated RT $n = 25$). In the 3-group randomization, in comparison with standard RT, median OS was significantly longer with TMZ (8.3 months [95% CI 7.1–9.5; $n = 93$] vs. 6.0 months [95% CI 5.1–6.8; $n = 100$], HR 0.70; 95% CI 0.52–0.93, $p = .01$), but not with hypofractionated RT (7.5 months [6.5–8.6; $n = 98$], HR 0.85 [0.64–1.12], $p = .24$). For all patients who received TMZ or hypofractionated RT ($n = 242$) OS was similar (8.4 months [7.3–9.4; $n = 119$] vs. 7.4 [6.4–8.4; $n = 123$]; HR 0.82, 95% CI 0.63–1.06; $p = .12$). For age older than 70 years, survival was better with TMZ and with hypofractionated RT than with standard RT (HR for TMZ vs. standard RT 0.35 [0.21–0.56], $p < .0001$; HR for hypofractionated vs. standard RT 0.59 [95% CI 0.37–0.93], $p = .02$). As expected, patients treated with TMZ with tumor *MGMT* promoter methylation had significantly longer survival than those without *MGMT* promoter methylation (9.7 months [95% CI 8.0–11.4] vs. 6.8 months [5.9–7.7]; HR 0.56 [95% CI 0.34–0.93], $p = .02$), but no difference was noted between those with methylated and unmethylated *MGMT* promoter treated with RT (HR 0.97 [95% CI 0.69–1.38]; $p = .81$). This trial therefore further suggests that both TMZ alone and hypofractionated RT alone produce equivalent survival in elderly patients with GBM, and both are superior to standard RT, but the trial does not address the role of concomitant CRT. The trial also further suggests that *MGMT* promoter methylation status might be a useful predictive marker for benefit from TMZ [35].

Final Recommendation

We first discussed the role of hospice with the patient, which she declined as she was categorical regarding her desire to seek active interventional therapy for her disease, as opposed to expectant symptom-management. Because the patient had a good performance status following an extensive resection, we recommended postoperative CRT to the patient on the basis of the premise that she would likely fall in the subgroup of elderly patients more likely to derive longer-term survival benefit from this approach, compared to either modality alone. Next, we discussed the duration of RT, and given the prevailing bias that a significant component of the benefit of TMZ is derived from its concomitant administration with RT, we discussed both abbreviated hypofractionation and conventionally fractionated RT, and the patient elected to pursue the latter. At the time of this discussion, the tumor *MGMT* status was pending. We next discussed the choice of centers for her treatment, including centers closer to home to reduce the transportation and parking burdens, but after understanding the complexity of issues such as pseudoprogression and the need for a multimodality team in making these decisions, as well as the possibility of re-resection and further clinical trial options in the event of progression, the patient opted to seek care at the larger tertiary care facility, in spite of her decision not to pursue a clinical trial. In this high-performing patient with a radical resection, aggressive options are reasonable; should her performance status have been much worse, any of the other options such as TMZ alone, short-course RT, or hospice would have been reasonable options.

ACADEMIC COMMENT

Igor J. Barani

As summarized, an elderly patient with a GBM and good performance status (KPS higher than

70) poses a unique therapeutic challenge given the variety of clinical data to support different treatment strategies. In my view, the most relevant questions in these patients relate to (a) the use of short- versus long-course (6 week) RT with concomitant TMZ chemotherapy, and (b) the unknown relative benefit of adjuvant TMZ chemotherapy following concurrent chemoradiation treatment.

The available data clearly demonstrate superior survival outcomes with the use of combined chemoradiation treatment than with either modality alone. For example, Brandes et al. treated 58 patients who were 65 years or older using conventional RT (60 Gy in 30 fractions over 6 weeks) plus continuous daily TMZ (75 mg/m^2), followed by 12 maintenance cycles of TMZ (150 mg/m^2 given once daily for 5 consecutive days every 28 days) [28]. This regimen mirrored that used by Stupp et al. (plus 6 adjuvant cycles of chemotherapy) in their seminal publication where patients with a median age of 56 years were treated (range 19–70 years) [15]. Brandes et al. reported a median survival time of 13.7 months, which compares favorably to 14.6 months observed in the Stupp et al. study in younger patients. Similar results were observed by Minniti et al. in a study of 30 patients older than 70 years who underwent chemoradiation therapy following extensive resection [27]. However, in the study by Brandes et al., 31% and 25% of patients experienced grade 1–2 and grade 3–4 mental status deterioration, respectively. In total, 10% of patients experienced leukoencephalopathy in follow up at as early as 6 months after treatment. While likely multifactorial in nature, the rates of neurocognitive toxicity are significant and debilitating, raising the question of whether both concurrent and adjuvant chemotherapy is necessary in these patients.

Select prospective studies in elderly patients suggest that surgical resection followed by definitive RT and adjuvant-only chemotherapy with TMZ offer a significant advantage over both RT alone and over radiotherapy followed by classic PCV in terms of PFS at 6 months and over RT alone in terms of OS [29]. The median survival of the adjuvant TMZ group in this nonrandomized, longitudinal study was a respectable 14.9 months. In addition, this treatment approach seems to be well tolerated and has a good safety profile. Unfortunately, this study by Brandes et al. from 2003 does not report the observed rates of neurologic and neucognitive toxicity that precludes a comparison of toxicity rates between concurrent and adjuvant-only TMZ regimens in the setting of postoperative

RT in the elderly. In the absence of this toxicity data, it is difficult to draw direct conclusions about the optimal treatment regimen; however, given the prevailing bias that concurrent TMZ administration is superior to the adjuvant-only treatment in terms of survival outcomes, it would seem reasonable to recommend treatment with postoperative concurrent chemoradiation therapy with TMZ without further adjuvant treatment. In fact, studies of this approach by Combs et al. and a retrospective study by Gerstein et al. reported respectable OS of 11 months and 11.5 months, respectively; however, patients in whom gross total resection was achieved, Combs et al. reported a median survival of 18 months (as in our case patient). Unfortunately, neurologic and cognitive outcomes were not reported in these studies to permit estimation of the quality of life and post treatment performance status. Pending the findings of the EORTC/NCIC phase 3 trial of short-course RT with and without TMZ, we would not recommend short-course RT with TMZ without documentation of the survival and toxicity impact of this approach.

A brief comment regarding the *MGMT* methylation status is perhaps also warranted. Just as in the younger population, *MGMT* methylation status was found to have both a prognostic and predictive value in the elderly [28]. However, the fact that TMZ is a well-tolerated oral drug, and that few highly efficacious alternatives are currently available, we would still opt to treat the patient with this drug, regardless of *MGMT* status. It is worth noting that even though *MGMT* promoter methylation was identified as the only molecular marker that was enriched in so-called long-term survivors of GBM (OS of longer than 36 months), prolonged survival can be seen without *MGMT* promoter hypermethylation, which indicates the existence of other factors conferring this favorable prognosis [36,37]. So, while testing currently provides powerful prognostic information, its role in guiding patient management is more tenuous.

To summarize, our recommendation for an elderly patient with good performance status (KPS of 70 or higher) following gross total resection is to undergo concurrent chemoradiation therapy with TMZ with or without continued adjuvant chemotherapy. In our opinion, a short course of accelerated RT (over 2 weeks) would be appropriate in elderly patients who have a KPS of lesser than 60 and who have undergone only biopsy (or minimal resection); hospice would also be a consideration in these patients. It would be our preference to treat and enroll the case patient in a clinical trial if one were available, and to follow her post-treatment course within the context of a tertiary care center where various salvage therapy trials are available along with the benefits of a case discussion at a multidisciplinary tumor board.

COMMUNITY PRACTITIONER COMMENT

Deepak Khuntia

As described in the Major Opinion section, a strong rationale may exist to consider slightly different treatment regimens for the elderly GBM patient. This group of patients varies from younger patients in several aspects. First of all, we know from the RTOG recursive partitioning analysis (RPA) that patients who are 50 years or older do considerably worse compared to those under the age of 50; in fact, this was the most important node within the RTOG RPA [8]. Elderly patients are more likely to present with de novo or primary GBM (as opposed to younger patients who have a higher frequency of secondary GBM, progressing from a lower grade glioma). Primary GBMs often will have epidermal growth factor receptor (*EGFR*) amplification without a p53 mutation as opposed to those with astrocytic progression, where the inverse is more apparent. Although not universally agreed on, *EGFR* amplification is considered a poor prognostic factor in GBM by some. Finally, compared to younger patients, elderly patients may have special needs related to transportation issues and daily care. Given these factors, it is not unreasonable to consider these patients separately when discussing management.

In the example of the 77-year-old patient discussed here, it is useful to personalize her management as not all 77-year-old patients are the same and, as described, therapy could vary from everything from hospice to concurrent CRT. The specifics of this case would argue strongly in favor of concurrent CRT with standard radiation to a dose of 60 Gy with TMZ and adjuvant TMZ. First of all, the patient has very good performance status. Her KPS is at least 70 and her comorbidities were not significant enough to preclude tumor resection. Age alone should not be the deciding factor in determining treatment. Further, she has the social resources that will allow her to make it to 6 weeks of therapy and she should be given the benefit of the doubt

that she could potentially be a long-term survivor. If her *MGMT* status was found to methylated, it would bias us even more toward standard radiation and TMZ. If she physically did not have the means for coming in for 6 weeks of therapy, it would be reasonable to consider hypofractionated RT of 40 Gy/15 fractions as per Roa and colleagues [22]. Given the lack of level 1 evidence with TMZ and abbreviated RT, we would not advocate the use of concurrent CRT with the 15 fraction regimen. We would reserve hospice for patients with poor KPS (of lower than 50).

SECTION EDITOR'S NOTE

Minesh P. Mehta

The aforementioned case represents a difficult scenario in which several treatment options are available to the patient. A lengthy discussion between the physician and patient is warranted to ascertain the patient's goals of treatments and to discuss realistic outcomes based on patient and tumor characteristics. Based on the patient's performance status and goals, I believe concurrent hypofractionated radiation and TMZ would be a beneficial primary treatment approach that best balances aggressive treatment and quality of life.

REFERENCES

1. Black PM, Loeffler JS. *Cancer of the Nervous System.* 2nd ed. Philadelphia: Lippincott Williams & Wilkins; 2005.
2. Wrensch M, Rice T, Miike R, et al. Diagnostic, treatment, and demographic factors influencing survival in a population-based study of adult glioma patients in the San Francisco Bay Area. *Neuro Oncol.* 2006;8(1):12–26.
3. Jukich PJ, McCarthy BJ, Surawicz TS, et al. Trends in incidence of primary brain tumors in the United States, 1985–1994. *Neuro Oncol.* 2001;3(3):141–151.
4. Chandler KL, Prados MD, Malec M, Wilson CB. Long-term survival in patients with glioblastoma multiforme. *Neurosurgery.* 1993;32(5): 716–720; discussion 720.
5. Fleury A, Menegoz F, Grosclaude P, et al. Descriptive epidemiology of cerebral gliomas in France. *Cancer.* 1997;79(6):1195–1202.
6. Chakrabarti I, Cockburn M, Cozen W, et al. A population-based description of glioblastoma multiforme in Los Angeles County, 1974–1999. *Cancer.* 2005;104(12):2798–2806.

7. Elia-Pasquet S, Provost D, Jaffré A, et al. Incidence of central nervous system tumors in Gironde, France. *Neuroepidemiology*. 2004;23(3):110–117.

8. Curran WJ Jr, Scott CB, Horton J, et al. Recursive partitioning analysis of prognostic factors in three Radiation Therapy Oncology Group malignant glioma trials. *J Natl Cancer Inst*. 1993;85(9):704–710.

9. Asai A, Matsutani M, Kohno T, et al. Subacute brain atrophy after radiation therapy for malignant brain tumor. *Cancer*. 1989;63(10):1962–1974.

10. Grant R, Liang BC, Page MA, et al. Age influences chemotherapy response in astrocytomas. *Neurology*. 1995;45(5):929–933.

11. Whittle IR, Denholm SW, Gregor A. Management of patients aged over 60 years with supratentorial glioma: Lessons from an audit. *Surg Neurol*. 1991;36(2):106–111.

12. Meckling S, Dold O, Forsyth PA, et al. Malignant supratentorial glioma in the elderly: Is radiotherapy useful? *Neurology*. 1996;47(4):901–905.

13. Iwamoto FM, Reiner AS, Nayak L, et al. Prognosis and patterns of care in elderly patients with glioma. *Cancer*. 2009;115(23):5534–5540.

14. Chaichana KL, Garzon-Muvdi T, Parker S, et al. Supratentorial glioblastoma multiforme: The role of surgical resection versus biopsy among older patients. *Ann Surg Oncol*. 2011;18(1):239–245.

15. Stupp R, Hegi ME, mason WP, et al. Effects of radiotherapy with concomitant and adjuvant temozolomide versus radiotherapy alone on survival in glioblastoma in a randomised phase III study: 5-year analysis of the EORTC-NCIC trial. *Lancet Oncol*. 2009;10(5):459–466.

16. Sijben AE, McIntyre JB, Roldán GB, et al. Toxicity from chemoradiotherapy in older patients with glioblastoma multiforme. *J Neurooncol*. 2008;89(1):97–103.

17. Laperriere NJ, Leung PM, McKenzie S, et al., Randomized study of brachytherapy in the initial management of patients with malignant astrocytoma. *Int J Radiat Oncol Biol Phys*. 1998;41(5):1005–1011.

18. Keime-Guibert F, Chinot O, Taillandier L, et al., Radiotherapy for glioblastoma in the elderly. *N Engl J Med*. 2007;356(15):1527–1535.

19. Scott J, Tsai YY, Chinnaiyapan P, Yu HH. Effectiveness of radiotherapy for elderly patients with glioblastoma. *Int J Radiat Oncol Biol Phys*. 2011 Sep 1;81(1):206–210.

20. Kita D, Ciernik IF, Vaccarella S, et al. Age as a predictive factor in glioblastomas: Population-based study. *Neuroepidemiology*. 2009;33(1):17–22.

21. Mohan DS, Suh JH, Phan JL, et al. Outcome in elderly patients undergoing definitive surgery and radiation therapy for supratentorial glioblastoma multiforme at a tertiary care institution. *Int J Radiat Oncol Biol Phys*. 1998;42(5):981–987.

22. Roa W, Brasher PM, Bauman G, et al. Abbreviated course of radiation therapy in older patients with glioblastoma multiforme: A prospective randomized clinical trial. *J Clin Oncol*. 2004;22(9):1583–1588.

23. Bleehen NM, Stenning SP. A Medical Research Council trial of two radiotherapy doses in the treatment of grades 3 and 4 astrocytoma. The Medical Research Council Brain Tumour Working Party. *Br J Cancer*. 1991;64(4):769–774.

24. Bauman GS, Gaspar LE, Fisher BJ, et al. A prospective study of short-course radiotherapy in poor prognosis glioblastoma multiforme. *Int J Radiat Oncol Biol Phys*. 1994;29(4):835–839.

25. Ford JM, Stenning SP, Boote DJ, et al. A short fractionation radiotherapy treatment for poor prognosis patients with high grade glioma. *Clin Oncol (R Coll Radiol)*. 1997;9(1):20–24.

26. Combs SE, Wagner J, Bischof M, et al. Postoperative treatment of primary glioblastoma multiforme with radiation and concomitant temozolomide in elderly patients. *Int J Radiat Oncol Biol Phys*. 2008;70(4):987–992.

27. Minniti G, Lanzetta G, Scaringi C, et al. Radiotherapy plus concomitant and adjuvant temozolomide for glioblastoma in elderly patients. *J Neurooncol*. 2008;88(1):97–103.

28. Brandes AA, Franceschi E, Tosoni A, et al. Temozolomide concomitant and adjuvant to radiotherapy in elderly patients with glioblastoma: Correlation with MGMT promoter methylation status. *Cancer*. 2009;115(15):3512–3518.

29. Brandes AA, Vastola F, Basso U, et al. A prospective study on glioblastoma in the elderly. *Cancer*. 2003;97(3):657–662.

30. Gerstein J, Franz K, Steinbach JP, et al. Postoperative radiotherapy and concomitant temozolomide for elderly patients with glioblastoma. *Radiother Oncol*. 2010;97(3):382–386.

31. Chinot OL, Barrie M, Frauger E, et al. Phase II study of temozolomide without radiotherapy in newly diagnosed glioblastoma multiforme in an elderly populations. *Cancer*. 2004;100(10):2208–2214.

32. Laigle-Donadey F, Figarella-Branger D, Chinot O, et al. Up-front temozolomide in elderly patients with glioblastoma. *J Neurooncol*. 2010;99(1):89–94.

33. Malmstrom A, Grønberg BH, Stupp R, et al. Glioblastoma (GBM) in elderly patients: A randomized phase III trial comparing survival in patients treated with 6-week radiotherapy

(RT) versus hypofractionated RT over 2 weeks versus temozolomide single-agent chemotherapy (TMZ). *J Clin Oncol.* 2010;28(18:supplement).

34. Wick W, Platten M, Meisner C, et al. Temozolomide chemotherapy alone versus radiotherapy alone for malignant astrocytoma in the elderly: The NOA-08 randomised, phase 3 trial. *Lancet Oncol.* 2012 Jul;13(7):707–715. Epub 2012 May 10.

35. Malmström A, Grønberg BH, Marosi C, et al. Temozolomide versus standard 6-week radiotherapy versus hypofractionated radiotherapy in patients older than 60 years with glioblastoma: The Nordic randomised, phase 3 trial. *Lancet Oncol.* 2012 Sep 1;13(9):916–926.

36. Krex D, Klink B, Hartmann C, et al. Long-term survival with glioblastoma multiforme. *Brain.* 2007;130(Pt 10):2596–606.

37. Murat A, Migliavacca E, Gorlia T, et al. Stem cell-related "self-renewal" signature and high epidermal growth factor receptor expression associated with resistance to concomitant chemoradiotherapy in glioblastoma. *J Clin Oncol.* 2008;26(18):3015–3024.

Low-Grade Glioma

CLINICAL PROBLEM

The best and most appropriate treatment for patients with low-grade glioma, especially in young patients with near-total resection, remains a matter of considerable debate and controversy. Although some aspects have been studied in randomized trials, many aspects about treatment remain highly variable. This dilemma has been accentuated by the recognition that patients with these tumors have survival rates considerably superior to those of patients with glioblastoma (GBM) and they appear to have excellent outcomes with a variety of different treatments, including surgery followed by observation. The exact timing, role, and risk–benefit ratio of adjuvant therapies remain inadequately defined. These issues will be elaborated on through this case.

CASE EXAMPLE

A 48-year-old male initially presented to his primary care doctor with occasional headaches, and an MRI of the brain suggested a benign cyst in the left frontal lobe. Five years later, the patient had progressively worsening memory loss and headaches and a repeat brain MRI showed a 6.6 × 4.4 cm solid lesion in the left frontal region with a 4.8 × 3.6 cm cystic component along the deep margin of the lesion. This mass caused marked mass effect on the ventricular system with moderate left-to-right subfalcine herniation. The patient underwent craniotomy and pathology demonstrated a moderate to densely cellular tumor with cortical involvement, extensive microcyst formation, microgemistocytic cytomorphology, and moderately increased cytologic pleomorphism. Mitotic index was low with a proliferation index of less than 5% overall, but the index was 5% to

10% in focal areas. No microvascular proliferation or necrosis was seen. Final pathology confirmed a World Health Organization (WHO) grade 2 oligodendroglioma. Cytogenetics by fluorescent in situ hybridization (FISH) showed the tumor was nondeleted for chromosomes 1p and 19q, as well as nondeleted for chromosome 10q. A postoperative MRI within 24 hours of his surgery showed no residual enhancing tumor. The patient had no adjuvant treatment and was lost to follow up.

Five years after this resection, the patient experienced loss of consciousness at home possibly due to a seizure and presented to the emergency department. Repeat brain MRI showed an area of T1 hypointense signal in the posteromedial margin of a large left frontal resection cavity with no appreciable enhancement in this area and no hydrocephalus. A few millimeters of left to right midline shift and partial effacement were noted. The patient had a repeat craniotomy with gross tumor resection; microscopically possible residual tumor was left behind where it faded into normal brain and where no clear resection borders could be defined. Pathology was consistent with recurrent diffuse astrocytoma, possible protoplasmic type, WHO grade 2. Rare mitotic figures were observed, cells had minimal nuclear atypia, proliferation index was 6%, no microvascular proliferation or necrosis was noted, and immunostains were consistent with a p53 mutation. Immediate postoperative MRI showed residual fluid attenuated inversion recovery (FLAIR) hyperintense signal along the posterior margin of the resection cavity measuring up to 16 mm in maximum dimension, as well as abnormal FLAIR signal in the anterior body of the corpus callosum measuring 18 mm in maximum dimension. Following the patient's second resection, he had no neurologic deficits on physical exam.

Management Decisions

• Should the patient be treated with immediate adjuvant therapy or is observation a better option with treatment reserved for recurrent/progressive disease?
• Should dose escalation be considered for this patient?
• What, if any, chemotherapy should be given with radiation?

MAJOR OPINION

Minesh P. Mehta and Haider A. Shirazi

Low-grade gliomas (LGG) are primary brain tumors separated into grade 1 (noninfiltrative) and grade 2 (infiltrative) by the WHO on the basis of factors such as atypia, proliferation, and so forth [1]. Grade 1 gliomas are rare in adults. Approximately 1800 cases of LGG are diagnosed in the United States annually, accounting for 10% of newly diagnosed primary brain tumors [2].

Controversy exists as to the optimal management of newly diagnosed LGG and whether these patients should have surgery, radiation, chemotherapy, or any combination of these. The role of observation alone following gross total resection was analyzed in the phase 2 portion of the Radiation Therapy Oncology Group (RTOG) 98-02 trial, which prospectively observed 111 patients under 40 years of age with low-risk LGG [3]. Tumor size and histology were predictive of outcome, with a 78% 5-year progression-free survival (PFS) for oligodendroglioma or oligo-dominant mixed oligoastrocytomas less than 4 cm, compared to 34% for diffuse astrocytomas or astro-dominant mixed oligoastrocytomas 4 cm or greater. These results suggest that a subset of LGG patients have a very high likelihood of early relapse, and may potentially benefit from adjuvant treatment. The European Organisation for Research and Treatment of Cancer (EORTC) 22845 was a phase 3 trial of 311 patients with supratentorial LGG, excluding pilocytic astrocytoma, randomized after surgery to immediate radiotherapy or observation (in effect, delayed radiotherapy) [4]. Patients who were randomized to radiation received a dose of 54 Gy in 1.8 Gy fractions to a localized field. Five-year overall survival (OS) was 68% for the radiation group compared to 66% for the observation group (p = .49). Median time to progression for the radiation group

was 4.8 years versus 3.4 years for the observation arm (p = .02), and PFS was also improved in the radiation arm. This study provides level 1 evidence in support of early radiotherapy to improve time-to-progression, but it has no impact on OS. Median survival following salvage radiation was 4 years.

The optimal dose of radiation for postoperative treatment of LGG was investigated in 2 phase 3 randomized trials [5,6]. EORTC 22844 randomized 379 patients with completely or incompletely resected WHO grade 2 astrocytoma, oligodendroglioma, or oligoastrocytoma, and incompletely resected grade 1 pilocytic astrocytoma, to a dose of 45 Gy in 25 fractions or 59.4 Gy in 33 fractions to a local field. No significant difference was noted in survival, with a 5-year survival rate of 58% for low-dose radiation and 59% for the higher dose. The North Central Cancer Treatment Group (NCCTG)-led Intergroup study randomized 211 patients with completely or incompletely resected grade 2 astrocytoma, oligodendroglioma, or oligoastrocytoma to a dose of 50.4 Gy or 64.8 Gy. The low-dose group had a 5-year survival of 72% versus 64% for the high-dose group, with no significant survival difference observed. When treatment failures were analyzed, 92% failed in-field, 3% had failures within 2 cm of the field, and 5% had failures more than 2 cm outside of the field edge. Radiation toxicity rates were significantly lower in the low-dose group compared to the high-dose group. Age, histology, and tumor size were the most important predictors of survival in the NCCTG study, and degree of resection did not significantly affect this end point. These two trials in combination do not support dose escalation for postoperative treatment of LGG.

Pignatti et al. proposed prognostic factors for LGG using patient data from 2 phase 3 trials, EORTC 22844 and EORTC 22845 [7]. Negative prognostic factors included age 40 years or older, astrocytoma histology, largest tumor dimension of 6 cm or more, tumor crossing midline, and presence of neurologic deficit before resection. Patients with 2 or fewer factors had a median survival of 7.7 years, while 3 factors or more predicted a worse outcome with a median survival of 3.2 years. Another study from Shaw et al. found that patients who received radiation doses of 53 Gy or more had significantly better survival than those who received less than 53 Gy [8]. This was reconfirmed in RTOG 91-10 [6].

Because of the relatively long life expectancy of patients diagnosed with LGG, quality of life (QoL) following treatment is an important end point. A companion study to EORTC 22844 did not show major differences between the high-dose and low-dose groups or between early and late radiotherapy [9]. The NCCTG study also assessed changes in cognitive function following radiotherapy using the Folstein mini-mental status exam (MMSE) [10]. In patients without tumor progression, deteriorations in MMSE scores were observed in 8%, 5%, and 5% of patients at 1, 2, and 5 years, respectively. Interestingly, this decrease in MMSE score was not related to radiation dose, age, sex, or tumor size.

The role of chemotherapy in management of LGG is also an area of active inquiry. The Southwestern Oncology Group (SWOG) ran a randomized trial of patients with subtotally resected supratentorial low-grade astrocytoma that terminated prematurely, with only 54 patients enrolled. Patients were randomized to radiotherapy with or without lomustine for up to 2 years [11]. The radiation dose was 55 Gy in both arms. Median survival for the radiation alone arm was 4.5 years versus 7.4 years for the combined modality arm, and on final analysis no significant benefit was observed with the addition of chemotherapy. The phase 3 portion of RTOG 98-02 randomized unfavorable LGG patients to radiation alone or radiation followed by procarbazine, lomustine, and vincristine (PCV). PFS was improved in grade 2 patients who received combination radiation and chemotherapy, but no effect on OS was observed. Beyond 2 years, the combination treatment reduced progression by 55% and death by 48% consistent with a delayed benefit to chemotherapy [12]. This chemotherapy regimen was utilized partially on the basis of data from RTOG 94-02. Patients with anaplastic oligodendroglioma and anaplastic oligoastrocytoma were randomized to radiation alone or postoperative radiation followed by PCV. No difference in OS between the groups was noted, but PFS for the combined modality group was 2.6 years versus 1.7 years for radiation alone ($p = .004$), albeit with increased toxicity in the chemotherapy arm [13].

Recently, as a consequence of positive results reported by Stupp et al. for temozolomide in GBM, temozolomide is being increasingly used in LGG as well [14]. Brada et al. published a phase 2 study of primary temozolomide at 200 mg/m^2/day for 5 days every 28 days for 6 to 12 cycles in patients with grade 2 gliomas and noted 3-year PFS and OS of 66% and 82%,

respectively, along with modest improvement in QoL and seizure control [15]. Kesari et al. studied daily temozolomide at 75 mg/m^2 7 weeks on and 4 weeks off and observed a median PFS of 39.4 months [16]. The EORTC has completed a phase 3 trial for patients with newly diagnosed high-risk supratentorial LGG that compared postoperative radiation alone to a dose of 50.4 Gy or temozolomide 75 mg/m^2/day alone for 21 days every 28 days until progression; the results of that trial are pending. A second trial that will help determine the benefit of adding chemotherapy to radiation is an Eastern Cooperative Oncology Group (ECOG)-led Intergroup study randomizing adults with grade 2 gliomas to radiation with or without temozolomide given for 5 days every 28 days for 12 cycles or until disease progression.

Genetic characterization of LGG has shown some predictive benefit. The most common genetic alteration in low-grade astrocytomas is p53. A study by Chozick et al. noted that patients with grade 2 astrocytomas who had overexpression of p53, indicating a p53 mutation, had a 4-year OS of 25% compared to 87% for those who did not overexpress p53 [17]. Although 1p and 19q codeletion is an important prognostic factor for anaplastic oligodendrogliomas, a correlation also exists between codeletion and outcome for LGG. Jenkins et al. analyzed 98 patients with newly diagnosed LGG and found that those with 1p19q codeleted had a median survival of 11.9 years compared to 8.1 years in those without this codeletion [18]. The role of methylguanine DNA methyltransferase (*MGMT*) promoter methylation in predicting outcome in LGG continues to be investigated. The phase 2 study by Kesari et al. noted that patients with methylated *MGMT* promoter had a longer OS ($p = .008$) [16].

Final Recommendation

This 53-year-old male who was originally diagnosed with a WHO grade 2 oligodendroglioma greater than 6 cm in size with cytogenetics showing 1p19q non-codeletion and gemistocytic morphology, underwent a gross total resection. The patient had a high-risk LGG and could possibly have benefited from postoperative radiation, and possibly chemotherapy, in terms of PFS; my personal recommendation would have been to consider up-front radiotherapy. Moreover, the presence of the gemistocytic element according to Krouwer et al. is a poor prognostic sign and may indicate that the tumor could behave more like an anaplastic astrocytoma [19]. After his tumor recurred 5 years later, the tumor was found to be a diffuse grade 2 astrocytoma, and p53 was overexpressed, indicative of a possibly worse prognosis than a tumor with normal p53, although this has never been validated prospectively. Radiotherapy at time of recurrence to a dose of 54 Gy in 1.8 Gy fractions was recommended with concurrent daily temozolomide at 75 mg/m^2 followed by temozolomide at 150 mg/m^2 for 5 days every 28 days. No level 1 evidence for this recommendation exists and, in part, it represents an extrapolation of data from RTOG 98-02 [12].

ACADEMIC COMMENT

Igor J. Barani

The most important negative prognostic factors to emerge from the literature include increasing age, astrocytic histology, large tumor diameter (larger than 4–6 cm), tumors crossing the midline, neurologic deficits, and poor performance status. In contrast, presentation with seizures, which generally occur in patients who are otherwise neurologically intact, often is identified as a positive prognostic factor. In 2002, Pignatti et al. described a simple scoring system to account for these important prognostic factors so that physicians could better counsel patients and stratify patients for subsequent trials [7]. Based on a multivariate analysis of data from one prospective EORTC trial and validated on the basis of the data from another, they assigned one point each for age 40 years and above, astrocytoma histology, maximal tumor diameter of 6 cm and above, tumor crossing the midline, and presence of neurologic deficit before surgery. Low-risk patients (scores 0–2) had a median OS of 7.7 years, compared to 3.2 years for high-risk patients (scores 3–5). The University of California at San Francisco (UCSF) group introduced a more recent LGG scoring system that uses a 4-point scoring system to predict OS and PFS, assigning 1 point each for age 50 years and above, KPS of 80 and lesser, maximum tumor diameter of 4 cm or more, and tumor involvement of eloquent brain [20]. When stratified into groups according to risk, low (scores 0–1), medium (score 2), and high (scores 3–4), 5 year OS was 97%, 81%, and 56%, respectively. The 5-year PFS was 76%, 49%, and 18%, respectively. The unique feature of the UCSF system is the inclusion of eloquent brain location as an adverse prognostic factor. The

eloquent location may result in higher likelihood of neurologic deficits, and may limit the possible extent of resection. The UCSF prognostic model has not been externally validated.

The impact of increasing age on LGG prognosis has received particular attention more recently because older patients (aged 55–60 years or more) are increasingly being diagnosed with LGG. Older patients also have a poorer prognosis with a 5-year OS of 30% to 40% [21,22]. Moreover, each additional year of age has a negative prognostic impact that suggests that analysis of age as a binary variable rather than a continuous variable may underestimate the impact of increasing age on outcomes.

To what extent molecular markers such as 1p/19q codeletion status, isocitrate dehydrogenase (*IDH*) mutation status, and the presence or absence of *MGMT* promoter hypermethylation, which is a prognostic factor in GBM outcome, predict responsiveness to specific therapies or to overall prognosis remains uncertain. The presence of 1p/19q deletion seems to portend a better prognosis in LGG, although its favorable impact is weaker than in grade 3 gliomas. Small studies have suggested that *MGMT* methylation status may predict improved OS, but the small size of these studies and a potential confounding correlation between *MGMT* methylation and 1p/19q codeletion require larger studies to resolve this question [16]. Similarly, in univariate analyses, *IDH-1* mutations conferred improved OS in low-grade and anaplastic gliomas as well as in GBMs, but it is unclear whether mutational status retains prognostic significance when other prognostic markers are incorporated into multivariate models [23]. It appears that *IDH-1* mutations are an early event in LGG pathogenesis. *IDH-1* catalyzes the oxidative decarboxylation of isocitrate to alpha-ketoglutarate, reducing NADP to NADPH. *IDH-1* is found in the cytoplasm and the peroxisome. It has long been recognized that most LGGs harbored 1 of 2 mutually exclusive genetic changes: (a) *p53* mutations in most low-grade astrocytomas, and (b) deletions of chromosomes 1p and 19q in most pure low-grade oligodendrogliomas [24]. Low-grade mixed gliomas tend to have either *p53* mutation or 1p/19q codeletion. However, recent studies have demonstrated the presence of *IDH-1* mutations in 59% to 90% of grade 2 astrocytomas, 68% to 85% of grade 2 oligodendrogliomas, and 50% to 83% of grade 2 oligoastrocytomas [23,25]. The fact that *IDH-1* mutations are seen at similar frequencies in tumors with *p53* mutation and 1p/19q codeletion suggests that they may precede other genetic changes. The mechanism by which *IDH-1* mutations increase predisposition to gliomagenesis is unknown, but it is known that the mutated protein is metabolically less active and that the mutation is associated with improved survival. These molecular parameters—p53, 1p/19q, and *IDH*—do not, as of yet, have proven therapeutic relevance in grade 2 gliomas.

The optimal role for radiation therapy (RT) in the management of patients with LGG is not entirely clear. EORTC 22845 reported longer PFS and increased rates of seizure control in patients who received up-front RT to a dose of 54 Gy (30 fractions over 6 weeks) compared with patients who were treated at the time of progression (PFS 5.3 vs. 3.4 years, $p < .0001$; seizure control rate 75% vs. 59%, $p = .0329$) [4]. OS in this trial was not significantly different between the 2 groups (7.4 vs. 7.2 years). Despite its efficacy in terms of improving PFS and seizure control, the authors of the study concluded that RT could still be deferred in patients with LGG who are "in a good condition." Part of the reason for this sentiment is the fact that QoL was not thoroughly studied (a subset was studied) and, therefore, it is not clear what the "cost" is to patients to realize the PFS and seizure control benefit without realizing any gains in OS. Moreover, by delaying RT, 35% of patients in the group who did not receive up-front RT (median follow-up of 7.4 years) did not receive RT, which spared them potential adverse effects of RT.

Recent studies are therefore more focused on the QoL outcomes after RT to better define its role in managing patients with LGG. Douw et al. recently reported on a nonrandomized, longitudinal study of 65 patients with LGG, 1/2 of whom received RT [26]. With a mean follow-up of 12 years, 27% of patients who had not been irradiated had significant cognitive deficits in at least 5 of 18 neuropsychological test parameters, whereas 53% of patients who received RT had significant cognitive deficits. Even though studies such as this support clinical efforts to explore the role of chemotherapy-only treatments for patients with LGG in the up-front setting, it is worth noting that nonrandomized studies are subject to significant effects from selection bias (eg, patients who received RT likely did so because of the concerning tumor or patient factors) that could significantly impact the study findings.

With respect to chemotherapy, most of the recent focus has been on temozolomide, an oral agent that has a favorable toxicity profile. Phase 2 clinical studies indicate that temozolomide, given on either a standard 5-day schedule or a dose-dense, metronomic schedule (3 weeks on/1 week off, or 7 weeks on/4 weeks off) is active against both previously irradiated and unirradiated progressing LGGs [16,27,28]. There are 3 major questions relating to temozolomide in LGGs: (a) Can temozolomide be substituted for RT, (b) can temozolomide be substituted for PCV, and (c) is there a benefit from combining these 2 modalities in high-risk patients? Clinical trials addressing 2 of these questions have been launched. In Europe and Canada, a phase 3 clinical trial randomly assigned patients with LGG to receive either standard RT or temozolomide with patients being stratified according to chromosome 1p status. PFS is the primary end point, and the study includes both neurocognitive and QoL end points. RTOG 0424 recently completed accrual to a phase 2 clinical trial that evaluated the combination of RT and temozolomide in previously untreated high-risk patients with LGGs; the results are expected to mature after several years of follow up. ECOG recently also launched a phase 3 trial (ECOG E3F05) that randomly assigned patients with LGG to either standard RT with concurrent and 1 year of adjuvant temozolomide versus RT alone. This trial is built upon RTOG 0424 and is complementary to the European study; it is expected that the 2 studies will more comprehensively address the role of temozolomide in the management of LGG patients.

In summary, the management of LGG patients is evolving with well-planned clinical trials that are at present accruing patients to address many of the outstanding primary management questions. The case study patient clearly met the high-risk criteria by virtue of advanced age and tumor size at initial presentation, and could probably have benefited from adjuvant therapy at that time. At recurrence, the patient was 58 years old and underwent extensive resection with persistent FLAIR signal abnormality, likely representing residual tumor, at the margin of the resection cavity and extending across the midline. The resected tumor did not exhibit chromosome 1p/19q deletions, and so it may be useful to obtain *IDH-1* mutation status. In my view, the patient is clearly at high-risk for further disease progression and needs definitive adjuvant treatment. My recommendation would be for aggressive combined modality treatment with RT to a dose of 54 Gy (30 fractions over 6 weeks) with temozolomide given concurrently

(75 mg/m² daily during RT) and adjuvantly for 6 cycles (150–200 mg/m² every 5 days of a 28 day cycle). This recommendation is unsupported by the published clinical data and is based solely on the high-risk features of the patient and the tumor at the time of second recurrence. If *IDH-1* mutation was identified, one may consider treatment with RT alone, followed by close observation with temozolomide being reserved for salvage treatment in combination with re-resection if possible, although this recommendation is also not evidence based.

COMMUNITY PRACTITIONER COMMENT

Deepak Khuntia

In this interesting case, we have a 48-year-old male who presented with what later proved to be a LGG. He underwent gross total resection and observation at age 53. As described earlier, a strong case could have been made to actually deliver adjuvant therapy at the time of the initial resection. He has several risk factors as described earlier. In addition to the gemistocytic features mentioned earlier, he also was over the age of 40. In Shaw's original retrospective review of LGG, patients over 40 years of age did worse than those under 40 years of age [3]. RTOG 91-10 also reconfirmed age under 40 as a good prognosticator [6]. These studies set the foundation for RTOG 98-02 in which only patients under the age of 40 with gross total resection were observed (the phase 2 component of the study); all other patients were required to have radiotherapy. From a community physician's standpoint, from the fact that all patients over the age of 40 were not observed (ie, they were randomized to radiation with or without PCV), radiation would be the de novo RTOG standard of care for the patient presented here. Further, nearly 50% of all patients who were observed in the favorable group (ie, less than 40 years old, less than 4 cm, and gross totally resected tumors) had progression at 5 years arguing for a potentially even offering of adjuvant therapy up front in this group. That being said, he was observed and has subsequently developed a recurrence.

There are no level 1 data that suggest a standard of care for recurrent LGG. It is very reasonable to address the recurrence surgically, as was done here. However, adjuvant therapy is more controversial. If the pathology from his recurrence were in fact similar to the original presentation, we would offer radiotherapy and I see little reason why it would not be offered here. We would treat to a dose of 54 Gy in 1.8 Gy fractions. The question of chemotherapy is a bit more challenging. Little randomized data exist that use chemotherapy in this setting and even less data that use temozolomide. RTOG 98-02 showed that the addition of PCV did improve PFS, but it did not increase OS. Given that he has recurred once already, it would be reasonable to add systemic therapy to radiation in order to further improve PFS given that second recurrences are usually more difficult to salvage.

The discussion on agents of choice is also complicated. PCV has been found to be more toxic than temozolomide and as a result, temozolomide is generally the favored systemic first-line chemotherapeutic agent. However, little prospective data exist on this topic. RTOG 0424 should shed light on this difficult question. In this study, patients with high-risk LGG were given RT (54 Gy in 30 fractions) along with temozolomide and continued temozolomide for an additional 12 cycles. High-risk patients included 3 of the following: age over 40 years, tumor size of 6 cm or more, tumor crosses midline, astrocytic dominant, and neurologic function greater than 1. Results are pending at present. The randomized trial that will help address this question is ECOG E3F05 that randomized postoperative high-risk LGG patients to either radiation alone or temozolomide concurrently with radiation plus an additional 12 cycles. In the patient presented here, we would likely give temozolomide with radiation and continue this for an additional 12 cycles recognizing that this is a recurrence and there is no clear standard. If this were his original presentation, I would try to enroll the patient on E3F05 (an RTOG-endorsed study) but if he refuses, I would do radiation alone as he was 1p19q intact. If he were 1p19q deleted, we would offer postoperative radiation with concurrent temozolomide with an additional 12 cycles of temozolomide.

SECTION EDITOR'S NOTE

Minesh P. Mehta

An argument could have been made at the time of the original diagnosis for adjuvant treatment based on current data and the patient's tumor characteristics. In the setting of recurrence, I concur with the author's recommendation and recommend external beam RT to a dose of 54 Gy with concurrent temozolomide.

REFERENCES

1. Kleihues P, Burger PC, Scheithauer BW. *Histological Typing of Tumours of the Central Nervous System*, 2nd ed. Berlin: Springer; 1993.

2. *Statistical Report: Primary Brain Tumors in the United States, 1998–2002.* 2005: Central Brain Tumor Registry of the United States.

3. Shaw EG, Berkey B, Coons SW, et al. Recurrence following neurosurgeon-determined gross-total resection of adult supratentorial low-grade glioma: Results of a prospective clinical trial. *J Neurosurg.* 2008;109(5):835–841.

4. van den Bent MJ, Afra D, de Witte O, et al. Long-term efficacy of early versus delayed radiotherapy for low-grade astrocytoma and oligodendroglioma in adults: The EORTC 22845 randomised trial. *Lancet.* 2005;366(9490): 985–990.

5. Karim AB, Maat B, Hatlevoll R, et al. A randomized trial on dose-response in radiation therapy of low-grade cerebral glioma: European Organization for Research and Treatment of Cancer (EORTC) Study 22844. *Int J Radiat Oncol Biol Phys.* 1996;36(3):549–556.

6. Shaw E, Arusell R, Scheithauer B, et al. Prospective randomized trial of low- versus high-dose radiation therapy in adults with supratentorial low-grade glioma: Initial report of a North Central Cancer Treatment Group/Radiation Therapy Oncology Group/Eastern Cooperative Oncology Group study. *J Clin Oncol.* 2002;20(9):2267–2276.

7. Pignatti F, van den Bent M, Curran D, et al. Prognostic factors for survival in adult patients with cerebral low-grade glioma. *J Clin Oncol.* 2002;20(8):2076–2084.

8. Shaw EG, Daumas-Duport C, Scheithauer BW, et al. Radiation therapy in the management of low-grade supratentorial astrocytomas. *J Neurosurg.* 1989;70(6):853–861.

9. Kiebert GM, Curran D, Aaronson NK, et al. Quality of life after radiation therapy of cerebral low-grade gliomas of the adult: Results of a randomised phase III trial on dose response (EORTC trial 22844). EORTC Radiotherapy Co-operative Group. *Eur J Cancer.* 1998;34(12): 1902–1909.

10. Laack NN, Brown PD, Ivnik RJ, et al. Cognitive function after radiotherapy for supratentorial low-grade glioma: A North Central Cancer Treatment Group prospective study. *Int J Radiat Oncol Biol Phys.* 2005;63(4): 1175–1183.

11. Eyre HJ, Crowley JJ, Townsend JJ, et al. A randomized trial of radiotherapy versus radiotherapy plus CCNU for incompletely resected low-grade gliomas: A Southwest Oncology Group study. *J Neurosurg.* 1993;78(6):909–914.

12. Shaw EG, Wang M, Coons SW, et al. Final report of Radiation Therapy Oncology Group (RTOG) protocol 9802: Radiation therapy (RT) versus RT + procarbazine, CCNU, and vincristine (PCV) chemotherapy for adult low-grade glioma (LGG). *J Clin Oncol.* 2008 May 20; 26:(Suppl, abstract 2006).

13. Cairncross G, Berkey B, Shaw E, et al. Phase III trial of chemotherapy plus radiotherapy compared with radiotherapy alone for pure and mixed anaplastic oligodendroglioma: Intergroup Radiation Therapy Oncology Group Trial 9402. *J Clin Oncol.* 2006;24(18):2707–2714.

14. Stupp R, Mason WP, van den Bent MJ, et al. Radiotherapy plus concomitant and adjuvant temozolomide for glioblastoma. *N Engl J Med.* 2005;352(10):987–996.

15. Brada M, Viviers L, Abson C, et al. Phase II study of primary temozolomide chemotherapy in patients with WHO grade II gliomas. *Ann Oncol.* 2003;14(12):1715–1721.

16. Kesari S, Schiff D, Drappatz J, et al. Phase II study of protracted daily temozolomide for low-grade gliomas in adults. *Clin Cancer Res.* 2009;15(1):330–337.

17. Chozick BS, Pezzullo JC, Epstein MH, Finch PW. Prognostic implications of p53 overexpression in supratentorial astrocytic tumors. *Neurosurgery.* 1994;35(5):831–837; discussion 837–838.

18. Jenkins RB, Blair H, Ballman KV, et al. A t(1;19)(q10;p10) mediates the combined deletions of 1p and 19q and predicts a better prognosis of patients with oligodendroglioma. *Cancer Res.* 2006;66(20):9852–9861.

19. Krouwer HG, Davis RL, Silver P, Prados M. Gemistocytic astrocytoma: A reappraisal. *J Neurosurgery.* 1991;74(3):399–406.

20. Chang EF, Smith JS, Chang SM, et al. Preoperative prognostic classification system for hemispheric low-grade gliomas in adults. *J Neurosurg.* 2008;109(5):817–824.

21. Pouratian N, Mut M, Jagannathan J, et al. Low-grade gliomas in older patients: A retrospective analysis of prognostic factors. *J Neurooncol.* 2008;90(3):341–350.

22. Schomas DA, Laack NN, Brown PD. Low-grade gliomas in older patients: Long-term follow-up from Mayo Clinic. *Cancer.* 2009;115(17): 3969–3678.

23. Ichimura K, Pearson DM, Kocialkowski S, et al. IDH1 mutations are present in the majority of

common adult gliomas but rare in primary glioblastomas. *Neuro Oncol.* 2009;11(4):341–347.

24. Schiff D, Brown PD, Giannini C. Outcome in adult low-grade glioma: The impact of prognostic factors and treatment. *Neurology.* 2007;69(13):1366–1373.

25. Yan H, Parsons DW, Jin G, et al. IDH1 and IDH2 mutations in gliomas. *N Engl J Med.* 2009;360(8):765–773.

26. Douw L, Klein M, Fagel SS, et al. Cognitive and radiological effects of radiotherapy in patients with low-grade glioma: Long-term follow-up. *Lancet Neurol.* 2009;8(9):810–818.

27. Kaloshi G, Benouaich-Amiel A, Diakite F, et al. Temozolomide for low-grade gliomas: Predictive impact of 1p/19q loss on response and outcome. *Neurology.* 2007;68(21):1831–1836.

28. Pouratian N, Gasco J, Sherman JH, et al. Toxicity and efficacy of protracted low dose temozolomide for the treatment of low grade gliomas. *J Neurooncol.* 2007;82(3):281–288.